theclinics.com

RHEUMATIC DISEASE CLINICS OF NORTH AMERICA

Pain Mechanisms and Management in the Rheumatic Diseases

GUEST EDITOR
Mary-Ann Fitzcharles, MB, ChB, FRCP(C)

May 2008 • Volume 34 • Number 2

SAUNDERS
An Imprint of Elsevier, Inc.
PHILADELPHIA LONDON TORONTO MONTREAL SYDNEY TOKYO

W.B. SAUNDERS COMPANY

A Division of Elsevier Inc.

1600 John F. Kennedy Boulevard • Suite 1800 • Philadelphia, Pennsylvania 19103-2899

http://www.theclinics.com

RHEUMATIC DISEASE
CLINICS OF NORTH AMERICA
May 2008
Editor: Rachel Glover

Volume 34, Number 2
ISSN 0889-857X
ISBN 13: 978-1-4160-6047-5
ISBN 10: 1-4160-6047-2

Rheumatic Disease Clinics of North America (ISSN 0889-857X) is published quarterly by Elsevier Inc., 360 Park Avenue South, New York, NY 10010-1710. Months of issue are February, May, August, and November. Business and editorial offices: 1600 John F. Kennedy Boulevard, Suite 1800, Philadelphia, PA 19103-2899. Customer Service offices: 6277 Sea Harbor Drive, Orlando, FL 32887-4800. Periodicals postage paid at New York, NY and additional mailing offices. Subscription prices are USD 226 per year for US individuals, USD 370 per year for US institutions, USD 113 per year for US students and residents, USD 267 per year for Canadian individuals, USD 448 per year for Canadian institutions, USD 297 per year for international individuals, USD 448 per year for international institutions and USD 149 per year for Canadian and foreign students/residents. To receive student/resident rate, orders must be accompanied by name of affiliated institution, date of term, and the *signature* of program/residency coordinator on institution letterhead. Orders will be billed at individual rate until proof of status received. Foreign air speed delivery is included in all *Clinics* subscription prices. All prices are subject to change without notice. **POSTMASTER:** Send address changes to *Rheumatic Disease Clinics of North America*, Elsevier Journals Customer Service, 6277 Sea Harbor Drive, Orlando, FL 32887-4800. **Customer Service: 1-800-654-2452 (USA). From outside of the USA, call (+1) 407-563-6020. Fax: 1-407-363-9661. E-mail: JournalsCustomerService-usa@elsevier.com.**

Reprints. For copies of 100 or more of articles in this publication, please contact the Commercial Reprints Department, Elsevier Inc., 360 Park Avenue South, New York, New York, 10010-1710; Tel.: (+1) 212-633-3813, Fax: (+1) 212-462-1935, and E-mail: reprints@elsevier.com.

Rheumatic Disease Clinics of North America is covered in *MEDLINE/PubMed (Index Medicus), Current Contents/Clinical Medicine, Science Citation Index, ISI/BIOMED*, and *EMBASE/Excerpta Medica*.

Printed in the United States of America.

GUEST EDITOR

MARY-ANN FITZCHARLES, MB, ChB, FRCP(C), Associate Professor of Medicine, Pain Centre, Montreal General Hospital, McGill University Health Centre; and Division of Rheumatology, McGill University, Montreal, Quebec, Canada

CONTRIBUTORS

FABRIZIO BENEDETTI, MD, Professor of Physiology, Department of Neuroscience, University of Turin Medical School; and National Institute of Neuroscience, Turin, Italy

LESLIE G. CLELAND, MBBS, MD, FRACP, Director, Rheumatology Unit, Royal Adelaide Hospital, Adelaide, Australia

SHEENA DERRY, MA, Senior Research Officer, Nuffied Department of Anaesthetics, University of Oxford, John Radcliffe Hospital, Headington, Oxford, United Kingdom

PAUL DIEPPE, MD, Honorary Professor of Musculoskeletal Sciences, Nuffield Department of Orthopaedic Surgery, University of Oxford, Oxford, United Kingdom

ANDY DRAY, PhD, AstraZeneca Research and Development, Montreal, Quebec, Canada

EDZARD ERNST, MD, PhD, FRCP, FRCPEd, Complementary Medicine, Peninsula Medical School, Universities of Exeter and Plymouth, Exeter, United Kingdom

MARY-ANN FITZCHARLES, MB, ChB, FRCP(C), Associate Professor of Medicine, Pain Centre, Montreal General Hospital, McGill University Health Centre; and Division of Rheumatology, McGill University, Montreal, Quebec, Canada

MICHAEL J. JAMES, PhD, Chief Medical Scientist, Rheumatology Unit, Royal Adelaide Hospital, Adelaide, Australia

ROSE-MARIE JAVIER, MD, Service de Rhumatologie, Hopital Hautepierre, Strasbourg, Paris, France

WARREN A. KATZ, MD, Clinical Professor of Medicine, University of Pennsylvania School of Medicine; Attending and Former Chief, Rheumatology Division, Penn-Presbyterian Medical Center; and Associate, Rothman Institute, Philadelphia, Pennsylvania

FRANCIS A. KEEFE, PhD, Professor of Medical Psychology, Duke Medical Center, Department of Psychiatry and Behavioral Sciences, Duke Pain Prevention and Treatment Research Program, Durham, North Carolina

FRANÇOISE LAROCHE, MD, Centre d'Evaluation et de Traitment de la Douleur, Hopital St. Antoine, Paris, France

CLAIRE LE JEUNNE, MD, Professor, Service de Médicine Interne et Thérapeutique, Hotel Dieu, Université Paris Descartes, Paris, France

MARY E. LYNCH, MD, Pain Management Unit, Queen Elizabeth II Health Sciences Centre; and Department of Anesthesiology, Psychiatry, and Pharmacology, Dalhousie University, Halifax, Nova Scotia, Canada

FIONA MacKICHAN, MSc, PhD Candidate, Department of Social Medicine, University of Bristol, Bristol, United Kingdom

SERGE MARCHAND, PhD, Director of the FRSQ CRC-CHUS Pain Axis, Faculty of Medicine, Department of Neurosurgery, University of Sherbrooke, Axe Douleur CRC-CHUS, Sherbrooke, Quebec, Canada

LYNN M. MARTIRE, PhD, Associate Professor of Psychiatry, Department of Psychiatry, University of Pittsburgh School of Medicine, University Center for Social and Urban Research, Pittsburgh, Pennsylvania

MARC MARTY, MD, Service de Rhumatologie, Hopital Henri Mondor, Créteil, Paris, France

HENRY J. McQUAY, MA, DM, FRCA, FRCP (Edin), Professor of Clinical Anaesthetics, Pain Research, Nuffied Department of Anaesthetics, University of Oxford, John Radcliffe Hospital, Headington, Oxford, United Kingdom

R. ANDREW MOORE, MA, DPhil, CChem, FRSC, DSc, Senior Research Fellow, Nuffied Department of Anaesthetics, University of Oxford, John Radcliffe Hospital, Headington, Oxford, United Kingdom

SERGE PERROT, MD, PhD, Service de Médicine Interne et Thérapeutique, Consultation de la Douleur, Hotel Dieu, Université Paris Descartes, Paris, France

ANTONELLA POLLO, MD, Assistant Professor of Physiology, Department of Neuroscience, University of Turin, Faculty of Pharmacy; and National Institute of Neuroscience, Turin, Italy

SUSANNA M. PROUDMAN, MBBS, FRACP, Senior Rheumatologist, Rheumatology Unit, Royal Adelaide Hospital, Adelaide, Australia

TAMARA J. SOMERS, PhD, Post Doctoral Fellow, Duke Medical Center, Department of Psychiatry and Behavioral Sciences, Duke Pain Prevention and Treatment Research Program, Durham, North Carolina

YORAM SHIR, MD, Pain Centre, Montreal General Hospital, McGill University Health Centre, Montreal, Quebec, Canada

VIKKI WYLDE, BSc, Research Assistant, University of Bristol, Bristol Implant Research Centre, Avon Orthopaedic Centre, Southmead Hospital, Bristol, United Kingdom

CONTENTS

Emerging therapies are directed to targeting inflammatory mediators, ligand and voltage regulated ion channels, as well as increasing inhibition through monoaminergic modulation. Finally, neurotrophic abnormalities may be restored through the modulation of specific neurotrophins. These developments are supported by increasing emphasis on the clinical understanding of the neurologic changes in pain patients to enable confident translation to clinical application.

FORTHCOMING ISSUES

August 2008

Osteoarthritis
David J. Hunter, MD, *Guest Editor*

November 2008

Sjogren's Syndrome
Steven E. Carsons, MD, *Guest Editor*

RECENT ISSUES

February 2008

Scleroderma
Fredrick M. Wigley, MD, *Guest Editor*

November 2007

Vasculitis
John H. Stone, MD, MPH, *Guest Editor*

August 2007

Pediatric Rheumatology
Ronald M. Laxer, MD, FRCPC, *Guest Editor*

ELSEVIER
SAUNDERS

Rheum Dis Clin N Am
34 (2008) xi–xii

RHEUMATIC
DISEASE CLINICS
OF NORTH AMERICA

Preface

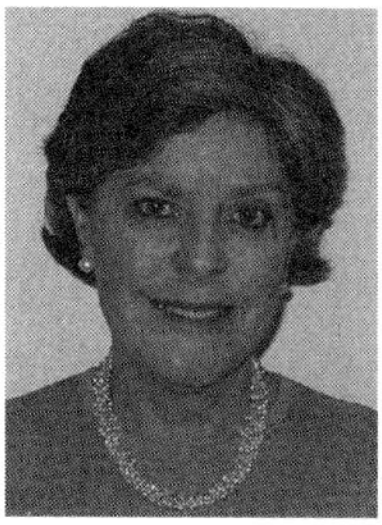

Mary-Ann Fitzcharles, MB, ChB, FRCP(C)
Guest Editor

Fred, a lowland gorilla in the St. Louis Zoo, died of pain [1]. One day he crawled into a corner of his cage and turned his back on life, as the pain of osteoarthritis of his hips was too great to bear. Ten years later, the medical community has acknowledged the importance of pain by its inclusion as the fifth vital sign in clinical medicine. Pain, especially of musculoskeletal origin, is prevalent and impacts greatly on quality of life. The experience of pain, unique for each individual, is influenced by the specific characteristics of the pathology, as well as factors such as genetic makeup, psychologic status, previous pain experience, and psychosocial environment.

The bread and butter of rheumatology practice have always been the management of conditions causing pain. For the last century, physician-prescribed management for musculoskeletal pain has focused mainly on pharmacologic treatments such as anti-inflammatory medications and simple analgesics. Although the understanding of both inflammatory as well as degenerative arthritic disease has progressed rapidly, no absolute cure for either is in sight in the foreseeable future and pain will therefore remain an ongoing and important symptom. The primary focus for the management of inflammatory disease is the modulation of the underlying disease process by the use of disease-modifying antirheumatic medications, whereas there is no disease-modifying treatment for patients who have osteoarthritis. In parallel with scientific progress in the rheumatic field, there have been impressive advances within the discipline of pain, with improved knowledge of pain mechanisms and also pain treatments. It is therefore timely to integrate the current science of pain from both the mechanism and the treatment perspective into the rheumatic domain.

doi:10.1016/j.rdc.2008.05.001

In this issue of the *Rheumatic Disease Clinics of North America*, which is devoted to rheumatic pain, rheumatologists will read articles that, at first glance, may seem beyond the mainstream of standard rheumatology practice and may move us out of our traditional comfort zone. We will learn that rheumatic pain can no longer be simply categorized as a consequence of prostaglandin overload or be treated with a single anti-inflammatory pill. The experienced and respected authors that have contributed to this issue will broaden our appreciation of pain mechanisms and open the door for more diverse treatment concepts that will optimize care of our patients.

The stage is set with the article describing mechanisms of pain which invoke endogenous pain relieving factors, neurogenic sensitization with increase and perpetuation of pain, as well as the importance of our psyche. Thereafter follow articles addressing the concept of the placebo response, important to any well-designed study in rheumatic diseases, as well as an article discussing the challenges in measurement of the rheumatic disease patients' experiences of pain. Building on the foundation of pain mechanisms, we will better understand treatments that are described in subsequent articles that address use of medications such as opioids, antidepressants, topical agents, dietary interventions, complementary treatments, and psychogenic interventions. Finally, pharmacologic treatment options that are in the pipeline for pain management will stimulate our curiosity.

Pain should therefore be viewed as a distinct entity which parallels the specific musculoskeletal process and requires measurement, monitoring, and treatment. Goals regarding pain management must be realistic for the physician as well as for the patient. Complete pain relief is often idealistic, and therefore strategies focused towards modulation of pain in order to continue a meaningful life may often be the best compromise. The best success in pain treatment today will be achieved if all of these factors are addressed.

I would like to acknowledge the many years of scholarship of scientists and clinicians in the fields of rheumatic diseases as well as pain, which have contributed to the status of our knowledge today, and I would especially thank the authors of this issue for thoughtful and comprehensive synthesis of the state of the art.

Mary-Ann Fitzcharles, MB, ChB, FRCP(C)
Montreal General Hospital
1650 Cedar Avenue
Montreal, Quebec H3G 1A4, Canada

E-mail address: mary-ann.fitzcharles@muhc.mcgill.ca

Reference

[1] Atkinson JP. A remembrance of Fred, the lowland gorilla. Arthritis Rheum 1996;39:891–3.

ELSEVIER
SAUNDERS

Rheum Dis Clin N Am
34 (2008) 267–283

RHEUMATIC
DISEASE CLINICS
OF NORTH AMERICA

New Concepts in Rheumatic Pain

Mary-Ann Fitzcharles, MB, ChB, FRCP(C)[a,b,*],
Yoram Shir, MD[a]

[a]Pain Centre, Montreal General Hospital, McGill University Health Centre, 1650 Cedar Avenue, Montreal, Quebec H3G 1A4, Canada
[b]Division of Rheumatology, McGill University, Montreal, Quebec, Canada

The inclusion of pain as the fifth vital sign in clinical medicine underlines the importance of this symptom [1]. Pain that is consistently present in any rheumatic condition should today be considered a specific disease entity, rather than simply a concomitant symptom. Therefore, pain should be addressed on its individual merits and be actively managed in parallel with the rheumatic complaint. Rheumatic pain is the most prevalent pain syndrome worldwide and will be experienced by almost all persons at some time during their lifetime [2,3]. Pain results in a significant burden of suffering with impact upon overall well-being and associated effects on sleep, mood, and energy [4–6]. Understanding of pain mechanisms from the anatomic and molecular perspectives has advanced greatly in the last decade, prompting the use of more varied pain interventions beyond simple analgesic medications.

Although patients should no longer be expected to endure uncontrolled pain, they should also become active participants in their health care management and demonstrate a willingness to achieve better health. Attention to healthy lifestyle habits such as good diet, adequate exercise and weight control should be an integral part of every good pain management program. Patients increasingly use various non-pharmacologic interventions, many of which still need formal evaluation. Current pharmacologic treatments address pain from various perspectives, taking into account the knowledge of molecular mechanisms of pain, but the pain treatments are still suboptimal for many patients because of a myriad of unacceptable side effects. In addition, the barriers to good pain control that still exist, from both the

* Corresponding author. Pain Centre, Montreal General Hospital, McGill University Health Centre, 1650 Cedar Avenue, Montreal, Quebec H3G 1A4.
E-mail address: mary-ann.fitzcharles@muhc.mcgill.ca (M-A. Fitzcharles).

doi:10.1016/j.rdc.2008.03.005

patient's as well as the physician's perspective, will need to be whittled away over time [7]. Physicians must recognize the importance of pain in its own right; with better understanding of the mechanisms of pain, physicians will be able to implement appropriate treatment interventions.

Rheumatic pain will affect all individuals at some time during their lives, resulting in suffering and reduced quality of life [2]. All diseases of joints, whether inflammatory or degenerative, as well as soft tissue processes are associated with pain. The worldwide prevalence of musculoskeletal pain will inevitably increase because of the increasing age of populations and the associated development of osteoarthritis (OA) of peripheral and spinal joints [8]. For these reasons, the awareness of the symptom of pain and its management is of increasing importance to the practice of rheumatology.

To date, the main focus in caring for patients with musculoskeletal complaints has been to make an accurate diagnosis and develop a treatment plan that will affect the disease process as favorably as possible. However, even with astounding advances in the understanding of the pathogenesis of inflammatory arthritis (IA), as well as OA disease, there will likely be no cure for either disease in the near future. Consequently, patients will continue to suffer the effects of disease, with pain as a prominent symptom [9,10]. It is disappointing, therefore, that only limited attention has been paid so far to this specific symptom as part of the evaluation and treatment of patients with rheumatic diseases.

Pain, which is defined as "an unpleasant sensory and emotional experience associated with actual or potential tissue damage or described in terms of such damage" is a debilitating symptom of arthritic as well as soft tissue musculoskeletal disease [11]. The pain of arthritis has important negative consequences for overall health and is associated with poorer functional outcome and worse quality of life when compared with other chronic illnesses [12]. Indeed, pain is likely the most important factor in functional limitation and its successful management has a significant impact upon well-being and outcome.

Acute pain mostly serves a protective function, but chronic pain, as in arthritis, has negative effects that are detrimental to health. There are four important associations that should be addressed in any patient presenting with ongoing pain:

1. Impaired function and quality of life
2. Sleep disturbance
3. Fatigue
4. Mood disturbance

Although the paradigm for pain treatments for the busy rheumatologist has until now mostly been the prescription of a nonsteroidal anti-inflammatory medication (NSAID) or the addition of a simple analgesic such as acetaminophen, an effective approach to pain control must also take the aforementioned factors into consideration. As a result, good pain management will encompass a variety of both pharmacologic as well as nonpharmacologic treatments [7].

Prevalence of rheumatic pain

Chronic pain affects between 20%–50% of individuals worldwide, with musculoskeletal conditions being the most common causes of nonmalignant chronic pain [13–15]. Doctor-diagnosed arthritis was reported in more than 21% of adults in the United States according to a recent survey [16]. It is currently estimated that arthritis affects at least 50% of individuals over the age of 65 years [16] and it is predicted that up to 40% of the general population will be affected by musculoskeletal complaints within the next 25 years [8]. This accelerated increase in arthritis is caused by the increasing age of the population and an associated increase in OA. The consequences of arthritic disease are far-reaching with arthritis and rheumatism identified as the current leading causes of disability in the United States [2]. Back pain is probably the most ubiquitous arthritic pain syndrome with a positive response in over 80% of individuals for lifetime pain [17] and over a quarter of individuals reported back pain lasting at least a full day in the previous 3 months [18].

Pain complaint is more prevalent today than in the past. In a recent population survey in Great Britain, Harkness and colleagues [19] reported that pain complaint is two to three fold greater than 40 years ago. A number of factors may explain this worrisome increase. It is possible that there is a true change in the prevalence of conditions causing pain; populations are aging and the prevalence of pain conditions in individuals over the age of 50 years is prominent. On the other hand, there may be an increased tendency to report pain symptoms because of cultural and social changes. Regardless of the reason for the increased prevalence of chronic pain, it is important that physicians be able to accurately assess pain and recommend appropriate treatment.

The anatomy of rheumatic pain pathways

The periphery

With the exception of healthy cartilage, all joint structures are richly innervated with sensory neurons, which can mediate the pain response [20,21]. Any process affecting joints may involve structures such as cartilage, synovial membrane, subchondral bone, bone marrow, and connective tissues such as ligaments and tendons [22]. Under normal circumstances, the structures of the joint are not sensitive to strong pressure or even vigorous movement. In contrast, diseased joints that have been primed by inflammatory molecules develop sensitivity to seemingly benign movements, and these joints have a low threshold of activation to noxious stimuli. This exaggerated response is defined as hyperalgesia (a greater pain response to a normally painful stimulus) and allodynia (pain induced by a usually innocuous stimulus). These are the first steps toward the complex perpetuation of chronic musculoskeletal pain.

Sensory neurons are classified according to their function, anatomy and speed of impulse conductivity. Pain is initially conducted through nociceptive fibers, either the small diameter myelinated Aδ fibers (causing the acute, sharp initial pain) or the slower conducting, non-myelinated C fibers (the subsequent dull throbbing pain) [23]. Large diameter myelinated Aβ fibers conduct stimuli such as pressure and limb movement under normal circumstances. Although nociceptive fibers constitute up to 80% of the joint innervation in animal studies, these fibers typically have a high threshold of activation to noxious stimulation [24–26]. Silent or sleeping nociceptors may also be activated by inflammation, thereby allowing more pain input into the nervous system. In the disease setting, Aβ fibers, which are usually responsive to low intensity mechanical stimuli, may be phenotypically changed to transmit pain with joint movement.

Persistent firing of peripheral afferent fibers results in temporal summation and cumulative depolarization, which is also known as windup and reflects a hyper responsiveness of the periphery to stimulation. Peripheral sensitization represents an increased sensitivity of pain sensitive neurons.

Spinal cord

The dorsal horn laminae of the spinal cord are the first relay points of input from the periphery to higher pain centers in the thalamus and somatosensory cortex. The primary sensory neurons synapse at this level with a variety of neurons including connecting interneurones, descending inhibiting neurons, as well as those from the sympathetic nervous system [27]. Pain messages that are carried along primary afferents from the periphery do not simply flow in a continuous bombarding stream, but are rapidly modulated and attenuated by a number of mechanisms. Melzack and Wall [28] were the first to suggest that modulation at the dorsal horn functions as a gate to the central flow of noxious sensory information. Not only does the dorsal horn attenuate the pain messages, but it is also the location of increased sensitization to incoming stimuli. An important feature of central sensitization is the increased excitability of dorsal horn neurons from inputs from peripheral nociceptors as well as responses to Aβ fiber stimuli that normally transmit pressure sensation only. Central sensitization occurs following intense or prolonged noxious stimulation that causes alterations in patterns of gene expression, altering the phenotype of the neuron and providing the nervous system with a substantial degree of neuroplasticity [29,30]. Central sensitization represents an increase in spinal neuron excitability to painful stimuli or to stimuli that are usually not painful. Central sensitization is the end result of a combination of increased excitability with decreased inhibition.

Brain

Ascending nociceptive information is integrated in the thalamus, which relays information to the somatosensory cortex and the limbic system, which is crucial in relaying the emotional aspects of pain. Neurons projecting from the periaqueductal gray matter act as the descending inhibitory mechanism and the neurons control many of the antinociceptive and autonomic responses that follow noxious stimuli [27].

The pain pathway stimulus may be summarized as: the immediate nociceptive response associated with A-δ and C fiber input; subsequent changes in the excitability of nerve fibers in the dorsal horn of the spinal cord; peripheral and central sensitization that takes place in an hour or two; and thereafter, changes in intracellular signal molecules and gene expression, taking place over many hours. In addition, there is disinhibition as well as A-β mediated pain stimulation. The contribution of disinhibition to the persistence of chronic pain is an important phenomenon; disinhibition likely plays a role in complex pain conditions such as the fibromyalgia syndrome. All of these impulses represent a series of neurobiological events that activate, modulate, and modify the nervous system response to the sensory input.

Chemical mediators of rheumatic pain

Damaged and inflamed tissues release molecules such as H^+, K^+ and ATP, capable of activating inflammatory cells. These, in turn, produce inflammatory cytokines that can initiate a response in the primary sensory neuron [20]. Other chemical mediators of pain such as substance P and serotonin are intrinsic to the neuron. Neuronal firing is achieved by activation of ion-channel-linked receptors, which can become sensitized in the presence of ongoing inflammation and contribute to the spontaneous pain frequently reported in chronic joint disease.

The primary excitatory neurotransmitter at the level of the dorsal horn is the amino-acid glutamate according to Westlund and colleagues [31], whereas γ-aminobutyric acid (GABA) is an important inhibitory molecule. Glutamate preferentially binds to α-amino-3-hydroxy-5-methyl-4-isoxazole-proprionic acid (AMPA) or N-methyl-D-aspartate (NMDA) ligand-gated sodium and calcium channels [32]. Activation of these receptors depolarizes the membrane and results in fast excitatory postsynaptic potentials.

The afferent pathways are greatly influenced by descending neuron projections that synapse in the laminae of the dorsal horns. These descending impulses are mostly sent forth from the periaqueductal gray region of the brain, and are mediated by serotonin, norepinephrine, endogenous opioids, and cannabinoids. Therefore the excitability of neurons can be modulated by a variety of pre- and postsynaptic opioids (μ, κ, δ) and anti- noradrenergic (α-1, α-2) and muscarinic receptors.

Inflammatory mediators also increase the production of nerve growth factor (NGF), which regulates the expression of neuropeptides, receptors and ion channels [33]. The inflammatory response may be further augmented by molecules such as substance P and calcitonin gene reactive protein (CGRP), which induce vasodilatation and extravasation of fluid from capillaries [30,34]. This neuroactive and inflammatory milieu lowers the firing threshold of high threshold nociceptors to mechanical, thermal or chemical stimuli, and a cycle of pain is set in motion.

Mechanistic approach to rheumatic pain: a change in paradigm

Traditionally, pain arising in areas of tissue damage has mostly been categorized as nociceptive, whereas pain that is associated with specific nerve damage was regarded as neurogenic. The concept of inciting molecules at a peripheral site as the sole cause of rheumatic pain is, however, too simplistic; recent research has identified a more complex path of events that becomes operative especially in the chronic pain setting of musculoskeletal origin. The distinct divide between nociceptive and neurogenic pain no longer exists; clear evidence points to considerable overlap between the two types of pain. Recent studies have highlighted the importance of neurogenic mechanisms in arthritic disease [30,34,35]. The mechanistic understanding of rheumatic pain therefore has far-reaching implications for treatments and it opens the arena for novel treatment choices that have previously been outside the rheumatology domain.

Rheumatic pain can be divided into acute pain caused by an active inflammatory process or chronic pain that is a result of tissue destruction and mechanical changes to cartilage, bone and soft tissues. In the acute stage of a rheumatic process, the major stimulus initiating the pain response is the soup of inflammatory molecules at the local site [20]. These inflammatory cytokines, which are key players in the pathogenic mechanisms of IA, are also important for the generation of pain [20]. Treatments that directly modulate this inflammation are most appropriate and are usually successful at this stage. The success of the numerous NSAIDS used during the last century can be attributed to the importance of inflammatory mechanisms in most acute rheumatic pain settings.

In contrast, pain in the chronic setting is sustained by activation of neurogenic mechanisms. Peripheral and central sensitization that occurs in the setting of persistent pain stimulus contributes to the chronic nature of the pain and it also has implications with respect to the response to pain treatments [29,36]. For these reasons, the management of chronic pain is more challenging and often less successful than the management of acute pain.

Pain-generation mechanisms may differ depending upon the stage of disease, irrespective of the underlying primary rheumatic diagnosis. Successful pain management should therefore take into account the underlying mechanism of pain generation, rather than simply the specific rheumatologic diagnosis. This approach results from the fact that, even in the realm of well-defined taxonomy of rheumatic diseases, a strategy that is directed at examining, classifying and then treating pain on the basis of the underlying disease can be surprisingly limited. This concept of mechanism and/or symptom-based approach to chronic pain, rather than treating specific syndromes or disease, was proposed a decade ago for neuropathic pain conditions and the concept has greatly improved treatment approaches [37,38]. Lessons learned in the neuropathic pain domain can be used to facilitate the approach to chronic rheumatic pain, whereby the pain symptom becomes a disease in its own right.

The pathogenic mechanisms operative in both IA and OA have similarities; both demonstrate various degrees of inflammation and structural tissue damage at various stages of the disease process. Although the most prevalent IA is RA, other arthritic conditions such as psoriatic arthritis, inflammatory spondyloarthritis, and reactive arthritis, to name just a few, have equally negative effects on quality of life and well-being. The pathogenic mechanisms with regard to generation of pain are probably somewhat similar in the various inflammatory conditions. For example, although IA has a more pronounced inflammatory phase compared with OA (ie, dense synovial infiltration with immune cells, leading to invasion of ligaments, cartilage and bone), structural changes occur in both IA and OA with time [39,40]. Indeed, radiographic erosions are indicative of structural damage in IA, whereas subchondral sclerosis and osteophyte formation are seen in OA.

Anatomic associations in rheumatic pain

Because bone, bone marrow, and periosteum are richly innervated, these tissues are likely the origin of much of the pain experienced in arthritis. Changes in juxta-articular bone, bone marrow edema, and vascular stasis, therefore, all play a part in pain generation. Changes in these tissues have been observed on MRI scans in both IA and OA. Pain in OA has been associated both with bone marrow edema as well as synovial thickening [41,42]. In the setting of persistent pathologic change, neurogenic mechanisms are activated and contribute to pain perpetuation. Neurophysiologic studies have demonstrated cutaneous hyperalgesia, as well as a reduced pain threshold to mechanical and thermal stimulation, in the area of a painful OA joint, but not in the absence of pain.

Vascular pathology

Vascular pathology likely plays an important role in the pathogenesis of OA and IA [43,44]. Bone marrow edema in early OA is associated with pain and progressive cartilage loss leading to structural damage of OA joints over time [41,42,45–48]. Although the primary focus of pathology in IA is the synovium, bone marrow edema is correlated with synovial inflammation, bone erosion, and DAS28 in early disease [44]. In the setting of bone marrow edema, there is increased intra-osseous pressure in the rigid bony compartment [43], secondary to reduced venous drainage. Increased pressure in turn results in poor circulation of nutrients, impaired removal of waste metabolic products, and compromise of bony tissue with accelerated apoptosis of osteocytes, activation of osteoclasts, and breakdown of bony supporting structure. The rich sensory innervation of bone marrow is likely an important mediator of this pressure-induced pain. In addition, impaired blood flow in the subchondral bone, as a result of venous stasis or occlusion by microemboli in subchondral blood vessels may be an important contributor to progressive cartilage damage in early OA.

Subchondral bone changes

Subchondral bone is increasingly recognized as playing a key role in the maintenance of healthy cartilage. MRI studies have demonstrated that some of the earliest changes in OA occur at the highly vascularized subchondral site [41]. Bony changes that have been long recognized include sclerosis of subchondral bone, cysts, and osteophytes formation. Elevation of bone markers in progressive OA points toward increased turnover of bone as a component of a disease previously believed to be based primarily in cartilage [10]. Subchondral bone is richly innervated with sensory fibers and as a result, it could become a source of pain.

The clinical domain

Quality of life issues for patients with rheumatic pain

Increasing attention is being paid to factors that are important from the patient's perspective regarding health [49]. Physical function and health-related quality of life (HRQOL) are more immediately relevant to a patient's perception of health and control of disease than are the traditional laboratory or clinical measures used by clinicians [50–52].

Pain is an important component of all measurements of HRQOL. Even seemingly small changes in pain intensity may have a large impact upon perceived health in patients with rheumatic diseases. A recent study of pediatric rheumatology patients has demonstrated that even a minimal change in pain score is associated with meaningful improvement in HRQOL [53]. The concept of "minimally clinically important difference" addresses changes in health status that are considered worthwhile from the patient perspective [54]. Improvements in HRQOL have far-reaching effects upon the physical, emotional and social well-being of patients who have rheumatic diseases.

The way in which pain affects HRQOL is complex and multifaceted. Chronic pain has characteristics of intensity and also quality, as well as impacts on sleep, mood and the ability to function in social, work, and leisure activities. Pain is highly correlated with the standard measures of health status in RA such as the "Health Assessment Questionnaire" (HAQ) [55] and the "Disease Activity Score" (DAS28) [56]. It has even been suggested that the simple measurement of pain may serve as a substitute for measures of general health or disease status [56]. Patients who have inflammatory arthritis and an associated pain syndrome of fibromyalgia report higher DAS scores than those without the associated pain syndrome [57].

The ability to function as close to normal as possible is a criteria that can be used to identify health. In the rheumatic diseases, function is influenced by pain, fatigue, mood disturbance, and eventually musculoskeletal dysfunction. In the early stages of IA, functional status is closely associated with the degree of inflammation and joint damage [58,59]. Inflammation, in turn, correlates with the severity of pain. Therefore, it may be construed that the intensity of pain has an important effect upon function. Pain, particularly in the chronic setting, is, however, a highly individual experience that is influenced by many factors other than simply the disease process. Psychological status, previous pain and health experience, and the social and cultural environment all play important roles in the individual perception of pain.

The pain complaint

Fluctuations in pain intensity

Pain in rheumatic conditions is subject to considerable variability and fluctuation within an individual patient's experience. Recent study has demonstrated up to 20% variation in OA pain, both within a week and from week to week [60]. These usual fluctuations in pain levels would be sufficiently large to be considered clinically significant in a treatment efficacy study setting [61,62]. Therefore, single measurements at specific time points may not accurately reflect an intervention's true treatment effects (see article by Dieppe). Pain level fluctuations correlated with changes in mood, as well as with HRQOL, which emphasizes the importance of pain [60].

Effect of weather conditions

It is not rare to encounter patients attributing their rheumatic pain aggravation or suppression to weather conditions. Actually, it is somewhat rare to meet patients who do not associate weather conditions with their miseries. It is surprising that only a meager research has been done in this field. In one of the only prospective studies done, Guedj and colleagues [63] showed that most patients with a variety of rheumatic diseases (RA, OA, other IA conditions, and fibromyalgia) reported changes in their arthritic symptoms that were dependent on weather conditions. This association was more prevalent in women than in men. In OA, for example, pain symptoms were significantly associated with changes in all three examined parameters: temperature, barometric pressure, and rain. In another longitudinal analysis of pain reports from a three-month clinical trial among individuals with knee OA dispersed across the United States, there were consistent associations of pressure change and ambient temperature with pain severity [64].

Is the pain caused by chronic joint damage or is there a superimposed inflammatory component?

In the setting of long-standing inflammatory disease it may be difficult to identify the exact cause of pain. Articular changes may be established with permanent soft tissue and bony changes; inflammatory markers such as sedimentation rate and C-reactive protein may not necessarily be reflective of activity of the disease process. A simple therapeutic intervention that can help to rule out uncontrolled active inflammation is the administration of a short course of corticosteroids for 7–10 days. Even without appreciable change on joint examination, a report of important improvement in symptoms indicates that at least some of the pain is of an inflammatory nature and attention should be paid to treating the underlying inflammatory disease process. A negative response supports the concept of nociceptive pain caused by chronic structural changes and can be addressed accordingly.

Associated complaints with pain

In the setting of continued pain, there is almost always associated sleep disturbance, fatigue, and mood disorder [65]. Each of these factors plays an important role in the continued suffering of patients with chronic pain. Although attention to these specific complaints has previously been out of the mainstream of rheumatologic practice, rheumatologists, in particular, and other physicians will now need to address these symptoms to achieve whole patient care.

Sleep disturbance

Pain is strongly associated with sleep disturbance. Sleep disturbance, in turn, affects mood and fatigue. A self-perpetuating cycle of closely interlinked symptoms develops: frequently disturbed sleep in the setting of a chronic illness results in fatigue, exhaustion, irritability, poor function, and a cycle of more pain [66]. Poor sleep, independent of mood status, has been associated with greater pain report in a population of chronic pain patients [67]. The added distress for a patient who is already suffering interferes with ability to function during the day. Sleep disturbance may manifest as difficulty falling asleep, interrupted sleep during the night, and awakening feeling unrefreshed [68]. Sleep disturbance may be caused by factors such as the presence of restless leg syndrome, inadequate pain control at night pain, underlying depression, or simply poor attention to good sleep hygiene. Therefore sleep disturbance should not immediately be treated with the prescription of a sleeping pill, but explored from the perspective of the nature of the sleep disturbance and its underlying cause. A few focused questions will help clarify the characteristics of the sleep complaint and direct the physician to appropriate management. This area of care for rheumatology patients has previously received limited attention in the past and it deserves further study.

Fatigue

The second important complaint commonly associated with pain is fatigue. Fatigue is present to some degree in almost all patients with chronic pain and it is extremely challenging [49]. This symptom, like pain, is purely subjective and solely measured by patients' report. Fatigue is perhaps the most challenging symptom to address in patients with chronic pain. Some causes of fatigue may include: inadequate control of the underlying systemic disease commonly seen in RA; systemic lupus erythematosis and ankylosing spondylitis; the effects of medications including NSAIDs, opioid analgesics and antidepressants; or depression. Increasing physical activity is the only intervention that has consistently shown some positive impact on fatigue. There are no current pharmacologic recommendations for fatigue, although occasional cautious off-label use of stimulants such as methylphenidate or modafinil may be considered in severe situations.

Mood disturbance

Pain is inevitably associated with some mood disturbance [69]. This important symptom and its treatment thereof will be addressed in other articles in this clinic (see articles by Keefe, Perrot). Depending upon the underlying personality of the individual, mood disturbance may play a role of greater or lesser importance for individual patients. Compounded with sleep disturbance and fatigue, depression and anxiety have important negative effects on quality of life.

Obstacles to optimal pain management

The main focus in the management of rheumatic diseases has been directed toward controlling the disease process especially for those with IA, with less attention to the symptom of pain. Specific management of pain in patients with rheumatic diseases has been somewhat neglected mainly because of barriers that exist from the perspective of both the physician as well as the patient [7,70–73].

Patient-related barriers

1. The misconception that pain should be a normal part of the rheumatic disease and pain management will mask the disease process
2. Poor adherence to treatment recommendations, eg, some studies report only 50% compliance with treatments
3. Fear and distrust of medications because of side effects, concerns about loss of efficacy of pain treatments, and risks of addiction
4. Lack of motivation and shift of locus of control away from personal involvement in health care

Physician-related barriers

1. Considering pain management of secondary importance to disease management
2. Additional time investment needed to effectively treat pain
3. Lack of basic and clinical training in pain treatment
4. The belief that patients will always report their pain honestly
5. Fear of regulatory scrutiny, particularly with regard to opioid prescriptions
6. Unjustified concerns about addiction and side effects of medications, especially opioids

Treatments

Effective pain management for the rheumatology patient can no longer be simply the prescription of a pill. Pain treatment should take into account the many factors that have been previously described, which affect patient wellbeing in the setting of chronic rheumatic disease. A treatment plan directed toward pain control should be developed in parallel with the best management of the underlying rheumatologic process. Physicians must actively assess the severity of pain, gauge the effect on daily life, explore features commonly associated with pain, and offer management appropriate to the individual patient (65). The tendency for modern society to be passive with respect to health care issues (ie, patients look toward pharmacologic treatments as a solution to most problems) should be superseded by the active participation of patients in their health management. Patients should be educated regarding their disease and encouraged to adopt healthy lifestyle practices.

The following articles of this clinic will expand upon treatments some of which, at first glance, may seem out of the mainstream of rheumatic disease practice, but which are now integral to the management of chronic pain. The placebo mechanism described by Benedetti and colleagues is without side effect and it will continue to play a role in pain control in many patients (see Benedetti's article). The authors of this article have already come to doubt the results of any randomized clinical trial that does not show a robust placebo response of 20%–30%. Placebo is, therefore, a powerful tool that has been underutilized in modern medicine.

Patients demonstrating active participation in their disease management frequently try dietary or complementary interventions independent of a physician's advice (see articles by Cleland, Ernst). This should be seen as an active and positive step by the patient toward health, and the physician should acknowledge that disclosure of this information strengthens the doctor-patient relationship. Many forms of complementary treatment have been used for years, often on the basis of hearsay and tradition rather than scientific rigor, but they should not be immediately discarded for want of evidence. Trust and empathy in the doctor-patient relationship may be as important as the prescription of a new designer molecule. Physicians should strive to understand the scientific evidence for these interventions as much as possible to advise patients appropriately and safely. These strategies are discussed in greater detail in specific articles in this volume (see articles by Marchand, Benedetti).

Psychological considerations play an increasingly important role in the management of patients with chronic diseases. Because most arthritic disease will not be cured in the foreseeable future, emphasis on coping strategies and locus of control will help patients to continue with a worthwhile life even in the setting of illness. Additional psychological stressors such as anxiety and depression impact greatly on wellbeing and on continued symptoms (see articles by Keefe, Perrot). The intricate relationship between the body's physiology and the psyche must be appreciated to adequately understand and treat a complaint of pain in an individual patient.

For centuries, anti-inflammatory treatments have been the mainstay of rheumatic disease medicinal management. Hippocrates wrote of the bitter powder from the willow bark that could ease rheumatic aches and pains. Salicin from the willow led to the development of salicylic acid and eventually to the variety of NSAIDS that constitute the focus of the modern day rheumatology pharmacopoeia. The NSAIDS remain the most frequently used medications for pain and inflammation in the rheumatic diseases, but, because rheumatic pain is no longer believed to be entirely dependent upon the inflammatory prostaglandin cascade, other drug treatment modalities are showing promise and should be explored. Because ingested medications are frequently associated with unacceptable side effects, other methods of administration such as topical application or buccal absorption are likely to offer alternate routes of use (see the article by Moore). Understanding the complexity of chronic pain mechanisms gives credibility to the use of these more diverse pharmacologic treatments. There is further discussion in ensuing articles in this volume about the use of opioids, cannabinoids, antidepressants, and specific channel blockers.

This greater understanding of mechanisms and the modulation of pain will lead the way to the development of more targeted and specific pain therapies that will be further addressed in this volume (see article by Dray). Important targets for pain modulation in the future will include: focusing on specific electrolyte channels of nerves; expanded use of NSAIDS, opioids, α-2 agonists for modulation of excitatory and inhibitory neuronal activity; and local anesthetics for suppression of electrical impulses. Identification of opioid, α-2 and prostaglandin receptors in the spinal cord as well as inflamed tissues argues in favor of the administration of molecules targeting these receptors at the local site. Administering drugs that promote spinal inhibitory mechanisms such as α-2 agonists may modify the consequences of disinhibition. Therefore, physicians may look forward to a broader scope of pharmacologic treatments for rheumatic pain in the future.

Summary

Rheumatic pain will affect almost every single person at some time during his or her life. The prevalence of rheumatic pain increases with aging of populations and the presence of chronic poorly controlled pain greatly affects wellbeing and global health. For these reasons, rheumatic pain deserves specific and directed attention. The symptom of pain has important consequences for daily function, sleep, energy, and mood, independent of the underlying disease process. Therefore, pain can even be considered an independent disease entity requiring treatment of equal importance and in parallel with that of the rheumatic disease. Although the clinical evaluation of pain still remains subjective, impressive progress has been made in the understanding of pain mechanisms—especially pertaining to chronic pain. This has led to the introduction of more diverse treatments that were previously unfamiliar to rheumatology practice. Successful pain management today can be achieved by combining the knowledge of molecular mechanisms with the art of medicine, and by tailoring treatments to the specific and unique needs of an individual patient.

References

[1] Phillips DM. JCAHO pain management standards are unveiled. JAMA 2000;284:428–9.
[2] Centers for Disease Control and Prevention (CDC). Prevalence of disabilities and associated health condition among adults- United States, 1999. MMWR Morb Mortal Wkly Rep 2001; 50:120–5.
[3] The burden of musculoskeletal conditions at the start of the millennium. World Health Organ Tech Rep ser 2003;919:1–218.
[4] Cooper RG, Booker CK, Spanswick CC. What is pain management, and what is its relevance to the rheumatologist? Rheumatology 2003;42:1133–7.
[5] Skevington SM. Investigating the relationship between pain and discomfort and quality of life, using the WHOQOL. Pain 1998;76:395–406.
[6] Fries JF, Spitz P, Young DY. The dimensions of health outcomes: the health assessment questionnaire, disability and pain scales. J Rheumatol 1982;9:789–93.
[7] Fitzcharles MA, Almahrezi A, Shir Y. Pain: understanding and challenges for the rheumatologist. Arthritis Rheum 2005;52:3685–92.
[8] Hootman JM, Helmick CG. Projections of US prevalence of arthritis and associated activity limitations. Arthritis Rheum 2006;54:226–9.
[9] Firestein GS. Evolving concepts of rheumatoid arthritis. Nature 2003;423:356–61.
[10] Krasnokutsky S, Samuels J, Abramson SB. Osteoarthritis in 2007. Bull NYU Hosp Jt Dis 2007;65:222–8.
[11] Merskey H, Bogduk N, editors. Classification of chronic pain. Seattle (WA): IASP Press; 1994.
[12] Sprangers MA, de Regt EB, Andries F, et al. Which chronic conditions are associated with better or poorer quality of life? J Clin Epidemiol 2000;53(9):895–907.
[13] Salaffi F, De Angelis R, Grassi W, et al. Prevalence of musculoskeletal conditions in an Italian population sample: results of a regional community-based study. I. The mapping study. Clin Exp Rheumatol 2005;23:819–28.
[14] Macfarlane GJ. Looking back: developments in our understanding of the occurrence, aetiology and prognosis of chronic pain 1954–2004. Rheumatology 2005;44(Suppl 4):23–6.

[15] Louw QA, Morris LD, Grimmer-Somers K. The prevalence of low back pain in Africa: a systematic review. BMC Musculoskelet Disord 2007;8:105.
[16] Helmick CG, Felson DT, Lawrence RC, et al. Estimates of the prevalence of arthritis and other rheumatic conditions in the United States part I. Arthritis Rheum 2008;58:15–25.
[17] Kelsey JL, White AA. Epidemiology and impact of low back pain. Spine 1980;5:133–42.
[18] Lawrence RC, Felson DT, Helmick CG, et al. Estimates of the prevalence of arthritis and other rheumatic conditions in the United States part II. Arthritis Rheum 2008;58(1):26–35.
[19] Harkness EF, Macfarlane GJ, Silman AJ, et al. Is musculoskeletal pain more common now than 40 years ago?: two population-based cross-sectional studies. Rheumatology 2005;44: 890–5.
[20] Kidd BL, Urban LA. Mechanisms of inflammatory pain. Br J Anaesth 2001;87:3–11.
[21] Kidd BL. Osteoarthritis and joint pain. Pain 2006;123:6–9.
[22] Haywood L, McWilliams DF, Pearson CI, et al. Inflammation and angiogenesis in osteoarthritis. Arthritis Rheum 2003;48:2173–7.
[23] Raja SN, Meyer RA, Ringkamp M, et al. Peripheral neural mechanisms of nociception. In: Wall PD, Melzack R, editors. Textbook of pain. London: Churchill Livingstone; 1999. p. 11–57.
[24] Langford LA, Schmidt RF. Afferent and efferent axons in the medial and posterior articular nerves of the cat. Anat Rec 1983;206:71–8.
[25] Heppelmann B, McDougall JJ. Inhibitory effect of amiloride and gadolinium on fine afferent nerves in the rat knee: evidence of mechanogated ion channels in joints. Exp Brain Res 2005; 167:114–8.
[26] McQueen DS. Inflammatory pain and the joint. In: Brain SD, Moore PK, editors. Pain and neurogenic inflammation. Basel (Switzerland): Birkhauser Verlag; 1999. p. 137–66.
[27] Basbaum AI, Fields HL. Endogenous pain control systems: brainstem spinal pathways and endorphin circuitry. Annu Rev Neurosci 1984;7:309–38.
[28] Melzack R, Wall PD. Evolution of pain theories. Int Anesthesiol Clin 1970;8:3–34.
[29] Coderre TJ, Katz J, Vaccarino AL, et al. Contribution of central neuroplasticity to pathological pain: review of clinical and experimental evidence. Pain 1993;52:259–85.
[30] Schaible HG, Del Rosso A, Matucci-Cerinic M. Neurogenic aspects of inflammation. Rheum Dis Clin North Am 2005;3:77–101.
[31] Westlund KN, McNeill DL, Coggeshall RE. Glutamate immunoreactivity in rat dorsal root axons. Neurosci Lett 1989;96:13–7.
[32] Dickenson AH, Sullivan AF. Evidence for a role of the NMDA receptor in the frequency dependent potentiation of deep rat dorsal horn nociceptive neurones following C-fibre stimulation. Neuropharmacology 1987;26:1235–8.
[33] Heppenstall PA, Lewin GR. Neurotrophins, nociceptors and pain. Curr Opin Anaesthesiol 2000;13:573–6.
[34] McDougall JJ. Arthritis and pain. Neurogenic origin of joint pain. Arthritis Res Ther 2006;8: 220–30.
[35] Xiao WH, Bennett GJ. Persistent low-frequency spontaneous discharge in A-fiber and C-fiber primary afferent neurons during an inflammatory pain condition. Anesthesiology 2007;107:813–21.
[36] Bolay H, Moskowitz MA. Mechanisms of pain modulation in chronic syndromes. Neurology 2002;59:S2–7.
[37] Woolf CJ, Bennett GJ, Doherty M, et al. Towards a mechanism-based classification of pain? Pain 1998;77:227–9.
[38] Finnerup NB, Otto M, Jensen TS, et al. An evidence-based algorithm for the treatment of neuropathic pain. MedGenMed 2007;9:36.
[39] Schett G. Joint remodelling in inflammatory disease. Ann Rheum Dis 2007;66(Suppl 3): 42–4.
[40] Tak PP, Bresnihan B. The pathogenesis and prevention of joint damage in rheumatoid arthritis: advances from synovial biopsy and tissue analysis. Arthritis Rheum 2000;43:2619–33.

[41] Felson DT, Chaisson CE, Hill CL, et al. The association of bone marrow lesions with pain in knee osteoarthritis. Ann Intern Med 2001;134:541–9.
[42] Felson DT, McLaughlin S, Goggins J, et al. Bone marrow edema and its relation to progression of knee osteoarthritis. Ann Intern Med 2003;139:330–6.
[43] Findlay DM. Vascular pathology and osteoarthritis. Rheumatology 2007;46:1763–8.
[44] Tamai M, Kawakami A, Uetani M, et al. Bone edema determined by magnetic resonance imaging reflects severe disease status in patient with early-stage rheumatoid arthritis. J Rheumatol 2007;34(11):2154–7.
[45] Hunter DJ, Zhang Y, Niu J, et al. Increase in bone marrow lesions associated with cartilage loss: a longitudinal magnetic resonance imaging study of knee osteoarthritis. Arthritis Rheum 2006;54:1529–35.
[46] Garnero P, Peterfy C, Zaim S, et al. Bone marrow abnormalities on magnetic resonance imaging are associated with type II collagen degradation in knee osteoarthritis: a three-month longitudinal study. Arthritis Rheum 2005;52:2822–9.
[47] Zhai G, Blizzard L, Srikanth V, et al. Correlates of knee pain in older adults: Tasmanian older adult cohort study. Arthritis Rheum 2006;55:264–71.
[48] Carrino JA, Blum J, Parellada JA, et al. MRI of bone marrow edema-like signal in the pathogenesis of subchondral cysts. Osteoarthritis Cartilage 2006;14:1081–5.
[49] Uutela T, Kautiainen H, Hakala M. Nottingham health profile questionnaire incorporates important aspects of the patient perspective into outcome assessment in rheumatoid arthritis. Clin Exp Rheumatol 2008;26:39–44.
[50] Tugwell P, Wells G, Strand V, et al. Clinical improvement as reflected in measures of function and health related quality of life: sensitivity and relative efficiency to detect a treatment effect in a 12 month placebo controlled trial comparing leflunomide with methotrexate. Arthritis Rheum 2000;43:506–14.
[51] Strand V, Cohen S, Crawford B, et al. Patient-reported outcomes better discriminate active treatment from placebo in randomized controlled trials in rheumatoid arthritis. Rheumatology 2004;43:640–7.
[52] Cohen S, Strand V, Aguilar D, et al. Patient versus physician-reported outcomes in rheumatoid arthritis patients treated with recombinant interleukin-1 receptor antagonist (anakinra) therapy. Rheumatology 2004;43:648–56.
[53] Dhanani S, Quenneville J, Perron M, et al. Minimal difference in pain associated with change in quality of life in children with rheumatic diseases. Arthritis Care Res 2002;47: 501–5.
[54] Kosinki M, Zhao SZ, Dedhiya S, et al. Determining minimally important changes in generic and disease-specific health-related quality of life questionnaires in clinical trials of rheumatoid arthritis. Arthritis Rheum 2000;43:1478–87.
[55] Häkkinen A, Kautiainen H, Hannonen P, et al. Muscle strength, pain, and disease activity explain individual subdimensions of the health assessment questionnaire disability index, especially in women with rheumatoid arthritis. Ann Rheum Dis 2006;65:30–4.
[56] Leeb BF, Haindl PM, Maktari A, et al. Disease activity score-28 values differ considerably depending on patient's pain perception and sex. J Rheumatol 2007;34:2382–7.
[57] Leeb BF, Andel I, Sautner J, et al. The DAS28 in rheumatoid arthritis and fibromyalgia patients. Rheumatology 2004;43:1504–7.
[58] Scott DL, Pugner K, Kaarela K, et al. The links between joint damage and disability in rheumatoid arthritis. Rheumatology 2000;39:122–32.
[59] Hazes JM. Determinants of physical function in rheumatoid arthritis: association with the disease process. Rheumatology 2003;42(Suppl 2):17–21.
[60] Hutchings A, Calloway M, Choy E, et al. The longitudinal examination of arthritis pain (LEAP) study: relationships between weekly fluctuations in patient-rated joint pain and other health outcomes. J Rheumatol 2007;34:2291–300.
[61] Farrar JT, Portenoy RK, Berlin JA, et al. Defining the clinically important difference in pain outcome measures. Pain 2000;88:287–94.

[62] Pham T, van der Heijde D, Altman RD, et al. OMERACT-OARSI initiative: osteoarthritis research society international set of responder criteria for osteoarthritis clinical trials revisited. Osteoarthritis Cartilage 2004;12:389–99.

[63] Guedj D, Weinberger A. Effect of weather conditions on rheumatic patients. Ann Rheum Dis 1990;49:158–9.

[64] McAlindon T, Formica M, Schmid CH, et al. Changes in barometric pressure and ambient temperature influence osteoarthritis pain. Am J Med 2007;120:429–34.

[65] Winfield JB. Pain and arthritis. N C Med J 2007;68:444–6.

[66] Wolfe F, Michaud K, Li T. Sleep disturbance in patients with rheumatoid arthritis: evaluation by medical outcomes study and visual analog sleep scales. J Rheumatol 2006;33: 1942–51.

[67] Morin CM, Gibson D, Wade J. Self-reported sleep and mood disturbance in chronic pain patients. Clin J Pain 1998;14:311–4.

[68] Cole JC, Dubois D, Kosinski M. Use of patient-reported sleep measures in clinical trials of pain treatment: a literature review and synthesis of current sleep measures and a conceptual model of sleep disturbance in pain. Clin Ther 2007;29:2580–8.

[69] Smith BW, Zautra AJ. The effects of anxiety and depression on weekly pain in women with arthritis. Pain, in press.

[70] Boulanger A, Clark AJ, Squire P, et al. Chronic pain in Canada: have we improved our management of chronic noncancer pain? Pain Res Manag 2007;12(1):39–47.

[71] Gardner-Nix J. Principles of opioid use in chronic noncancer pain. CMAJ 2003;169:38–43.

[72] Jovey RD, Ennis J, Gardner-Nix J, et al. Pain society. Use of opioid analgesics for the treatment of chronic noncancer pain–a consensus statement and guidelines from the Canadian pain society, 2002. Pain Res Manag 2003;8(Suppl A):3A–28A.

[73] Monsivais D, McNeill J. Multicultural influences on pain medication attitudes and beliefs in patients with nonmalignant chronic pain syndromes. Pain Manag Nurs 2007;8:64–71.

ELSEVIER
SAUNDERS

Rheum Dis Clin N Am
34 (2008) 285–309

RHEUMATIC
DISEASE CLINICS
OF NORTH AMERICA

The Physiology of Pain Mechanisms: From the Periphery to the Brain

Serge Marchand, PhD

Department of Neurosurgery, University of Sherbrooke, Axe Douleur CRC-CHUS, 3001, 12e Avenue Nord, Sherbrooke, QC J1H 5N4, Canada

Pain is a dynamic phenomenon. From the periphery to the brain, the nociceptive signal will be modulated at all levels of the central nervous system (CNS). This plasticity speaks to the ability to adapt and change within the nervous system. The current science regarding concepts of pain mechanisms also takes into account genetic and environmental factors that will influence the development of persistent pain. Moreover, the maintenance of chronic pain is not only the result of continued and increased nociceptive activity mostly arising at the peripheral site of pathology, but also depends on additional changes within the CNS, such as an increase of excitatory or reduction of inhibitory endogenous pain modulation mechanisms.

Multiple endogenous excitatory and inhibitory mechanisms have been identified [1]. This article introduces the scientific basis for the understanding of pain mechanisms and highlights the importance of endogenous excitatory and inhibitory controls within the CNS. These innate control systems have an impact on the evolution of chronic pain and may be manipulated to alter the pain process, and therefore have implications regarding treatment. Rheumatic pain, particularly as seen in longstanding osteoarthritis, may be considered the prototype of chronic pain. Additionally, inflammatory arthritic diseases also account for important pain complaints and suffering across all ages. Understanding neurophysiologic mechanisms involved in the development and maintenance of pain will help the clinician to devise a more effective treatment plan guided by pathophysiologic dysfunction.

From nociception to pain

A good way to understand the physiology of pain is to follow the nociceptive signal pathways from the periphery to the brain, with emphasis on

E-mail address: serge.marchand@usherbrooke.ca

doi:10.1016/j.rdc.2008.04.003

the integration and modulation of the nociceptive signal at different steps in the CNS (Fig. 1).

Mechanical, chemical, or thermal nociceptive stimulation will recruit peripheral nociceptors that conduct the nociceptive signal in the primary somatosensory neuron to the dorsal horn of the spinal cord. In the dorsal horn, the primary neuron will make a synaptic contact with the secondary or projection neuron. Secondary neurons form the spinothalamic (lateral) and spinoreticular (medial) tracts will immediately cross in the spinal cord and send afferent projections to higher centers. A large proportion of afferents will make a second synapse in the lateral and medial nuclei of the thalamus, which subsequently make synaptic contact with tertiary neurons. It is important to emphasize that the secondary neurons may also synapse with neurons in different nuclei of the brainstem, including the periaqueductal gray (PAG) and nucleus raphe magnus (NRM), areas involved in descending endogenous pain modulation. Tertiary neurons

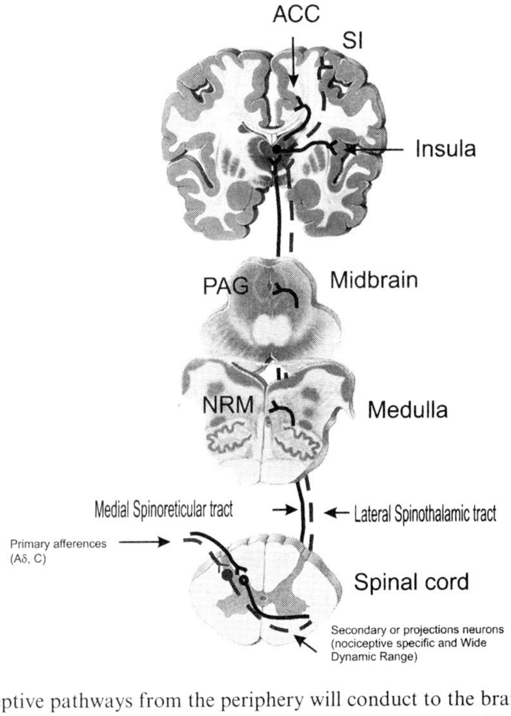

Fig. 1. The nociceptive pathways from the periphery will conduct to the brain after two synaptic relays. The Aδ and C-fibers will make their first synapse with the projection neurons in the dorsal horn of the spinal cord. The secondary neurons will decussate immediately in the cord and conduct to the thalamic nuclei, where they will make the second synaptic contact. The third neurons will finally project to the somatosensory cortices for the sensory-discriminative component of pain, and to limbic structures (anterior cingulated cortex and insula) for the motivational component of pain. ACC, anterior cingulate cortex; NRM, nucleus raphe magnus; SI, SII, somatosensory cortices; PAG, periaqueductal gray.

from the thalamus send afferents to the primary and secondary somatosensory cortices (SI, SII). The SI and SII are involved in the sensory quality of pain, which includes location, duration, and intensity. Tertiary neurons also project to limbic structures, including the anterior cingulate cortex (ACC) and the insula, which are involved in the affective or emotional component of pain.

The various synaptic contacts with excitatory and inhibitory neurons at all levels of the CNS are important integration regions that are the target of most pharmacologic approaches.

The periphery: the nociceptors

An injury that causes a potential risk for the organism will activate free nerve endings that respond to nociceptive stimulation (Fig. 2). Most of these fibers are polymodal and will respond to different modalities, including mechanical, thermal, and chemical stimulation [2].

A nociceptive stimulation will initiate a cascade of events. Pronociceptive inflammatory molecules will be released into the periphery and will produce

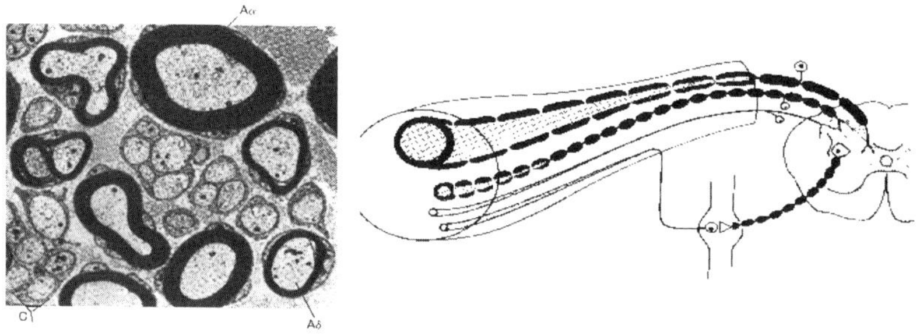

	Aβ	Aδ	C
Diameter	6 to 12 μ myelinated	1 à 5 μ myelinated	0,2 à 1,5 μ unmyelinated
Conduction	35 to 75 M/s	35 to 75 M/s	35 to 75 M/s
Role	Light touch, proprioception	Temperature, Nociception (mechanical, thermal)	Nociception (mechanical, thermal and chemical)

Fig. 2. The nociceptive afferent fibers can be separated according to their physical characteristics and conduction velocity. On this nerve section, where the myelin has been stained in black, one can see the large myelinated Aβ fibers, the smaller and myelinated Aδ fibers, and the unmyelinated C fibers. As seen in the table, the conduction velocity will increase with the diameter and thickness of the myelin sheet.

peripheral hyperalgesia. These pronociceptive inflammatory molecules originate in various blood cells (mastocytes, polymorphonuclear cells, and platelets) and include bradykinins, prostaglandins, histamine, serotonin, adenosine triphosphate, and also from immune cells which produce interleukins, interferon, and tumor necrosis factors [3–6]. Substance P and calcitonin gene related protein (CGRP), which act as neurotransmitters in the CNS, are also released into the periphery and act as proinflammatory factors in the periphery, favoring neurogenic inflammation [3].

Primary hyperalgesia: peripheral nociceptors hyperactivity

Injured tissues will release various substances, such as potassium, prostaglandins, histamine, or bradykinins that are pronociceptive, and will also invoke an immune response. These inflammatory and immune factors will sensitize the nociceptive receptors directly within the lesion and in the surrounding neurons [6]. Primary hyperalgesia, which follows the release of these factors, may be measured as a lowered pain threshold in and around the lesion. This has been demonstrated to occur in the area of arthritic joints both in animal studies and in human beings.

Sensory afference from periphery to spinal cord

Afferent fibers originating in the periphery fall into three groups: Ab fibers, C fibers, and Aδ fibers. The Ab fibers are large myelinated fibers that conduct at high speed and usually transmit non-nociceptive signals. They do, however, also participate in pain modulation, as will be explained later in this article. Nociceptor messages are mainly transmitted by the other two classes of fibers, the larger myelinated Aδ fibers and the thin unmyelinated C fibers. The nociceptors are frequently refer to by the characteristics of their fibers.

Myelination and increasing size of a nerve fiber facilitate the speed of conduction of the stimulus. The Aδ fibers conduct the signal relatively rapidly from the periphery to the spinal cord. Because of this rapid conduction velocity, they are responsible for the sharp localization of pain and for the rapid spinal response, which can be measured in the laboratory as the nociceptive reflex. In contrast, the C fibers, which have a slow conducting velocity, will mediate a second or dull aching pain.

Ab fibers

The Ab (or Aβ) fibers are principally involved in the conduction of non-nociceptive input, such as vibration, movement, or light touch. The Ab fibers are large myelinated fibers with a rapid conduction velocity (35 m–75 m per second). Besides conducting the non-nociceptive signal, the stimulation of Ab fibers will recruit inhibitory interneurones in the substantia gelatinosa of the dorsal horn of the spinal cord, which will inhibit nociceptive input at the same spinal segment. This mechanism is one of the fundamental components of the gate control theory, whereby an innocuous stimulus will reduce the nociceptive input from the same region [7]. Besides playing a dynamic inhibitory role when recruited, the Ab fibers seem also to play a tonic inhibitory role on the nociceptive input. Blocking the input from these large fibers will result in an increased response to nociceptive stimuli [8].

Aδ fibers

The Aδ fibers are relatively large myelinated fibers with slower conduction velocity than the Ab fibers, but faster (5 m–30 m per second) than the C fibers. They represent the majority of the myelinated fibers. Two types of Aδ fibers exist depending on the specificity of their responses to different stimulation [9]: the mechanonociceptors respond preferentially to intense and potentially harmful mechanical stimulation; the polymodal Aδ fibers respond to mechanical, thermal, and chemical stimulation. However, the mechanonociceptor Aδ fibers will also increase their discharge after intense thermal stimulation, a phenomenon known as hyperalgesia. Because of the rapid conduction velocity, the Aδ fibers are responsible for the first pain sensation, a rapid pinprick, sharp, and transient sensation.

C fibers

Because of their small caliber and lack of myelin, the conduction of the C fibers is relatively slow (0.5m–2 m per second). They represent three quarters of the sensory afferent input and are mostly recruited by nociceptive stimulation. However, they are also involved in non-nociceptive somatosensory information, such as in the sensation of pruritus [10], and paradoxically, in the perception of pleasant touch, as documented in a patient with a rare disease linked to a deafferentation of the myelinated sensory fibers [11].

First and second pain

The conduction velocity differences between the Aδ and C fibers can be appreciated when isolating the sensation of first and second pain (Fig. 3). Following a brief nociceptive stimulation, the Aδ fibers will rapidly transmit a brief and acute pinprick-like sensation, perceived to be precisely located at the point of stimulation. It is this precision and fast conduction that will result in the nociceptive withdrawal reflex. Following this activity, C fibers will transmit their information with a relatively long delay (100 milliseconds to a second, depending on the stimulus location). This second sensory input results in a more diffuse deep pain sensation.

It is possible to isolate first and second pain in the laboratory. Using a blood pressure cuff, one can temporarily block trophic factors present in the blood from localizing to the nerves. The first fibers that will show reduced activity are those with largest diameter, including the Aδ fibers. This allows the activity of C fibers to be isolated and independently studied. Following this procedure, a nociceptive stimulation, independent of the nature of the stimulation, hot, cold or mechanical, will be perceived with a certain delay as a deeper pain sensation.

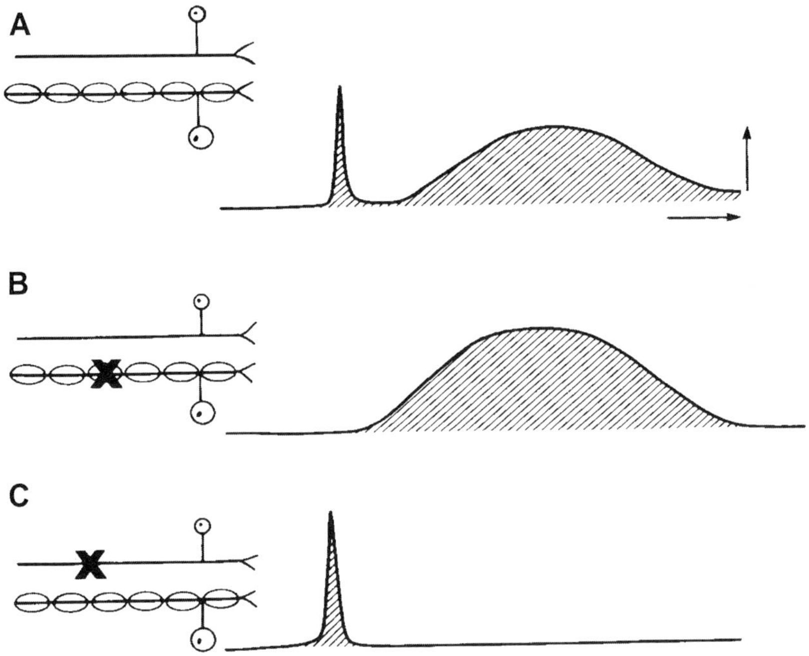

Fig. 3. Because of the differences in conduction velocity between the relatively rapid and slow C-fibers, a nociceptive stimulation will induce a first pain having the characteristics of a localized and sharp pinprick sensation related to the fast action of the fibers, and a second slower and more diffuse burning-like perception related to the slower activity of the C-fibers (*A*). Using a blood pressure cuff, one can temporarily block the activity of the fibers with largest diameter, including the Aδ fibers (*B*). This allows the activity of C-fibers to be isolated and independently studied. A nociceptive stimulus will only conduct the C-fiber activity, perceived as a diffuse burning sensation independently of the stimulation type (*B*). If the activity of the small C-fibers is blocked by using capsaicin, only the sharp pinprick perception will persist (*C*).

The application of capsaicin, the hot pepper extract, will produce a burning sensation because of the activation of the vallinoid receptors on the C fibers. However, at higher doses, the C fibers will be blocked as a result of a specific action on ionic calcium channels, with resulting isolation of the Aδ fibers at the skin surface. This time, the same nociceptive sensation will be perceived as a sharp pinprick-like sensation without the second burning pain sensation.

Secondary neurons in the spinal cord

When recruited, the Aδ and C fibers transport their signal to the spinal cord, where they will have a first synaptic contact with secondary neurons that are principally located in the superficial zones of the dorsal horn (I, II) and lamina V [12]. Both nociceptive and non-nociceptive afferents to the spinal cord will also have synaptic contact with an important network of inhibitory and excitatory interneurones that modulate the nociceptive signal before the secondary neuron projects to superior centers. The secondary neurons can be divided into two classes: the nociceptive specific neurons and the wide dynamic range (WDR) neurons [2,3,13].

Nociceptive specifics neurons

As indicated by their name, the nociceptive specific neurons respond only to nociceptive stimulation. They can be divided in two subclasses depending on their recruitment by Aδ or the combination of Aδ (or Ad) and C fibers.

Wide dynamic range neurons

WDR neurons respond gradually to stimuli ranging from innocuous to nociceptive. Their capacity to respond to both innocuous and nociceptive stimuli is related to the fact that they have received input from Aδ fibers, C fibers, and also Ab fibers (Fig. 4). Interestingly, the receptive field of WDR neurons is dynamic, as the name implies, and changes in conditions of persistent pain. Animal studies have shown that inflammatory pain will have multiple effects on the function of WDR neurons. Changes in the receptive field, the membrane permeability to ion exchange, and the discharge frequency of these neurons all suggest that they play a substantial role in the chronicity of pain [14].

Excitatory mechanisms: secondary hyperalgesia

Secondary hyperalgesia is a phenomenon that refers to sensitization that occurs within the CNS [13]. Repeated recruitment of C-fibers following an injury will produce central sensitization by changing the response properties of the membranes of secondary neurons. This will result in an increase of the firing rate, a phenomenon known as windup [15]. The high frequency recruitment of C fibers, either by increased repetitive stimuli or by a tonic stimulation [16], will then induce an increase of the perceived pain, even if the intensity of the stimulation remains constant. This spinal sensitization can persist for minutes, but can also be present for hours and even days [17]. The prolonged activation of the NMDA receptors will induce the transcription of rapidly expressed genes (c-fos, c-jun), resulting in sensitization of nociceptors. This neuronal plasticity of the secondary neuron will result in reduced recruitment threshold of secondary neurons in the spinal cord and produce hyperalgesic and allodynic responses that may persist even after the healing of the injury. Taking note of the impact of sensitization, an aggressive and early treatment plan to reduce pain will help in preventing ongoing chronic pain (see Fig. 4).

Excitatory mechanisms: temporal summation

The temporal summation paradigm is a good illustration of the importance of signal conduction in Aδ and C fibers [18]. In this paradigm, pain perception is compared with repeated stimulations at the same intensity

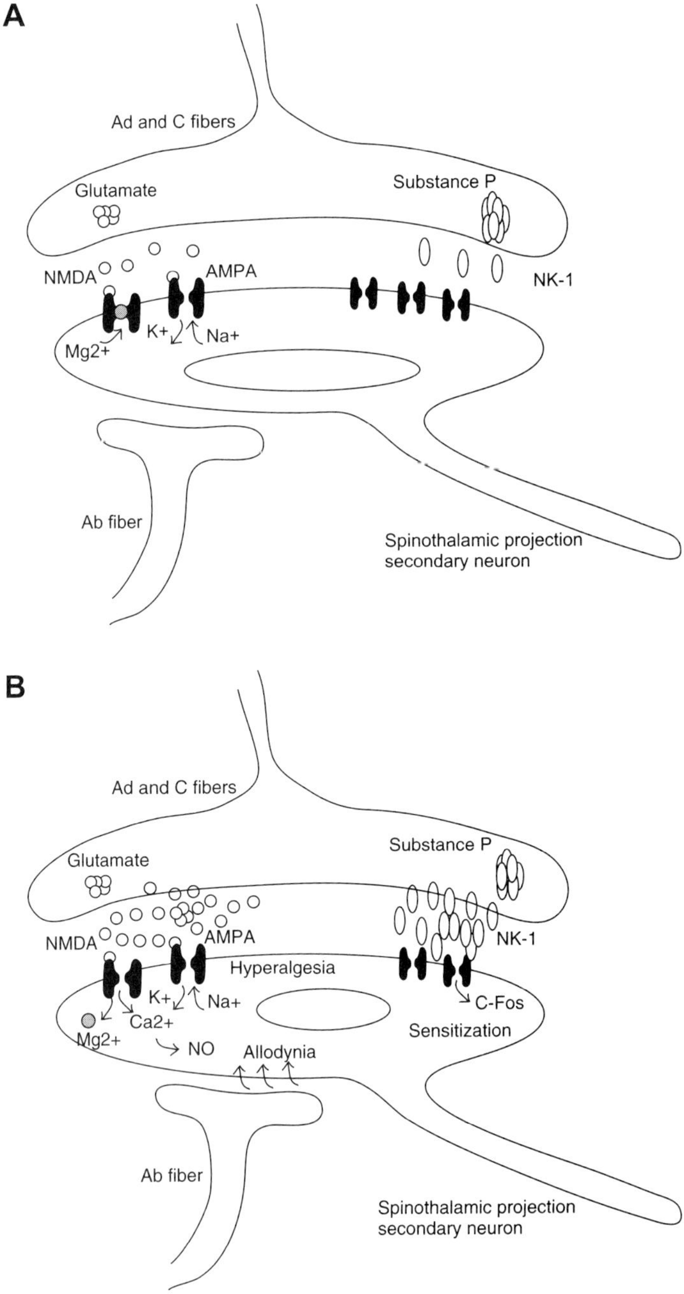
A
Ad and C fibers
Glutamate
Substance P
NMDA
AMPA
NK-1
K+
Na+
Mg2+
Ab fiber
Spinothalamic projection
secondary neuron
B
Ad and C fibers
Glutamate
Substance P
NMDA
AMPA
NK-1
Hyperalgesia
K+
Na+
Ca2+
Mg2+
NO
C-Fos
Sensitization
Allodynia
Ab fiber
Spinothalamic projection
secondary neuron

but at different rates. The rationale is that high frequency of stimulation will produce a temporal summation of the C-fiber activity, as a result of the relatively slow conduction of these fibers. This temporal summation results in an increase in the perceived intensity of the second pain, which is related to C-fiber activity, without changing the perception of the first pain, related to Aδ fibers [19]. The accumulation of nociceptive activity will produce a transient change in the excitability of the spinal cord second neuron, or windup, that may lead to central sensitization [20]. However, windup, a transient effect related to the frequency of discharge from the primary neuron, is different from central sensitization [17].

Central sensitization refers to a phenomenon whereby the second neuron membrane permeability changes and responds at higher frequency when recruited by nociceptive (hyperalgesia) and non-nociceptive primary input (allodynia). Central sensitization is defined as an increase of excitability and spontaneous discharge at the dorsal horn neurons with an associated increase in the receptive field for these neurons. This phenomenon will principally affect the WDR neurons from the dorsal horn (see next section on the spinal cord neurons) and is dependent on the activity of the NMDA receptors [21,22]. Central sensitization may persist for prolonged periods after termination of stimulation and has important effect on the persistence of pain.

Excitatory mechanisms: spatial summation

Another important phenomenon in the CNS is spatial summation. The stimulation of a large territory will recruit more nociceptors than when a smaller area is stimulated and will result in more intense pain perception. It is worth noting that increasing the surface area that is stimulated recruits both excitatory and inhibitory mechanisms [23].

Clinical implications of temporal and spatial summation. It is possible to study the relative role of endogenous pain excitatory and inhibitory mechanism dysfunction in certain chronic pain conditions using temporal [24] and spatial summation [25]. The author and colleagues have examined this spatial summation paradigm in patients with fibromyalgia (FM), and have

◀

Fig. 4. Spinal sensitization occurs when the secondary neurons of the spinal cord change their discharge frequency following a sustained recruitment from the primary nociceptive afferences. In this schematic representation, one can see that an acute discharge from the nociceptive primary afferences (C-fibers) will induce the release of peptide (substance P, CGRP) and glutamate that will produce the recruitment of the NK1 and AMPA receptors (*A*). A sustained discharge (*B*) will recruit the NMDA receptors and produce a sensitization of the secondary neurons that will now discharge at a higher frequency when recruited by nociceptive (hyperalgesia) and non-nociceptive stimulation (allodynia). This phenomenon is generally transitory, but may persist over a long time and participate in pain chronicization. AMPA, alpha-amino-3-hydroxy-5-methyl-4-isoxazolepropionic acid; Ca, calcium; K, potassium; Mg, magnesium; Na, sodium; NK1, neurokinin; NMDA, N-methyl-D-aspartate.

observed no differences in pain perception between the increasing or decreasing nociceptive area, suggesting a deficit of endogenous pain modulation. This deficit was not present in patients with low back pain, suggesting that the deficit of endogenous pain modulation is not present in all chronic pain conditions [25]. A chronic pain condition may therefore be related to either hyperactivity of nociceptive activity or, conversely, to hypoactivity of endogenous pain inhibitory mechanisms at different levels of the CNS. Exploring the role of excitatory and inhibitory mechanism dysfunction in different patient populations will help to better characterize the underlying deficit and facilitate treatment choices.

Pain pathways from the spine to the superior centers

The secondary neuron travels to superior centers by two main pathways: the spinothalamic tract, which sends afferents to the lateral nuclei of the thalamus, and the spinoreticular tract, which send afferents to the medial thalamus and nuclei of the brainstem, including the NRM and the PAG, two nuclei involved in descending pain modulation [26]. A third pathway, from the medial dorsal cord (lemniscal) is mostly associated with non-nociceptive afference, but also conducts nociceptive afference from the viscera [27,28].

Sensory spinothalamic tract

The spinothalamic tract comprises the lateral part of sensory input and projects directly to the lateral nuclei of the ventrobasal thalamus (ventroposterolateral or VPL; ventroposteromedian or VPM). The projection neurons from the spinothalamic tract are primarily from lamina I and IV to VI of the spinal cord [29], and project to the contra lateral nuclei of the thalamus.

The fibers of the spinothalamic tract conduct rapidly and the projection neurons have relatively small receptive fields, directed toward regions of the thalamus and somatosensory cortex that have defined somatotopic representation. The spinothalamic tract has all the characteristics for localization of a sensory pathway [26].

Affective spinoreticular tract

Most afference from the spinoreticular tract is from the deep lamina VII and VIII of the spinal cord and projects to the medial nuclei of the thalamus, as well as to structures of the brainstem involved in pain modulation, including the PAG and NRM [26]. Unlike the spinothalamic tract, the spinoreticular tract projects to neurons having large receptive fields that may cover wide areas of the body and play a role in the memory and affective component of pain [26].

Thalamic organization

The secondary neurons from the spinal cord project to the thalamus. The thalamic nociceptive neurons are localized in two groups of nuclei: the ventrobasal (VPL and VPM) and the centromedian nuclei. The ventrobasal nuclei project their tertiary neurons to the primary and secondary somatosensory cortices (SI, SII). The centromedian neurons project to structures of the limbic system. This simplified description of the thalamus projections suggests that the sensorial and motivational components of pain are organized early in the CNS.

Moreover, the thalamus also plays a role in certain chronic pain conditions. Upon stimulation of specific nuclei of the thalamus, patients have experienced memory recall of the sensory and affective component of a previous pain that had long since disappeared. This suggests that some thalamic neurons may conserve a past painful experience that can be masked by a circuitry of inhibitory interneurones [30]. It is therefore plausible that a localized stroke in the thalamus may destroy tonic inhibitory circuitry and unmask nociceptive activity, leading to the well-recognized painful clinical thalamic pain syndrome.

Brain and pain

Pain can only be experienced when nociceptive afference reaches the cortex. It is for this reason that the term nociception is used to describe the signal following a lesion, whereas pain is a complex perception requiring CNS activity.

A complex network of cortical structures is activated during pain perception. Similar to the thalamic nuclei, the cortex can be represented in a simplified way by subdivision into structures involved in either the sensory or the affective components of pain. Brain imaging has demonstrated four cortical structures important for the perception of pain [31,32]. There are the somatosensory cortex (SI) in the postcentral circumvolution of the parietal lobe, the secondary somatosensory cortex (SII) in the parietal operculum, the ACC above the corpus callosum circumvolution, and the insular cortex (IC) under the temporal and frontal lobes at the level of the Sylvian fissure. The first two structures (SI and SII) are mainly involved in the sensory discriminative aspect of pain, while the ACC and IC are associated with the affective component of pain.

Most brain imaging studies report an activation of the sensory and affective brain structures following a nociceptive stimulus, demonstrating that pain perception is a complex experience with emotion, cognitive factors, and previous experience playing an important role in perceived pain. It can therefore be understood why the clinician should address pain from both the physical as well as the emotional aspect.

Endogenous pain modulation mechanisms

As pain is a dynamic phenomenon, the nociceptive signal will be modulated at multiple levels of the CNS before pain is fully perceived. Because of the dynamic and plastic characteristics of the nervous system, pain perception, especially in a chronic pain condition, will change over time, dependent on different factors. Pain perception is the final outcome of complex mechanisms that modulate the nociceptive afferent signal. The modulation of the nociceptive signal starts at the periphery and involves several CNS structures, including excitatory and inhibitory mechanisms from the brainstem, the autonomic nervous system, and the cortical structures responsible for the emotional and cognitive aspect of pain perception.

Based on knowledge of the neurophysiology of pain, one can conclude that the development and maintenance of chronic pain is dependent upon several factors. Persistent pain can arise from the activity of nociceptive afference, but can also be related to a reduction of endogenous inhibition or augmentation of endogenous excitatory mechanisms. The literature on central sensitization supports the importance of endogenous pain excitatory circuitry on the development and maintenance of pain. The excitatory and inhibitory roles played by different structures of the brainstem have been well documented [33–35].

Endogenous excitatory mechanisms

Primary afferents are normally activated by nociceptive stimuli that can potentially induce an injury and by pronociceptive activation triggered by the inflammatory response.

Spinal excitatory mechanisms

As previously described, excitatory mechanisms can induce a central sensitization at the spinal level. Spinal sensitization is defined as an increase in the excitability and spontaneous discharge of the nociceptive spinal neurons, augmentation of the receptive field, and an accentuated response of spinal neurons to nociceptive (hyperalgesia) and non-nociceptive (allodynia) input. Spinal sensitization depends on the activation of the NMDA receptors of the spinal neurons, which are activated by a sustained released of glutamate [21,22,36]. These neurophysiologic and neurochemical mechanisms involved in spinal sensitization are responsible for modification of the spinal nociceptive circuitry and contribute to the maintenance of pain.

Descending excitatory mechanisms

It is now well documented that several supraspinal excitatory and inhibitory mechanisms play a major role in pain perception and, most probably, in certain chronic pain conditions [1]. The work of Fields and colleagues [37] describing activation of "ON" cells and inhibition of "OFF" cells in the brainstem during nociceptive activity has demonstrated the importance of excitatory mechanisms in amplifying the nociceptive response.

Recent studies have also demonstrated that certain physiologic conditions, such as nociceptive hyperactivity, may change the usual neuronal response to specific neurotransmitters. A particular example is the hyperalgesic effect that can be observed in some patients using opioid medications, mostly at higher doses [38]. Therefore, drugs with opioid activity could, under some circumstances, produce a completely opposite effect and enhance pain by producing an hyperalgesic response [38,39]. The same is also true for GABA, which has been clearly identified as an inhibitory neurotransmitter, but in certain conditions may cause hyperpolarization of neurons [40]. These observations support the concept of pain as a dynamic phenomenon. An understanding of these complex mechanisms can help explain the clinical variability of response to treatments in patients with chronic pain.

Endogenous inhibitory mechanisms

To better understand the role of endogenous pain inhibitory mechanisms in the development and treatment of pain, one should appreciate three levels of modulation in the CNS (Fig. 5): (1) spinal mechanisms producing localized analgesia; (2) descending inhibitory mechanisms from the brainstem producing diffuse inhibition and; (3) superior center effects that will either modulate descending mechanisms or change the perception of pain by reinterpreting the nociceptive signal.

Spinal mechanisms

Since the proposal of the gate control theory by Melzack and Wall [7], the modulation of nociceptive afference at entry into the spinal cord has been well documented. This input may be increased or decreased at the level of the spinal cord. The gate control theory hypothesizes that, among other mechanisms, selective activation of non-nociceptive afferent Ab fibers will recruit inhibitory interneurones in the substantia gelatinosa of the posterior spinal cord, producing a localized analgesia and decreasing pain perception. In contrast, in certain neuropathic pain conditions, the nociceptive secondary projection neurons will be recruited at high frequency to transmit a pain signal following an innocuous stimulation, a phenomenon known as allodynia and increased pain perception. Certain pain conditions may also result from a reduced efficacy of tonic inhibitory controls within the spinal cord [41,42].

Diffuse noxious inhibitory controls

A few years after the gate control theory was proposed in 1965, Reynolds [43] demonstrated that stimulation of the PAG produced a strong inhibition. The role of the rostroventral medulla in the modulation of pain has since been well documented [33,44]. Regions, such as the PAG and the NRM, have been identified as important serotoninergic and noradrenergic descending inhibitory pathways. These inhibitory pathways then recruit enkephalinergic interneurones in the spinal cord to produce the analgesic response.

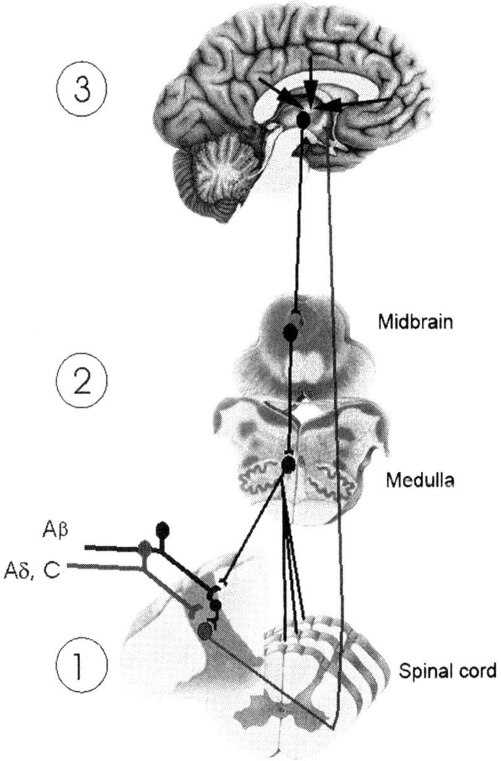

Fig. 5. Endogenous pain modulation. This schematic representation of the main three levels of endogenous pain modulation presents: (1) the spinal, (2) descending from the brainstem, and (3) higher center inhibitory mechanisms. As described in this article, better understanding these mechanisms helps in developing a mechanistic approach for the treatment of some chronic pain conditions that are related to a deficit of these mechanisms. Serotonin and noradrenalin are two neurotransmitters implicated in diffuse noxious pain inhibitory mechanims (DNIC). However, other neurotransmitters, such as dopamine, are also implicated. The spinal interneuron is proposed to be enkephalinergic, but other inhibitory interneurons, such as gamma-aminobutyric acid (GABA), are also implicated. The secondary projection neurons have NMDA receptors that are implicated in the persistancy of certain neurogenic chronic pain conditions. The PAG in the mesencephalon and the NRM are two regions implicated in descending inhibition.

It was not until the end of the 1970s before a model, known as DNIC, was proposed. This model is based on the observation that a localized nociceptive stimulation can produce a diffuse analgesic effect over the rest of the body, an analgesic approach known as counter-irritation. In the DNIC model, Le Bars and colleagues [35,45] proposed that a nociceptive stimulus will send input to superior centers, but will also send afference to the PAG and NRM of the brainstem, recruiting inhibitory output at multiple levels of the spinal cord.

Animal studies demonstrate that a lesion of the dorsolateral funiculus, the main descending inhibitory pathway, will produce hyperalgesia, suggesting a role for tonic descending inhibition under normal conditions [46–48]. Certain clinical conditions are related to reduced endogenous inhibition. For example, the low concentration of serotonin and noradrenaline in the cerebrospinal fluid of patients with FM [49] suggests a deficit of DNIC, with increasing evidence corroborated by other studies [25,50–52].

Documenting the role of descending inhibitory mechanisms will help to better understand certain chronic pain conditions, such as FM. It will also help toward understanding the mechanism of action of pharmacologic approaches, such as the use of antidepressants in chronic pain conditions. Therefore, two key neurotransmitters involved in the DNIC response are those subserving the serotoninergic and noradrenergic mechanisms.

Superior control centers

There has been an increased appreciation of the role of supra-spinal centers in pain and pain modulation. Several cortical regions receive input from the spinothalamic tract and interact to produce the multidimensional experience of pain perception [53]. The use of brain imaging techniques has shown robust activation of certain cortical regions, including the primary and secondary somatosensory cortices, related to the sensory aspect of pain, and the ACC and IC for the affective component of the pain experience [54].

There is no doubt that cognitive manipulations, such as distraction, hypnosis, and expectation influence pain perception [54]. Hypnosis has been demonstrated to change both the sensory and affective component of pain perception. Subjects given the same nociceptive stimulus perceived both intensity as well as unpleasantness of pain differently, depending upon the suggestion given [55]. Using positron emission tomography to obtain brain activity images, activity of the primary somatosensory cortex was proportional to the perceived intensity of pain [56], whereas cingulate cortex activity reflected unpleasantness of pain [57]. These data confirm that a simple suggestion can change the brain activity related to pain perception. These concepts will be further described in the article by Keefe and colleagues on psychologic mechanisms, found elsewhere in this issue.

In a recent study, the author and colleagues were able to demonstrate that manipulating the expectation related to an analgesic procedure can totally reverse the analgesic effect of endogenous pain modulation and the related pain experience. By suggesting that a procedure that is normally analgesic would produce more pain, subjects indeed reported more pain. Therefore, suggestion was able to totally block the administered analgesic effect. Suggestion was also able to reverse the inhibition of the spinal nociceptive reflex (RIII) and of the brain activity measured by somatosensory evoked potential [58]. These results support the idea that cognitive information can modulate the efficacy of endogenous pain modulation and emphasize the importance of the patient's expectations regarding analgesia. This will be further addressed in the article by Pollo and Benedetti on placebo mechanisms found elsewhere in this issue.

Risk factors for developing chronic pain

Understanding factors other than the primary disease process that are involved in the development and maintenance of pain will help toward prevention of a chronic pain state. Three factors have been proposed to play a role in the chronicity of pain: personal predisposition, environmental factors, and psychologic factors. Paying attention to these elements will facilitate the management of patients with chronic pain.

Individual predisposition to chronic pain

Individual predisposition refers to the characteristics of a person that will influence their predisposition to pain and which are either acquired or innate. Under this category, are the role of gender and biological sex, the role of age, and the role of endogenous pain modulation responses.

Gender and sex

Women are more frequently affected by chronic pain syndromes than are men. The reason for this predisposition is probably multifactorial, with sex hormones likely playing an important role. Animal research supports differential responses between the sexes and supports the effect of sex hormones on pain experience. For instance, females show greater nociceptive responses than do males for the same stimulus, but this difference disappears after gonadectomy [59]. Moreover, if gonadectomized rats receive replacement hormones of the opposite sex, females receiving testosterone and males receiving estrogen and progesterone, they demonstrate the same nociceptive behavior attributable to the sex hormone status [60]. Interestingly, this influence of sex hormones seems also to be true in human beings, as differences in response to pain between men and women appears only after puberty and disappears after menopause or andropause [61,62].

Age

Even if we know that an increase in the prevalence of chronic pain among older individuals is partly because of progressive musculoskeletal degeneration that accompanies aging, decline in the efficacy of endogenous pain control systems may contribute to the high prevalence of pain in the elderly. Studies have shown a deficit of endogenous mechanisms with aging [63,64] and also a significant decrease of DNIC, which can occur as early as 50 years of age [65]. This reduction in endogenous pain control with age probably contributes to the higher prevalence of chronic pain in the older population.

Endogenous pain modulation

The efficiency of the endogenous inhibitory system, which can be measured by DNIC, has been shown to be a good predictor for the development of chronic pain. More effective inhibitory control was correlated with less clinical pain [66]. The deficit of DNIC in FM but not in low back pain [25] also supports the role of DNIC in chronic pain, but may also be specific to certain pathologies.

Genetic predisposition

There is increasing evidence that some individuals are more prone to the development of chronic pain than others. Genetic predisposition to the development of pain and to the response to pain treatments is now well documented in the literature [67,68]. This genetic predisposition helps toward understanding the differential response between individuals to the development of chronic pain following an injury. The persistence of pain following an injury, which at times may be without objective pathology, such as occurs in whiplash injury, may be influenced by genetic factors. The same applies for certain treatments. It is well recognized by clinicians that different patients respond differently to individual analgesic medications with regard to both efficacy as well as side-effect profile.

Environmental factors

External stressors, history of previous pain [69], or abuse [70] are also good predictors of the development of chronic pain. For instance, it has been demonstrated that children born prematurely, receiving painful clinical interventions, will be more sensitive to pain later in life [71–73]. The mechanism by which these children may be sensitized to pain can be partly explained by deficits in pain inhibitory mechanisms. The author and colleagues have recently reported that children born prematurely and exposed to repeated painful clinical procedures will demonstrate a deficit of DNIC when tested in later childhood [71].

Psychologic factors

Finally, psychologic factors, such as anxiety, depression, and catastrophizing are also important predictors of pain chronicity [74–77]. Psychologic factors will not only predict the reactions to a pain experience or the ability to cope with the pain, but will also affect the evolution of the chronic pain symptoms. The treatment of pain should always take into consideration the role of psychologic factors as an important predictor for a risk of pain chronicity (discussed in the article by Keefe and colleagues in this issue).

Mechanistic approach to pain treatment

Based on the understanding of pain neurophysiology, treatment plans for pain management in the clinical setting may be devised. Treatments could be aimed toward either reducing excitatory mechanisms or enhancing inhibitory activity. The first goal is to identify as best as possible the mechanism's operative. For a nociceptive acute pain, depending on the nature of the injury, topical or systemic anti-inflammatory (NSAIDs) or analgesic treatments would be primarily indicated. However, even if the nociceptive activity is clearly identified to be peripheral, central sensitization may also have occurred.

Chronic pain is even more difficult to manage because of the complexity of pain mechanisms and the evolution of the pathology over time. As a central component to the pain will almost always be present, the use of opioid, anticonvulsant, or antidepressant drugs could be included in pharmacologic treatment.

Types of pain

The different types of pain may be divided into two categories and five subcategories: nociceptive (somatic, visceral, and inflammatory) and neurogenic (causalgia and functional) [78] (Table 1). A purely psychogenic pain may exist, but this is both rare and controversial because of multiple factors influencing pain perception [79]. Caution is needed before diagnosing isolated psychogenic pain.

Nociceptive pain

Nociceptive pain is generally transitory in response to nociceptive stimuli that could be mechanical, thermal, or chemical. Nociceptive pain plays an important protective role and is normally present for as long as the protection of the organism is necessary. However, in certain situations the pain will persist even after healing of the initial injury. Clinicians are currently unable to predict which patients will develop a persistent pain following an acute pain, such as in the case of postsurgical pain, and several factors are implicated. It is for this reason that early treatment of acute pain is so important in the prevention of chronic pain.

The recommended treatments for nociceptive pain are analgesics, NSAIDs, and sodium channels blockers. Opioids also have an important place in the treatment of acute pain, as peripheral opioid receptors are up-regulated following an inflammatory response [80,81]. Persistent acute pain that may have a nociceptive origin may require treatment strategies similar to those used for neuropathic pain to prevent central sensitization.

It is important to differentiate somatogenic versus viscerogenic nociceptive pain that can, in certain cases, present a comparable clinical picture. It is known that referred pain from the internal organs, such as the gut, liver,

Table 1
Mechanistic classification of pain and overview of categories and characteristics

Type of pain		Characteristics	Mechanisms	Example of pharmacologic treatments
Nociceptive	Somatic (tissue injury)	Superficial (skin) or deep pain (muscle, fascia, tendon)	Mechanical, thermal or chemical stimuli	Acetaminophen Na+ blockers NSAID, steroids, opioids
	Visceral (irritable bowel, cystitis)	Constant or cramping, poor localization. Autonomic responses	Visceral distension	NSAID, antispasmodics
	Inflammatory (musculoskeletal)	Localized or diffuse pain hyperalgesia, allodynia.	Associated with localized inflammation	NSAID, steroids
Neurogenic	Causalgia (neuralgia, radiculopathy, CNS lesions)	Spontaneous, paroxysmal pain. allodynia, hyperalgesia.	Peripheral or CNS lesions	Anticonvulsivants, opioids, antidepressants
	Functional (FM, thalamic syndromes, irritable bowel syndrome)	Diffuse deep pain, hyperalgesia, allodynia	Dysregulation of excitatory or inhibitory mechanisms in CNS	Antidepressants, anticonvulsivants, opioids, cannabinoids.

ovaries, or bladder will induce a pain perception localizing in somatic territories, giving the impression of a purely somatic pain. For example, pain arising in the abdominal cavity can mimic low back pain. Appropriate diagnosis and management is dependent upon understanding the concept of referred pain.

Inflammatory pain

Inflammatory pain is associated with the healing process following a lesion. Inflammation is a natural protective reaction of the organism following an injury. Inflammatory substances are released into the periphery by cells in the area of damaged tissue but can also arise from hyperactivity of the nociceptive neurons in the CNS, a phenomenon know as neurogenic inflammation [82]. In that the molecules released during inflammation are pronociceptive, the use of NSAIDs will reduce this nociceptive activity. NSAIDs have well-known peripheral effects, but inhibition of cyclooxygenase can also occur centrally in the spinal cord and the brain, and may thereby participate in reducing neurogenic inflammation [83].

Neurogenic pain

Neurogenic pain is defined by the International Association for the Study of Pain as pain arising as a direct consequence of diseases affecting the somatosensory system [84]. The mechanisms involved and treatments are different depending on whether the pain originates peripherally (vascular, mechanical, or chemical lesion affecting the nerve) or centrally (spinal or supraspinal hyperactivity). Neurogenic pain, even of a peripheral origin, is frequently associated with sensitization of the CNS. Pharmacologic approaches to treatment of neurogenic pain aim to reverse or reduce the hyperactivity of the nociceptive neurons. Commonly used agents include opioids, anticonvulsivants, antiarrhythmics, antidepressants, and even NMDA receptors antagonists (eg, ketamine).

Functional neurogenic pain

Functional neurogenic pain is a subcategory of neurogenic pain occurring in the absence of a defined anatomic lesion within the nervous system, but rather representing a dysfunction of pain modulation mechanisms. This may occur as a result of central activation of endogenous excitatory systems that will amplify the nociceptive signal or by a dysfunction of endogenous inhibitory mechanisms.

An example of central hyperactivity is the thalamic syndrome following a lesion of thalamic nuclei as a result of a cerebral event. This lesion will produce hyperactivity of thalamic neurons that are normally inhibited by a complex interneuron network. A small lesion within the thalamus may result in intense pain over a large body area, frequently involving almost half of the body. In contrast, another pain syndrome, namely FM, may be at least partly explained by a deficit of descending endogenous pain inhibitory mechanisms [25]. In this condition the hyperalgesia is related to lack of inhibition, rather than just hyperactivity of the nociceptive neurons.

Therefore, strategies for the treatment of functional neurogenic pain will be either focused toward reduction of nociceptive hyperactivity or activation of endogenous inhibition. Anticonvulsants will reduce sensory input by effect on ion channels, whereas antidepressant medications will augment inhibition by effect on serotonin and noradrenergic systems.

Summary of the mechanistic approaches to the treatment of pain

Based on one's knowledge of the neurophysiology of pain and the specific mechanisms involved, therapeutic strategies may be selected.

- Nociceptive pain arising in the periphery may be treated by reduction of inflammation (NSAID), blocking the activity of the nerve fibers (ion channels blockers), or by acting on the C-fiber receptors by using an agent such as capsaicin.
- If there is reason to suspect hyperactivity of spinal neurons following a sensitization of the CNS (allodynia, hyperalgesia), then anticonvulsant or antiarrhythmic agents are used to reduce neuronal hyperactivity. NMDA antagonists could also be used to reverse this hyperactivity. It is also possible that the prophylactic use of these agents, such as during surgery, may prevent chronic pain.
- If the descending inhibitory mechanisms are implicated, the use of serotoninergic and noradrenergic agonists, as in the antidepressants, may help to recruit and modulate these systems.
- Finally, antidepressant medications, opioids, and the anticonvulsant drugs would also have an effect on the higher centers influencing the motivational aspect of pain.
- Cognitive manipulation can also play a role in pain modulation. Harnessing these mechanisms from higher cerebral centers by use of distraction, relaxation, suggestion, and positive support will facilitate pain management.

These pharmacologic and nonpharmacologic examples, based on the neurophysiologic characteristics of the pain, demonstrate that a better understanding of the mechanisms of pain generation will influence therapeutic approaches and facilitate treatments.

Summary

This article has described the complexity of the pain phenomenon and explained mechanisms involved in the development and maintenance of pain conditions. This knowledge is a strong foundation on which to develop a therapeutic guide for the treatment of pain. Although there is commonality in the nociceptive pathways of our patients, each individual will respond differently to pain as a result of genetic and environmental background. This variability in perception and response to pain may lead to physician bias or even misinterpretation of an individual patient's symptoms. Keeping in mind the heterogeneity of the pain response and the unique characteristics of an individual patient will lead to better patient care. Understanding the neurophysiologic mechanisms underlying the development and maintenance of pain will help focus treatments more efficiently toward the specific abnormality causing pain. The knowledge of the science of pain has provided an opportunity to address pain from a mechanistic approach, with the objective of reinforcing inhibitory mechanisms or reducing the hyperactivity of the nociceptive response.

References

[1] Millan MJ. Descending control of pain. Prog Neurobiol 2002;66(6):355–474.
[2] Meyer RA, Ringkamp M, Campbell JN, et al. Peripheral neural mechanisms of nociception. In: McMahon SB, Koltzenburg M, editors. Wall and Melzack's texbook of pain. 5th edition. Philadelphia: Elsevier Limited; 2006. p. 3–34.
[3] Guilbaud G, Besson J-M. Physiologie du circuit de la douleur. In: Brasseur L, Chauvin M, Guilbaud G, editors. Douleurs. Paris: Maloine; 1997. p. 7–22.
[4] Levine J, Taiwo Y. Inflammatory pain. In: Wall PD, Melzack R, editors. Texbook of pain. New York: Chruchill Livingston; 1994. p. 45–56.
[5] Marchand S. Le phénomène de la douleur. Montréal (Canada): Chenelière McGraw-Hill et Masson; 1998. p. 311.
[6] Byers MR, Bonica JJ. Peripheral pain mechanisms and nociceptor plasticity. In: Loeser JD, editor. Management of pain. New York: Lippincott Williams & Wilkins; 2001. p. 26–72.
[7] Melzack R, Wall PD. Pain mechanisms: a new theory. Science 1965;150:971–9.
[8] Price DD. Primary afferent and dorsal horn mechanisms of pain. In: Price DD, editor. Psychological mechanisms of pain and analgesia. New York: Raven Press; 1999. p. 71–96.
[9] Treede RD, Meyer RA, Campbell JN. Myelinated mechanically insensitive afferents from monkey hairy skin: heat-response properties. J Neurophysiol 1998;80(3):1082–93.
[10] Stander S, Steinhoff M, Schmelz M, et al. Neurophysiology of pruritus: cutaneous elicitation of itch. Arch Dermatol 2003;139(11):1463–70.
[11] Olausson H, Lamarre Y, Backlund H, et al. Unmyelinated tactile afferents signal touch and project to insular cortex. Nat Neurosci 2002;5(9):900–4.
[12] Fields HL. Pain. New York: McGraw-Hill Book Company; 1987. p. 354.
[13] Terman GW, Bonica JJ. Spinal mechanisms and their modulation. In: Loeser JD, editor. Management of pain. 3rd edition. New York: Lippincott Williams & Wilkins; 2001. p. 73–152.
[14] Le Bars D. The whole body receptive field of dorsal horn multireceptive neurones. Brain Res Brain Res Rev 2002;40(1–3):29–44.
[15] Mendell LM. Physiological properties of unmyelinated fiber projections to the spinal cord. Exp Neurol 1966;16(3):316–32.
[16] Granot M, Granovsky Y, Sprecher E, et al. Contact heat-evoked temporal summation: tonic versus repetitive-phasic stimulation. Pain 2006;122(3):295–305.
[17] Woolf CJ. Windup and central sensitization are not equivalent. Pain 1996;66(2–3): 105–8.
[18] Price DD, Dubner R. Mechanisms of first and second pain in the peripheral and central nervous systems. J Invest Dermatol 1977;69(1):167–71.

[19] Vierck CJ Jr, Cannon RL, Fry G, et al. Characteristics of temporal summation of second pain sensations elicited by brief contact of glabrous skin by a preheated thermode. J Neurophysiol 1997;78(2):992–1002.
[20] Li J, Simone DA, Larson AA. Windup leads to characteristics of central sensitization. Pain 1999;79(1):75–82.
[21] Eide PK. Wind-up and the NMDA receptor complex from a clinical perspective. Eur J Pain 2000;4(1):5–15.
[22] Woolf CJ, Thompson SW. The induction and maintenance of central sensitization is dependent on N-methyl-D-aspartic acid receptor activation; implications for the treatment of post-injury pain hypersensitivity states. Pain 1991;44(3):293–9.
[23] Marchand S, Arsenault P. Spatial summation for pain perception: interaction of inhibitory and excitatory mechanisms. Pain 2002;95(3):201–6.
[24] Staud R, Vierck CJ, Cannon RL, et al. Abnormal sensitization and temporal summation of second pain (wind-up) in patients with fibromyalgia syndrome. Pain 2001;91(1–2): 165–75.
[25] Julien N, Goffaux P, Arsenault P, et al. Widespread pain in fibromyalgia is related to a deficit of endogenous pain inhibition. Pain 2005;114(1–2):295–302.
[26] Willis WD. Nociceptive pathways: anatomy and physiology of nociceptive ascending pathways. Philos Trans R Soc Lond B Biol Sci 1985;308(1136):253–70.
[27] Palecek J, Paleckova V, Willis WD. Fos expression in spinothalamic and postsynaptic dorsal column neurons following noxious visceral and cutaneous stimuli. Pain 2003;104(1–2): 249–57.
[28] Palecek J, Willis WD. The dorsal column pathway facilitates visceromotor responses to colorectal distention after colon inflammation in rats. Pain 2003;104(3):501–7.
[29] Willis WD, Kenshalo DR Jr, Leonard RB. The cells of origin of the primate spinothalamic tract. J Comp Neurol 1979;188(4):543–74.
[30] Lenz FA, Gracely RH, Romanoski AJ, et al. Stimulation in the human somatosensory thalamus can reproduce both the affective and sensory dimensions of previously experienced pain. Nat Med 1995;1(9):910–3.
[31] Coghill RC, Talbot JD, Evans AC, et al. Distributed processing of pain and vibration by the human brain. J Neurosci 1994;14(7):4095–108.
[32] Talbot JD, Marrett S, Evans AC, et al. Multiple representations of pain in human cerebral cortex. Science 1991;251(4999):1355–8.
[33] Basbaum AI, Fields HL. Endogenous pain control mechanisms: review and hypothesis. Ann Neurol 1978;4(5):451–62.
[34] Fields HL, Heinricher M. Anatomy and physiology of a nociceptive modulatory system. Philos Trans R Soc Lond B Biol Sci 1985;308(1136):361–74.
[35] Le Bars D, Dickenson AH, Besson JM. Diffuse noxious inhibitory controls (DNIC). 1. Effects on dorsal horn convergent neurones in the rat. Pain 1979;6(3):283–304.
[36] Woolf CJ, Salter MW. Neuronal plasticity: increasing the gain in pain. Science 2000; 288(5472):1765–9.
[37] Fields HL, Malick A, Burstein R. Dorsal horn projection targets of ON and OFF cells in the rostral ventromedial medulla. J Neurophysiol 1995;74(4):1742–59.
[38] Simonnet G, Rivat C. Opioid-induced hyperalgesia: abnormal or normal pain? Neuroreport 2003;14(1):1–7.
[39] Davis MP, Shaiova LA, Angst MS. When opioids cause pain. J Clin Oncol 2007;25(28): 4497–8.
[40] Coull JA, Boudreau D, Bachand K, et al. Trans-synaptic shift in anion gradient in spinal lamina I neurons as a mechanism of neuropathic pain. Nature 2003;424(6951):938–42.
[41] Millan MJ. The induction of pain: an integrative review. Prog Neurobiol 1999;57(1):1–164.
[42] Traub RJ. Spinal modulation of the induction of central sensitization. Brain Res 1997; 778(1):34–42.
[43] Reynolds DV. Surgery in the rat during electrical analgesia. Science 1969;164(878):444–5.

[44] Fields HL, Basbaum AI. Anatomy and physiology of a descending pain control system. In: Bonica BJ, editor. Advances in pain and research and therapy. New York: Raven Press; 1979. p. 427–40.
[45] Le Bars D, Dickenson AH, Besson JM. Diffuse noxious inhibitory controls (DNIC). II.Lack of effect on non-convergent neurones, supraspinal involvement and theoretical implications. Pain 1979;6(3):305–27.
[46] Abbott FV, Hong Y, Franklin KB. The effect of lesions of the dorsolateral funiculus on formalin pain and morphine analgesia: a dose-response analysis. Pain 1996;65(1):17–23.
[47] Davies JE, Marsden CA, Roberts MH. Hyperalgesia and the reduction of monoamines resulting from lesions of the dorsolateral funiculus. Brain Res 1983;261(1):59–68.
[48] Wei F, Dubner R, Ren K. Dorsolateral funiculus-lesions unmask inhibitory or disfacilitatory mechanisms which modulate the effects of innocuous mechanical stimulation on spinal Fos expression after inflammation. Brain Res 1999;820(1–2):112–6.
[49] Russell IJ. Neurochemical pathogenesis of fibromyalgia. Z Rheumatol 1998;57(2):263–6.
[50] Kosek E, Hansson P. Modulatory influence on somatosensory perception from vibration and heterotopic noxious conditioning stimulation (HNCS) in fibromyalgia patients and healthy subjects. Pain 1997;70(1):41–51.
[51] Lautenbacher S, Rollman GB. Possible deficiencies of pain modulation in fibromyalgia. Clin J Pain 1997;13(3):189–96.
[52] Staud R, Robinson ME, Vierck CJ, et al. Diffuse noxious inhibitory controls (DNIC) attenuate temporal summation of second pain in normal males but not in normal females or fibromyalgia patients. Pain 2003;101(1–2):167–74.
[53] Price DD. Psychological and neural mechanisms of the affective dimension of pain. Science 2000;288(5472):1769–72.
[54] Apkarian AV, Bushnell MC, Treede RD, et al. Human brain mechanisms of pain perception and regulation in health and disease. Eur J Pain 2005;9(4):463–84.
[55] Rainville P, Carrier B, Hofbauer RK, et al. Dissociation of pain sensory and affective dimensions using hypnotic modulation. Pain 1999;82(2):159–71.
[56] Hofbauer RK, Rainville P, Duncan GH, et al. Cortical representation of the sensory dimension of pain. J Neurophysiol 2001;86(1):402–11.
[57] Rainville P, Duncan GH, Price DD, et al. Pain affect encoded in human anterior cingulate but not somatosensory cortex. Science 1997;277:968–71.
[58] Goffaux P, Redmond WJ, Rainville P, et al. Descending analgesia—when the spine echoes what the brain expects. Pain 2007;130(1–2):137–43.
[59] Gaumond I, Arsenault P, Marchand S. The role of sex hormones on formalin-induced nociceptive responses. Brain Res 2002;958(1):139–45.
[60] Gaumond I, Arsenault P, Marchand S. Specificity of female and male sex hormones on excitatory and inhibitory phases of formalin-induced nociceptive responses. Brain Res 2005;1052(1):105–11.
[61] Robinson JE, Short RV. Changes in breast sensitivity at puberty, during the menstrual cycle, and at parturition. Br Med J 1977;1(6070):1188–91.
[62] Von Korff M, Dworkin SF, Le Resche L, et al. An epidemiologic comparison of pain complaints. Pain 1988;32:173–83.
[63] Edwards RR, Fillingim RB, Ness TJ. Age-related differences in endogenous pain modulation: a comparison of diffuse noxious inhibitory controls in healthy older and younger adults. Pain 2003;101(1–2):155–65.
[64] Washington LL, Gibson SJ, Helme RD. Age-related differences in the endogenous analgesic response to repeated cold water immersion in human volunteers. Pain 2000;89(1):89–96.
[65] Larivière M, Goffaux P, Marchand S, et al. Change in pain perception and DNIC start at middle age in healthy adults. Edmonton (AB): Clinical Journal of Pain 2007;23(6):506–10.
[66] Edwards RR, Ness TJ, Weigent DA, et al. Individual differences in diffuse noxious inhibitory controls (DNIC): association with clinical variables. Pain 2003;106(3):427–37.

[67] Stamer UM, Stuber F. Genetic factors in pain and its treatment. Curr Opin Anaesthesiol 2007;20(5):478–84.
[68] Buskila D. Genetics of chronic pain states. Best Pract Res Clin Rheumatol 2007;21(3): 535–47.
[69] Turner JA, Dworkin SF. Screening for psychosocial risk factors in patients with chronic orofacial pain: recent advances. J Am Dent Assoc 2004;135(8):1119–25.
[70] Linton SJ. A population-based study of the relationship between sexual abuse and back pain: establishing a link. Pain 1997;73(1):47–53.
[71] Goffaux P, Lafrenaye S, Morin M, et al. Preterm births: can neonatal pain alter the development of endogenous gating systems? Eur J Pain 2008;130(1–2):137–43.
[72] Grunau RE, Holsti L, Peters JW. Long-term consequences of pain in human neonates. Semin Fetal Neonatal Med 2006;11(4):268–75.
[73] Buskila D, Neumann L, Zmora E, et al. Pain sensitivity in prematurely born adolescents. Arch Pediatr Adolesc Med 2003;157(11):1079–82.
[74] Gauthier N, Sullivan MJ, Adams H, et al. Investigating risk factors for chronicity: the importance of distinguishing between return-to-work status and self-report measures of disability. J Occup Environ Med 2006;48(3):312–8.
[75] Currie SR, Wang J. Chronic back pain and major depression in the general Canadian population. Pain 2004;107(1–2):54–60.
[76] Pincus T, Burton AK, Vogel S, et al. A systematic review of psychological factors as predictors of chronicity/disability in prospective cohorts of low back pain. Spine 2002;27(5): E109–20.
[77] Auerbach SM, Laskin DM, Frantsve LM, et al. Depression, pain, exposure to stressful life events, and long-term outcomes in temporomandibular disorder patients. J Oral Maxillofac Surg 2001;59(6):628–33.
[78] Woolf CJ. Pain: moving from symptom control toward mechanism-specific pharmacologic management. Ann Intern Med 2004;140(6):441–51.
[79] Turk DC, Okifuji A. Psychological aspect of pain. In: Warfield CA, Bajwa ZH, editors. Principle and practice of pain medicine. 2nd edition. New York: McGraw-Hill; 2004. p. 139–47.
[80] Lawrence AJ, Joshi GP, Michalkiewicz A, et al. Evidence for analgesia mediated by peripheral opioid receptors in inflamed synovial tissue. Eur J Clin Pharmacol 1992;43(4):351–5.
[81] Walker JS. Anti-inflammatory effects of opioids. Adv Exp Med Biol 2003;521:148–60.
[82] Leis S, Weber M, Schmelz M, et al. Facilitated neurogenic inflammation in unaffected limbs of patients with complex regional pain syndrome. Neurosci Lett 2004;359(3):163–6.
[83] Samad TA, Moore KA, Sapirstein A, et al. Interleukin-1beta-mediated induction of Cox-2 in the CNS contributes to inflammatory pain hypersensitivity. Nature 2001;410(6827):471–5.
[84] Treede RD, Jensen TS, et al. Neuropathic pain: redefinition and a grading system for clinical and research purposes. Neurology 2008;70(18):1630–5.

ELSEVIER
SAUNDERS

Rheum Dis Clin N Am
34 (2008) 311–330

RHEUMATIC
DISEASE CLINICS
OF NORTH AMERICA

The Assessment of Musculoskeletal Pain in the Clinical Setting

Fiona MacKichan, MSc[a,*], Vikki Wylde, BSc[b], Paul Dieppe, MD[c]

[a]*Department of Social Medicine, University of Bristol, Canynge Hall, Whiteladies Road, Bristol, BS8 2PR, UK*
[b]*University of Bristol, Bristol Implant Research Centre, Avon Orthopaedic Centre, Southmead Hospital, Bristol, BS10 5NB, UK*
[c]*Nuffield Department Orthopaedic Surgery, University of Oxford, Oxford, OX3 7LD, UK*

Musculoskeletal pain is a universal phenomenon: everyone experiences it. There are three main causes of musculoskeletal pain—everyday activities, trauma, and disease—but the nature, severity and impact of the pain that may arise from muscles, bones, joints and periarticular tissues varies considerably. As anyone with arthritis knows, the pain it causes is very different from the everyday aches and pains in the spine and elsewhere.

The main problem with the assessment of pain is that it is a subjective phenomenon, and as such it is both hard to describe and difficult to measure. When patients with arthritis are asked about the symptoms of their condition, they usually stress pain, stiffness (or "gelling") of the joints, and fatigue, but they find each of these symptoms hard to describe. When asked to talk about their pain, most people will tell you about its interrelationship with activities and its impact on function and life, rather than talking about the pain itself [1]. They may also use a variety of adjectives to describe the pain, but these may have little meaning for the health care professional. Similarly, when asked to rate how bad the pain is, people will often tell you that this depends on the time of day, what they are doing, and on other variables that can affect perception of pain and how much we focus on it (or are distracted from it). Finally, the relationships between pain, stiffness, and fatigue seem unclear to many patients, and the possible effects of comorbidities, such as depression, is equally difficult to understand or

* Corresponding author.
E-mail address: fiona.mackichan@bristol.ac.uk (F. MacKichan).

doi:10.1016/j.rdc.2008.03.002

assess. It has been suggested that the sensation of joint stiffness may be part of the pain experience [2], and many patients tell us that their fatigue results from their pain. Anxiety and depression are common in people with chronic arthritis, and are known to affect pain perception [3], but it is very difficult to know the direction of causality in any individual or the amount of the pain experience that may be "explained" by anxiety or depression. So, the assessment and measurement of pain in arthritis is complex, difficult, and, as outlined further below, cannot be adequately dealt with by the use of a simple self-assessment measure of pain severity at a single time point—the measure we usually employ.

Mainstream medical practitioners and researchers have been more concerned with diseases of the musculoskeletal system than with the symptoms that they cause. This may explain why, in comparison with the major advances seen in disease assessment and management, we have seen relatively few recent developments in the assessment of pain in arthritis, despite the importance of pain in clinical decision-making. But things are now changing for the better and new approaches are emerging, as this issue of *Clinics* illustrates. We need to be able to assess musculoskeletal pain for three main reasons:

- It is the problem of the most concern to many of our patients.
- It is necessary to assist with routine patient management, and in particular to help us understand whether our advice and interventions have helped the patient.
- It is necessary for research. For example, the primary outcome measure in many clinical trials is pain. As the relationship between joint damage (impairment), pain, and disability are far from either clear or perfect in most rheumatic diseases, health care practitioners need robust ways of assessing the pain, in addition to the measures of disease activity and joint damage.

This article reviews some of the standard approaches used to assess pain in musculoskeletal diseases—both in research and routine clinical care—and outlines some of their limitations. The authors then discuss how else one might be able to approach the problem of gaining a good understanding of patients' experiences, as well as being able to dissect out different pain mechanisms and assess the severity and impact of the symptoms. The discussion is limited to pain in adults who have a rheumatologic disease, with an emphasis on osteoarthritis (OA), as most of the authors' own experience is in that field. The authors have not addressed the separate issues of assessment of pain in children, nonspecific spinal pain, or pain associated with trauma.

What measures are currently used in rheumatology?

Pain self-report measures

Because pain is a subjective experience, it could be argued that the most valid and meaningful method of measuring the pain experience is by patient self-report. Self-report measures of pain are widely used and are a cost-effective and efficient method of gaining information of the pain experience, with the added advantage of being minimally intrusive. The use of validated patient-report outcome measures is becoming more common and numerous questionnaires exist. These can be categorized into generic, disease-specific, or joint-specific measures.

Generic pain measures

Pain severity

One of the most widely used and simple measures of pain severity is the visual analog scale (VAS) (Fig. 1). The pain VAS is a one-dimensional measurement of pain severity, most commonly consisting of a 100-mm horizontal line that is anchored at either end with pain descriptors, such as "no pain" and "worst pain imaginable." Respondents are required to place a mark along the line at a location that they feel reflects their pain intensity. Variants of the simple VAS have been developed, using a variety of markings on the 100-mm line to aid respondents.

The VAS has been found to be a valid and reliable method of measuring the intensity of clinical and experimental pain [4]. It has also been shown to be more responsive than other pain measures, such as the Numerical Rating Scale (NRS). However, the VAS has received criticism on both a conceptual and practical level.

Another simple generic pain measure, which has been found to be highly correlated with the VAS for assessing pain in OA, is the Likert scale [5]. This scale involves patients rating the severity of their pain using a check box scale labeled with pain descriptors at each response level, ranging from "no pain" to "extreme pain." It has been claimed that no more than seven response levels should be used because patients are unable to discriminate beyond these levels [6]. Rheumatology patients have been found to prefer using the Likert scale over the 100-mm VAS because they find it easier to rate pain in terms of words than through numbers or lines [7].

Likert scale and VAS have limited use in patients with language difficulties or cognitive impairment; in this group of patients, picture or face scales can be useful for assessing pain severity (Fig. 2) [8]. These tools use illustrations of facial impressions of people experiencing different levels of pain and the respondent has to indicate which face best illustrates their own pain experience. Picture scales have been found to correlate with the VAS and the Likert scale and are responsive to changes in pain in OA patients [9].

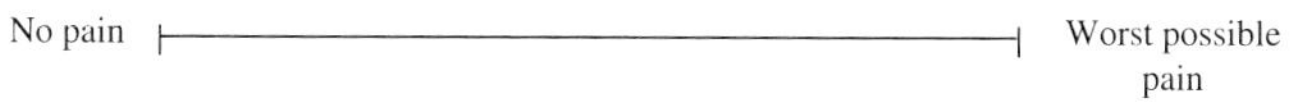

Fig. 1. Example of a visual analog scale.

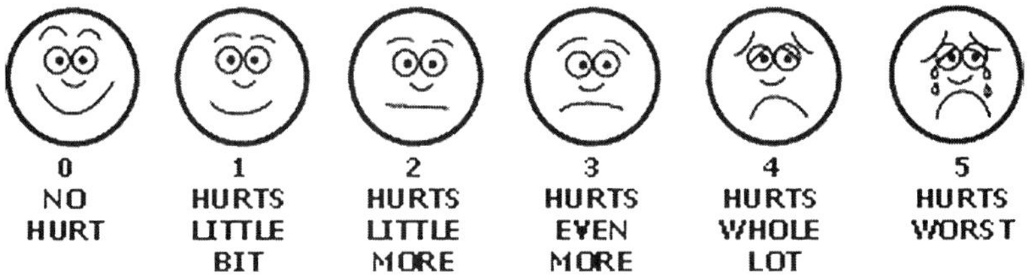

Fig. 2. Example of a face scale.

Pain disability and distress

Pain is inextricably linked with function [1] and distress [10], as such multidimensional measures that assess both pain severity and disability or distress are useful. Being widely used in cancer research, the Brief Pain Inventory (BPI) [11] was developed to assess pain severity and pain interference. To measure pain severity, respondents rate their worst, least, average, and current pain intensity, and to assess pain interference, respondents rate the degree to which pain interferes with seven domains of functioning on a scale of 0 to 10. A modified version of the BPI, known as the modified BPI short form [12], has also been validated for use in OA patients. This tool has three different scales: severity of pain, impact of pain on mood, and impact of pain on activity.

A similar pain self-report measure is the seven item Chronic Pain Grade questionnaire, which was developed to measurement three dimensions of chronic pain: persistence, intensity and disability [13]. This questionnaire enables chronic pain patients to be classified into one of four hierarchical categories according to pain severity and disability. Originally validated in a cross-sectional sample, the Chronic Pain Grade questionnaire has also been shown to be a valid questionnaire for measuring change in pain severity over time [14].

Pain qualities

Many pain self-report questionnaires, although multidimensional, do not explore the qualities and characteristics of pain. The McGill Pain Questionnaire (MPQ) [15], however, consists of 78 descriptors of pain that are grouped into three major classes to reflect the sensory, affective, and evaluative dimensions of pain. The MPQ has been extensively used in rheumatology research, and has demonstrated sensitivity in differentiating pain characteristics between arthritic conditions, such as OA, rheumatoid arthritis (RA), and fibromyalgia [16]. In response to the practical limitations of completing the lengthy MPQ in a clinical situation, the 15-item short-form MPQ was developed [17], which consists of 13 sensory pain descriptors and 3 affect pain descriptors.

Questionnaires that assess pain qualities can aid the diagnosis of specific painful conditions. For example, the Neuropathic Pain Questionnaire

(NPQ) was developed as a diagnostic tool to identify people with neuropathic pain. Because neuropathic pain of different etiologic causes is often described using similar pain symptoms, such as burning, numbness, and increased sensitivity to touch, it is possible to use the NPQ to discriminate between neuropathic and non-neuropathic pain, with an accuracy of 76% [18]. A short-form version of the 12-item NPQ has been developed, which contains three items from the original questionnaire, assessing numbness, tingling pain, and increased pain caused by touch [19].

Distribution of pain

Pain drawings are the most commonly used method of self-report for assessing the sensory distribution of pain. These can be full body pain mannequins, such as in the MPQ, or joint-specific drawings that provide a more detailed localization of pain. Using a standard drawing of the knee, knee OA has been found to take on two common patterns: generalized and medial [20]. Reliability properties of pain drawings have been shown to be high, with good repeatability even over long time periods [21].

Disease-specific pain measures

The Western Ontario and McMaster University Osteoarthritis Index (WOMAC) [22] is the most commonly used disease-specific outcome measure for OA pain assessment and is recommended by the World Health Organization to measure the progression of OA [23]. The WOMAC is a validated 24-item multidimensional measure of pain, function, and stiffness. The severity of pain over the past 4 weeks is rated on a 100-mm VAS or a 5-point Likert scale ("none" to "extreme"). Because of the distinctive characteristics of OA pain, such as exacerbation of pain during activity, the WOMAC separates the assessment of pain into five functional dimensions: when walking, climbing stairs, during the night, at rest, and upon standing. Recently, modifications of WOMAC for use to assess hip or knee OA have been developed—the hip disability and osteoarthritis outcome score (HOOS) [24] and knee injury and osteoarthritis outcome score (KOOS) [25].

An example of a widely used disease-specific measure used to assess pain in RA is the Arthritis Impact Measurement Scale (AIMS) [26]. Containing 46-questions, this tool has nine scales, with one scale focused on pain assessment. The pain scale consists of four questions exploring pain severity, pain frequency, stiffness, and pain in multiple joints. However, as outlined below, most instruments used to assess RA are composites, in which pain is either absent or replaced by joint tenderness.

Joint-specific pain measures

Generic and disease-specific measures do not limit assessment of pain to a specific joint; therefore, joint-specific questionnaires have been developed in rheumatology research to increase measurement specificity and sensitivity. The Oxford hip score [27], Oxford knee score [28], and Oxford shoulder score [29], are examples of 12-item joint-specific questionnaires that were validated to assess pain and function in patients undergoing arthroplasty surgery. Similar to the WOMAC, the Oxford questionnaires ask about average pain and function over the past 4 weeks, which patients can find difficult because of the variable nature of arthritic pain [30]. Responses are on a 5-Likert scale and are summed to produce an overall score of 12 to 60 (low to high pain and functional limitations). A recently validated joint-specific pain questionnaire is the Joint-Specific Multidimensional Assessment of Pain (J-MAP) [31], which consists of a six-item pain sensory scale and a four-item pain affect scale. Developed for use in patients with knee OA, this questionnaire is yet to be validated for use in patients with OA involvement in other joints.

Joint tenderness and composite scores

Tenderness as a proxy measure of pain

The assessment of joint tenderness as well as (or instead of) pain is popular in rheumatology. For example, the standard measures used to assess rheumatoid arthritis (eg, the disease activity score [32]) use counts of tender joints rather than pain as a key clinical parameter, and the assessment of fibromyalgia relies on the assessment of the standard tender spots [33]. The use of tenderness measurements, rather than trying to assess pain severity or distress, seems to be based on the belief that tenderness scores might be more objective than pain ratings, and the concept that tenderness reflects pathology in or around the joints.

However, dependence on this approach warrants debate. It has been known for a long time that referred tenderness (as well as referred pain) is a real phenomenon [34], and tenderness can reflect central pain sensitization rather than peripheral pathology, as is probably the case in fibromyalgia. In addition, tenderness, like pain, is a subjective experience, and health care practitioners rarely standardize the amount of pressure used to detect it (although this can be done with the help of algometers [35]).

Composite scores

Another common phenomenon in rheumatology is the use of composite scores, combining pain with a number of quite different domains. For example, one of the first measures used to assess the severity of OA was the Lequesne algofunctional index [36], which, as the name implies, combines pain and function to provide a single score. Similarly, in the assessment of inflammatory forms of arthritis it is common to combine pain (or tenderness) with other measures, such as blood tests, that reflect the amount of inflammation in the body. The authors believe that this approach also needs further discussion, as the combination of such different phenomena as pain perception and the blood level of a chemical, such as C-reactive protein, seems to ignore the complexity of the reporting of pain severity by our patients and implies that pain must be caused by pathology, rather than considering the pain as a problem in itself.

Some limitations of standard pain measures

Gaining an understanding of the limitations of standardized measures is important, given the extent of their use in clinical encounters. The subjective, multidimensional nature of pain (and the attributes of those multiple dimensions), pose significant challenges to measurement. By definition, standardized measures force the pain experience into static, grounded dimensions, which may not reflect the patient's reality. The face validity of measurement tools is rarely considered outside of expert panels [37]; however, the way people make sense of measures—the meanings attributed to their upper and lower endpoints, each increment, and even the distance between increments—differs from person to person. Data, primarily from qualitative and mixed method studies, including cognitive interviewing and the "Questerview" technique [37] (where the cognitive processes involved in item selection are explored), have provided valuable insight into a number of key issues.

Variations in pain

The majority of measures used to assess musculoskeletal pain fail to capture the dynamic nature of pain, yet patients often report significant variations in their pain over the course of the day, week, month, or longer. The large-scale Pain in Europe survey [38] found that 54% of the 46,394 respondents classed their pain as intermittent, as opposed to continuous. Smith and colleagues [39] highlight the failure of many definitions of chronic pain to acknowledge this distinction. Study of annotations to the Oxford hip score by Wylde and colleagues [30] found that the measure was limited by the significant variation in pain noted by nearly a quarter of respondents. Similar findings are reported by Gooberman-Hill and colleagues [1], who found that respondents described variations in pain both across time and by activity. Variations of this type inhibit a patient's ability to recall pain in the manner required by standardized measures.

The reliability of measurement may also be biased by the tendency to recall the most severe pain (peak effect) or most recent pain (end effect) in a given period [40]. Additionally, it has been suggested that accurate recall is more successful when questions relate to emotionally neutral events [41], which is often not the case in the context of pain. However, while recall bias can be problematic, numerous studies have found recall to be reliable. Baumgarten and colleagues [42], for example, reported an 82% agreement between verbal reports and records.

Comorbidities and "pain elsewhere"

Failure to account for comorbidities and the existence of pain in multiple sites can be a limiting factor of many measures. People tend to take a holistic view of their pain and find it difficult to tease apart their relative pains, and it is likely that few disease and site-specific measures are, in reality, "pure": that is, capturing the experience of pain in one site alone. Clinically, pain is generally considered in terms of a specific site and pathology, yet the prevalence of "pain elsewhere" can be high. Of the respondents in a recent study of knee pain by Croft and colleagues [43], 57% reported pain in at least two additional joints. Furthermore, the incidence of pain in multiple sites was linked to poor physical functioning and increased distress. In a focus group study where the HOOS [24] and KOOS [25] were completed, participants reported finding it difficult to answer questions that required them to reflect on pain in a single site alone [1].

Patients may also have difficulty distinguishing pain according to different conditions. Many measures are disease-specific, yet the prevalence of comorbidities in musculoskeletal patients is high [44] and comorbidities can have significant bearing on treatment outcome [45]. Thus, in a similar way to "pain elsewhere," the prevalence of comorbidities in people with chronic pain and the fact that they might not be able to distinguish between morbidities when asked about their pain, make it plausible that many measures are contaminated by outside factors, even in joint-specific assessment tools that are sensitive to functional status [46].

Attributing meaning to scores

The meaning attributed to increments on scales varies significantly from person to person and is relative to each individual's subjective baseline. Various issues impact the extent to which one can say that scores reflect reality. McMurray and colleagues [47] found that participants were concerned that drug treatments masked their pain experience and, additionally, that given the often extended trajectory, people learned to "live with" the pain. This notion is conceptualized in the coping literature in various guises: as response shift (where a problem is redefined, different values are attached to it, or new internal standards of measurement are applied) [48], avoidance [49], accommodation [50], and acceptance [51]. These all are likely to have a significant mediating effect on pain reporting but may mask the significantly deleterious impact of pain.

One of the primary issues is the fact that, although pain is now understood to be multidimensional, there is no agreement regarding what those dimensions are [52]. Partly because of this, one-dimensional scales such as the VAS or NRS have become almost ubiquitous in any pain assessment context, despite the fact that they may be difficult to understand—the upper limit of "worst pain imaginable" on the VAS may be outside the realm of experience for many patients, for example. When exploring how their sample responded to one-dimensional scales, Williams and colleagues [53] report that participants were inconsistent in their responses, and conclude that, "A representational model of measurement...generates expectations of consistency across scales, context and time, with a focus on a notional 'true pain'."

Other aspects of the pain experience

As we can see, the multifaceted nature of pain means that many aspects of the pain experience are enmeshed. The roles of pain-related distress [54] and function disability have particular bearing on the assessment of pain. Patients may not be able to unpick the relationship between the various aspects of experience when responding to measures, so it must be considered that questions about pain cannot be considered in isolation from other factors [1]. Studies of help-seeking behavior have found that pain severity alone may not be to best predictor of seeking a consultation for pain; living alone and previous experience have both been found to be significant predictors of consulting behavior [55]. Avoidance of activities that cause pain is common in people with arthritis [56], and this can result in uninterpretable negative responses to commonly used questions about pain related to certain activities.

Public versus private accounts

When analyzing the use of pain assessment tools, one must also consider the influence of the context in which measures are administered—the clinical setting. Through an ethnographic study of people living in East London, Jocelyn Cornwall [57] distinguished between two types of accounts of illness that people provide: public and private. Public accounts were conceptualized as morally acceptable responses to direct or formal questions; therefore, in a clinical encounter the person might provide answers that projected them as a "good" (legitimate) patient, reflecting to some extent the Parsonian sick role [58]. In contrast, private accounts were concerned with the context of illness, how it impacted on every aspect of the individual's life. In terms of assessment, it is plausible that all self-report measures, especially when administered by a health professional, are open to bias toward public accounts of pain, which fail to accurately reflect the lived experience.

What alternatives are there?

Narratives of pain

Williams and colleagues [53] suggest an alternative approach to current measurement, where appreciation for shared social meanings and the assessment context are recognized. They state that, "Sampling patient's experience of using current tools to describe their pain suggests that these [reflexive and social] elements are commonly overlooked, at a cost to our understanding." Listening to patients' narratives about pain can provide a unique opportunity to understand their experience. The principle that people make sense of the world through the use of stories is well established: in a clinical encounter, narratives provide context and quality of information that are not obtainable through other means.

Developing an ability to use a patient's narrative as a framework for assessment has specific advantages, enabling a holistic approach to care and eliciting detail that can direct treatment [59]. Despite time limitations, consultations, especially in secondary care, offer an opportunity for a clinician to gain valuable insight into a person's pain without the use of (or in addition to) standardized measures. The issue of patients providing only those stories that they feel the clinician will want to hear ("public" accounts), may be mediated by the use of more detailed questioning. To an extent, time constraints can be addressed through the use of semistructured interviews where open-ended questions can be asked. This form of assessment has certainly been found to be more appropriate in achieving a fuller picture of a person's pain in those with cognitive impairment (see "Measuring behaviors" section).

Quantitative sensory testing

Quantitative sensory testing (QST) is a psychophysical test that evaluates somato-sensory responses to quantified external stimuli that are administered under standardized conditions. QST can demonstrate the presence of an array of both peripheral and central somatosensory abnormalities and is frequently employed in both a clinical and research capacity, for example in the assessment and diagnosis of neuropathic pain syndromes [60,61]. QST can use a range of modalities to assess somatosensory functions, with thermal and mechanical stimuli being the most commonly used in pain assessment. Whereas pressure algometry (Fig. 3) stimulates pain in deep muscle tissues, thermal QST uses heat and cold to selectively activate C-fibers and A-δ pain fibers in the skin. Because of the noninvasive nature of QST, and its ability to provide evidence of abnormal pain fiber function, QST is now being employed in the field of rheumatology research.

Pain perception abnormalities

QST has the potential to diagnose pain perception abnormalities by comparing pain thresholds from patient groups to normative data from healthy controls. Measuring pain perception thresholds can indicate the presence of primary or secondary hyperalgesia. Primary hyperalgesia is sensitization of peripheral pain receptors at the site of tissue damage, such as an arthritic joint, resulting in reduced pain thresholds to further noxious stimuli. Prolonged peripheral sensitization, such as in chronic pain conditions, can in some cases lead to changes in central pain mechanisms, resulting in sensitization of pain receptors in the spinal cord, known as central sensitization

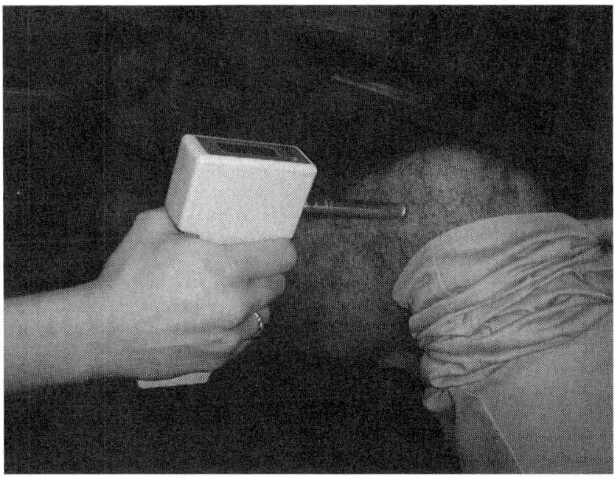

Fig. 3. QST and an algometer in use.

[62]. This involves reduced pain thresholds at sites distant from tissue damage or injury, known as secondary hyperalgesia. Whereas primary hyperalgesia is mediated by peripheral inflammation, secondary hyperalgesia is caused by central sensitization. Both peripheral and central sensitization usually diminish following the cessation of the nociceptive input [63,64], although central sensitization can become self-sustaining, resulting in a pathologic pain state [65].

Findings in some rheumatic diseases

There is strong evidence from QST that people with painful OA experience primary hyperalgesia. Pain perception thresholds in osteoarthritic joints have been found to be significantly lower than in healthy controls [63,66,67]. There is also evidence that OA can lead to the development of secondary hyperalgesia. Patients with hip OA had reduced pain thresholds over both the osteoarthritic hip and contralateral unaffected hip [63]. Patients with bilateral knee OA display pain sensitization at multiple body sites distant from the peripheral tissue damage cause by OA [66]. However, research has shown that central sensitization is not a phenomenon that develops in all patients with OA [67,68].

Similar to OA, fibromyalgia and RA subjects also have lower pain perception thresholds over affected joints than healthy controls, providing evidence of peripheral sensitization [69]. As well as pain sensitization at tender points, somatosensory abnormalities are generalized in fibromyalgia, suggesting a dysfunction of central pain mechanisms and the development of central sensitization [70,71].

Some of the limitations of quantitative sensory testing

QST has several methodologic limitations that need to be cknowledged. First, the relevance of experimental pain to clinical pain has been questioned, because experimental pain is nonthreatening and controllable, and will therefore evoke different psychologic reactions than clinical pain. Despite this, experimental pain responses are associated with the self-report of pain in the general population [72]. A second limitation of QST is that it is not an objective sensory test, such as a sensory nerve conduction test, and therefore it requires the active participation of the subject and is reliant on participant motivation, attention, and reaction times. A third drawback is that research suggests there is no uniform response to experimental painful stimuli of different modalities [73]. Because of this, it is advisable to use a range of modalities to identify pain perception abnormalities. Last, the reliability of QST is unclear, with conflicting reports of both high and low repeatability of QST in healthy controls and subject groups in the literature [74].

Measuring behavior

The idea that people engage in specific behaviors to communicate their pain, introduced by Fordyce [75], has been developed for use in pain assessment through various methods. Assessment might include observation of particular overt behaviors, including inactivity or resting, audible behavior (grunting, for example), guarding and bracing movements, touching or holding a painful site, and facial grimacing [76]. Keefe and colleagues [77] state that "behavioral analysis involves the use of assessment techniques that are more reliable and objective than those typically used to evaluate OA pain."

Behavioral assessment tools are also of particular use when self-report may not be an option: for example, in the case of cognitive impairment such as dementia. Given the high prevalence of pain in these populations and the potential consequences of having pain, effective assessment and treatment is vital. Accordingly, a growing literature base exists that considers alternatives to self-report [78–80], providing a number of options. Pain ratings relative to VAS or NRS can sometimes be achieved in nonverbal populations through blinking or using finger span to indicate more or less pain; however, people with cognitive impairment (often older adults) frequently have problems quantifying pain.

A wide range of behavioral assessment tools exist, varying in length and administration modality (eg, observational methods including videotaping; caregiver reports). In their detailed review of 12 instruments reported in 29 published papers, Zwakhalen and colleagues [81] concluded that, based on psychometric properties and clinical utility, the most appropriate behavioral assessment tools in the context of cognitive impairment were the Pain Assessment Checklist for Seniors with Limited Ability to Communicate (PACSLAC) [82], and the DOLOPLUS2 [83]. Further work by the same investigator found that the PACSLAC was considered the preferred instrument by those responsible for administering the measures [81].

Cognitive impairment can be a significant barrier to pain assessment. Cook and colleagues [79] cite a number of studies where failure to detect pain is given as the primary cause of under-treatment. As such, these alternatives are important elements of a clinician's "toolkit." However, it should also be noted that, although there is a tendency to under-report pain, in many cases those with cognitive impairment are still able to provide self-report data if it is elicited in a certain way. Ferrell and colleagues [84] assessed pain in 325 nursing home patients with cognitive impairments and found that their battery of self-rated pain assessment tools (including the MPQ, VAS, and the Present Pain Intensity scale), provided valid and reliable data when administered in the context of a semistructured interview, a conclusion that is reflected by an earlier large scale study [85].

Pain as a signal of danger: red and yellow flags

To the person in pain, their discomfort signifies danger, damage to the body, fear, and the need to take avoiding action and protect the body. But to the health care professional, it often means none of these things: we know that most musculoskeletal pain is relatively benign, and does not indicate serious disease or damage. However, reported pain can be a signal of a disease or of serious psychopathology. It can be important that, as part of their assessment of pain, health care professionals can quickly identify people in these categories. Those interested in back pain have led the way in this regard, with the introduction of the so-called "red and yellow flags" for pain (Box 1) [86]. Red flags signify the possible presence of serious pathology, such as malignancy or infection; yellow flags are indicative of psychopathology of the sort that predisposes to pain.

The premise that red flags require medical attention to explore pathology, but yellow flags require a refocusing of attention to illness behavior and therefore possibly cognitive or behavioral intervention rather than medical, is, however, not without problems. Yellow flags are primarily concerned with psychosocial factors, which are open to interpretation and bias based on the preconceptions of whomever is conducting the assessment; moving attention away from the possibility of medical intervention may lead to misdiagnosis or under-treatment. Main and Williams [87] suggest that, "for the vast majority of patients, the identification of contributory psychologic and social factors should be seen as an investigation of the normal range of reactions to pain rather than the seeking of psychopathology."

Imaging pain

The recent introduction of brain imaging, using either functional magnetic resonance imaging (fMRI) or positron emission tomography (PET), provides a powerful new window into the pain experience. It is now clear that pain is processed in the brain through a network of different structures, called the pain matrix [88]. The matrix includes two parallel systems: the

Box 1. Red and yellow flags for back pain

RED FLAGS: indicative of possible serious spinal pathology
- Age of onset less than 20 or greater than 55 years
- New pain that is quite different from previous back pain
- Severe pain at rest or at night
- Thoracic pain
- Fever or unexplained weight loss
- Bladder or bowel dysfunction
- History of cancer
- Ill health or the presence of other medical illness
- Progressive neurologic changes
- Disturbed gait or saddle anesthesia

YELLOW FLAGS: Psychosocial factors predicting chronic pain or long term disability
- Negative attitudes, such as presuming pain is harmful and disabling
- Fear avoidance and reduced activity
- An expectation that passive, rather than active intervention is needed
- Tendency to depression and social isolation
- History of previous pain disorders, such as fibromyalgia or irritable bowel syndrome
- Social or financial problems

Adapted from Samanta J, Kendall J, Samanta A. 10-minute consultation: chronic low back pain. BMJ 2003;326(7388):535; with permission.

medial system that is involved in affective (emotional) aspects of pain and the lateral system, which processes the discriminative and sensory aspects of pain (location, intensity, and so forth) [89]. Recent work has been published on imaging findings (fMRI and PET) in people with both RA and OA, and on the differences seen on their brain scans in response to experimental pain in comparison with their arthritis pain [90]. Such work has only just begun, but is likely to provide us with new insights into pain assessment.

Clinically significant change

Methods of testing clinical significance provide a way of exploring the impact of disease and its treatment in a tangible, socially meaningful way that is generally beyond the scope of methods involving tests of statistical significance alone [91]. This, and their ability to measure more than just effect size, makes them a good methodologic feature of outcome studies [92].

Various ways of assessing clinical significance exist; criteria may consist of a complete return to normal functioning (ie, the problem is eradicated) or a fixed level of improvement (eg, the minimal clinically important difference). One of the most robust methods of exploring clinical significance was proposed by Jacobson and Truax [93], who conceptualized the process as the degree to which an intervention has moved a person from the range of the clinical population into the range of the nonclinical population. Clinically significant change would be when the person, upon completing the intervention, provides outcome scores that lie nearer the nonclinical population mean than the clinical population mean.

Measuring clinical significance is reliant on determining a cut-off point for what constitutes "recovered." Following this, Jacobson and Truax [93] developed a method of calculating change, the reliable change index, which also takes into account the statistical significance of the change: when outcome measurement suggests that a patient is statistically more likely to be in the nonclinical population than the clinical population. Assuming normal distribution in both populations, this method is based on the probability of a patient's score ending up in one population as opposed to the other. Reliable change indices are calculated using temporal stability data to test if scores change to an extent that is beyond change that could be caused by measurement error. If a patient's score changes to a greater extent than the calculated criterion, then that patient can be described as "reliably improved" on the measure.

Assessing psychological status

The International Association for the Study of Pain definition of pain emphasizes the importance of both the sensory and affective aspects of pain. Many methods of self-reporting pain are one-dimensional and focus only on the sensory aspect of pain, neglecting the emotional and psychologic components of pain. The need to assess whether psychological problems are an important determinant of pain is particularly relevant when we see people in whom there does not appear to be much obvious pathology within the musculoskeletal system. This is often the case in chronic back pain and other regional pain syndromes, and in people with chronic widespread pain (including fibromyalgia).

A variety of relatively simple ways of assessing anxiety and depression are available, of which the Hospital Anxiety and Depression Score is probably the most widely used [94]. This well validated question self-assessment instrument can be completed in 5 to 10 minutes, and is therefore appropriate for use in clinical practice as well as research. Other tools that might help gain an understanding of the extent of psychologic sensitization to pain include measures of coping (eg, the Coping Strategies Questionnaire [95]), and pain catastrophising measures (eg, the Pain Catastrophizing Scale [96]).

Learning from other disciplines?

Specialists in musculoskeletal disease might be perceived to have been rather insular in their approach to pain and its assessment, developing their own disease specific or generic measures of pain, as described above, and investigating the phenomenon with relatively little appreciation of what is going on in other fields. The cancer field in general, and palliative care in particular, probably have the most to teach us about pain and its assessment, although other fields of medicine that are active in the field include neurology (headache and facial pain), gastronenterology (irritable bowel syndrome), gynecology (chronic pelvic pain), and of course, anesthesiology and health psychology.

In palliative care it is routine to assess the distress associated with pain, as well as its severity, through the utilization of generic instruments, such as the BPI [97], a measure that could easily be applied to musculoskeletal conditions. The concept of "breakthrough pain" is commonly used in this palliative care to indicate episodes of severe pain that occur in spite of analgesia. The authors' focus group work [1] indicated that people with arthritis experience similar phenomena, but the term "breakthrough pain" is not used. The authors talk about the ill-defined concept of flare-ups of arthritis, presumably because the authors think of pain as being the result of pathologic processes in joints, such as inflammation, rather than considering pain as a problem in its own right. The musculoskeletal health care professionals and researchers do not appear to have done much research to compare the experiences of their patients with those with cancer, or to explore possible explanations of these phenomena with their colleagues working in palliative care. The authors believe that there is much to be gained by working more closely with other disciplines.

Summary

Pain is a complex phenomenon involving peripheral nocioception, central sensitization, and cortical interpretation. At each level, a variety of factors can modify pain signaling and perception. Rheumatologists have tended to take what the authors view as a somewhat simplistic approach to the assessment of the pain their patients experience, usually limiting their measurement techniques to the use of self-report Likert or visual analog scales. These techniques have many limitations and clearly do not reflect the complexity of a patient's experience. A wide variety of alternative approaches are becoming available. The authors believe that these methods should be used more widely in rheumatologic practice and research.

References

[1] Gooberman-Hill R, Woolhead G, MacKichan F, et al. Assessing chronic joint pain: lessons from a focus group study. Arthritis Care Res 2007;57(4):666–71.

[2] Haigh RC, McCabe CS, Halligan PW, et al. Joint stiffness in a phantom limb: evidence of central nervous system involvement in rheumatoid arthritis. Rheumatology 2003;42(7):888–92.
[3] Covic T, Adamson B, Spencer D, et al. A biopsychosocial model of pain and depression in rheumatoid arthritis: a 12-month longitudinal study. Rheumatology 2003;42(11):1287–94.
[4] Price DD, McGrath PA, Rafii A, et al. The validation of visual analogue scales as ratio scale measures for chronic and experimental pain. Pain 1983;17:45–56.
[5] Bolognese JA, Schnitzer TJ, Ehrich EW. Response relationship of VAS and Likert scales in osteoarthritis efficacy measurement. Osteoarthritis Cartilage 2003;11:499–507.
[6] Streiner D, Norman G. Health measurement scales: a practical guide to their development and uses. 2nd edition. New York: Oxford University Press; 1995. p. 33–9.
[7] Clark P, Lavielle P, Martinez H. Learning from pain scales: patient perspective. J Rheumatol 2003;30:1584–8.
[8] Bierri D, Reeve RA, Champion GD, et al. The Faces Pain Scale for the self-assessment of the severity of pain experienced by children: development, initial validation, and preliminary investigation for ratio scale properties. Pain 1990;41:139–50.
[9] Frank AJ, Moll JM, Hort JF. A comparison of three ways of measuring pain. Rheumatol Rehabil 1982;21:211–7.
[10] McBeth J, Macfarlane GJ, Silman AJ. Does chronic pain predict future psychological distress? Pain 2002;96(3):239–45.
[11] Cleeland C. Measurement of pain by subjective report. In: Chapman C, Loeser J, editors. Advances in pain research and therapy. New York: Raven Press; 1989. p. 391–403.
[12] Mendoza T, Mayne T, Rublee D, et al. Reliability and validity of a modified Brief Pain Inventory short form in patients with osteoarthritis. Eur J Pain 2006;10(4):353–61.
[13] Von Korff M, Ormel J, Keefe FJ, et al. Grading the severity of chronic pain. Pain 1992;50(2): 133–49.
[14] Elliott AM, Smith BH, Smith WC, et al. Changes in chronic pain severity over time: the chronic pain grade as a valid measure. Pain 2000;88(3):303–8.
[15] Melzack R. The McGill Pain Questionnaire: major properties and scoring methods. Pain 1975;1:277–99.
[16] Nolli M, Ghirelli L, Ferraccioli GF. Pain language in fibromyalgia, rheumatoid-arthritis and osteo-arthritis. Clin Exp Rheumatol 1988;6(1):27–33.
[17] Melzack R. The short-form Mcgill Pain Questionnaire. Pain 1987;30(2):191–7.
[18] Krause SJ, Backonja MM. Development of a neuropathic pain questionnaire. Clin J Pain 2003;19(5):306–14.
[19] Backonja MM, Krause SJ. Neuropathic pain questionnaire–short form. Clin J Pain 2003; 19(5):315–6.
[20] Creamer P, Lethbridge-Cejku M, Hochberg MC. Where does it hurt? Pain localization in osteoarthritis of the knee. Osteoarthritis Cartilage 1998;6318–23.
[21] Ohnmeiss DD. Repeatability of pain drawings in a low back pain population. Spine 2000; 25(8):980–8.
[22] Bellamy N, Buchanan WW, Goldsmith CH, et al. Validation-study of WOMAC—a health-status instrument for measuring clinically important patient relevant outcomes to antirheumatic drug-therapy in patients with osteo-arthritis of the hip or knee. J Rheumatol 1988; 15(12):1833–40.
[23] Dieppe PA. Recommended methodology for assessing the progression of osteoarthritis of the hip and knee joints. Osteoarthritis Cartilage 1995;3(2):73–7.
[24] Nilsdotter AK, Lohmander LS, Klassbo M, et al. Hip disability and osteoarthritis outcome score (HOOS)–validity and responsiveness in total hip replacement. BMC Musculoskelet Disord 2003;24:41–8.
[25] Roos EM, Roos HP, Lohmander LS, et al. Knee injury and osteoarthritis outcome score (KOOS)–Development of a self-administered outcome measure. J Orthop Sports Phys Ther 1998;28(2):88–96.

[26] Meenan RF, Gertman PM, Mason JH. Measuring health-status in arthritis—arthritis impact measurement scales. Arthritis Rheum 1980;23(2):146–52.
[27] Dawson J, Fitzpatrick R, Carr A, et al. Questionnaire on the perceptions of patients about total hip replacement. J Bone Joint Surg Br 1996;78(2):185–90.
[28] Dawson J, Fitzpatrick R, Murray D, et al. Questionnaire on the perceptions of patients about total knee replacement. J Bone Joint Surg Br 1998;80(1):63–9.
[29] Dawson J, Fitzpatrick R, Carr A. Questionnaire on the perceptions of patients about shoulder surgery. J Bone Joint Surg Br 1996;78(4):593–600.
[30] Wylde V, Learmonth I, Cavendish V. The Oxford hip score: the patient's perspective. Health Qual Life Outcomes 2005;3(1):66.
[31] O'Malley KJ, Suarez-Almazor M, Aniol J, et al. Joint-specific multidimensional assessment of pain (J-MAP): factor structure, reliability, validity, and responsiveness in patients with knee osteoarthritis. J Rheumatol 2003;30(3):534–43.
[32] van der Heijde DM, van't Hof MA, van Reil PL, et al. Judging disease activity in clinical practice in rheumatoid arthritis. First step in the development of a disease activity score. Ann Rheum Dis 1990;49:916–20.
[33] Harris RE, Gracely RH, McLean SA, et al. Comparison of clinical and evoked pain measures in fibromyalgia. J Pain 2006;7(7):521–7.
[34] Kellgren JH. Observations on referred pain arising from muscle. Clin Sci 1938;3:175–90.
[35] Dunnett AJ, Roy D, Stewart A, et al. The diagnosis of fibromyalgia in women may be influenced by menstrual cycle phase. Journal of Bodywork and Movement Therapies 2007;11(2):99–105.
[36] Lequesne MG. The algofunctional indices for hip and knee osteoarthritis. J Rheumatol 1997;24(4):779–81.
[37] Adamson J, Gooberman-Hill R, Woolhead G, et al. "Questerviews": using questionnaires in qualitative interviews as a method of integrating qualitative and quantitative health services research. J Health Serv Res Policy 2004;9(3):139–45.
[38] Breivik H, Collett B, Ventafridda V, et al. Survey of chronic pain in Europe: prevalence, impact on daily life, and treatment. Eur J Pain 2006;10(4):287–333.
[39] Smith BH, Hopton JL, Chambers WA. Chronic pain in primary care. Fam Pract 1999;16(5):475–82.
[40] Jensen MP, Mardekian J, Lakshminarayanan M, et al. Validity of 24-h recall ratings of pain severity: Biasing effects of "Peak" and "End" pain. Pain, in press.
[41] Blane DB. Collecting retrospective data: development of a reliable method and a pilot study of its use. Soc Sci Med 1996;42(5):751–7.
[42] Baumgarten M, Siemiatycki J, Gibbs GW. Validity of work histories obtained by interview for epidemiological purposes. Am J Epidemiol 1983;118(4):583–91.
[43] Croft P, Jordan K, Jinks C. "Pain elsewhere" and the impact of knee pain in older people. Arthritis Rheum 2005;52(8):2350–4.
[44] Kadam UT, Jordan K, Croft PR. Clinical comorbidity in patients with osteoarthritis: a case-control study of general practice consulters in England and Wales. Ann Rheum Dis 2004;63(4):408–14.
[45] Greenfield S, Apalone G, McNeil BJ, et al. The importance of co-existent disease in the occurrence of postoperative complications and one-year recovery in patients undergoing total hip replacement. Comorbidity and outcomes after hip replacement. Med Care 1993;31(2):141–54.
[46] Harcourt WGV, White SH, Jones P. Specificity of the Oxford knee status questionnaire—the effect of disease of the hip or lumbar spine on patients' perception of knee disability. J Bone Joint Surg Br 2001;83(3):345–7.
[47] McMurray R, Heaton J, Sloper P, et al. Measurement of patient perceptions of pain and disability in relation to total hip replacement: the place of the Oxford hip score in mixed methods. Qual Saf Health Care 1999;8(4):228–33.

[48] Sprangers MAG, Schwartz CE. Integrating response shift into health-related quality of life research: a theoretical model. Soc Sci Med 1999;48(11):1507–15.
[49] Vlaeyen JW, Linton SJ. Fear-avoidance and its consequences in chronic musculoskeletal pain: a state of the art. Pain 2000;85(3):317–32.
[50] Brandtstadter J, Renner G. tenacious goal pursuit and flexible goal adjustment: explication and age-related analysis of assimilative and accommodative strategies of coping. Psychol Aging 1990;5(1):58–67.
[51] McCracken LM. Learning to live with the pain: acceptance of pain predicts adjustment in persons with chronic pain. Pain 1998;74(1):21–7.
[52] Morley S, Pallin V. Scaling the affective domain of pain: a study of the dimensionality of verbal descriptors. Pain 1995;62(1):39–49.
[53] Williams AC, Davies HTO, Chadury Y. Simple pain rating scales hide complex idiosyncratic meanings. Pain 2000;85(3):457–63.
[54] Linton S. Review of psychological risk factors in back and neck pain. Spine 2000;25(9): 1148–56.
[55] Jordan K, Jinks C, Croft P. A prospective study of the consulting behaviour of older people with knee pain. Br J Gen Pract 2006;56(525):269–76.
[56] Heuts PHTG, Vlaeyen JWS, Roelofs J, et al. Pain-related fear and daily functioning in patients with osteoarthritis. Pain 2004;110(1–2):228–35.
[57] Cornwell J. Hard-earned lives: accounts of health and illness from East London. London: Tavistock; 1984.
[58] Parsons T. The Social System. New York: Free Press; 1951.
[59] Greenhalgh T, Hurwitz B. Narrative based medicine: why study narrative? BMJ 1999; 318(7175):48–50.
[60] Berglund B, Harju E-L, Lindblom U. Psychophysical testing of somatosensory functions in neuropathic-pain patients. In: Jensen MP, Turner JA, Wiesenfeld-Hallin Z, editors. Progress in pain research and management, volume 8. Seattle (Washington): IASP Press; 1997. p. 435–47.
[61] Levy D, Abraham R, Reid G. A Comparison of 2 methods for measuring thermal thresholds in diabetic neuropathy. J Neurol Neurosurg Psychiatry 1989;52(9):1072–7.
[62] Woolf CJ, Salter MW. Neuroscience—Neuronal plasticity: Increasing the gain in pain. Science 2000;288(5472):1765–8.
[63] Kosek E, Ordeberg G. Abnormalities of somatosensory perception in patients with painful osteoarthritis normalize following successful treatment. Eur J Pain 2000;4(3):229–38.
[64] O'Driscol SL, Jayson MIV. Pain threshold analysis in patients with osteoarthrosis of hip. BMJ 1974;3(5933):714–5.
[65] Coderre TJ, Katz J, Vaccarino AL, et al. Contribution of central neuroplasticity to pathological pain–review of clinical and experimental-evidence. Pain 1993;52(3):259–85.
[66] Bradley LA. Recent approaches to understanding osteoarthritis pain. J Rheumatol Suppl 2004;3:154–60.
[67] Hendiani JA, Westlund KN, Lawand N, et al. Mechanical sensation and pain thresholds in patients with chronic arthropathies. J Pain 2003;4(4):203–11.
[68] Martinez V, Fletcher D, Bouhassira D, et al. The evolution of primary hyperalgesia in orthopedic surgery: quantitative sensory testing and clinical evaluation before and after total knee arthroplasty. Anesth Analg 2007;105(3):815–21.
[69] Maquet D, Croisier JL, Demoulin C, et al. Pressure pain thresholds of tender point sites in patients with fibromyalgia and in healthy controls. Eur J Pain 2004;8(2):111–7.
[70] Desmeules JA, Cedraschi C, Rapiti E, et al. Neurophysiologic evidence for a central sensitization in patients with fibromyalgia. Arthritis Rheum 2003;48(5):1420–9.
[71] Kosek E, Ekholm J, Hansson P. Sensory dysfunction in fibromyalgia patients with implications for pathogenic mechanisms. Pain 1996;68(2–3):375–83.
[72] Edwards RR, Sarlani E, Wesselmann U, et al. Quantitative assessment of experimental pain perception: multiple domains of clinical relevance. Pain 2005;114(3):315–9.

[73] Janal MN, Glusman M, Kuhl JP, et al. On the absence of correlation between responses to noxious heat, cold, electrical and ischemic Stimulation. Pain 1994;58(3):403–11.
[74] Chong DP, Cros DP. Technology literature review: quantitative sensory testing. Muscle Nerve 2004;29(5):734–47.
[75] Fordyce WE. Behavioural methods in chronic pain and illness. St. Louis (MO): Mosby; 1976.
[76] Moores LL, Watson PJ. The development of a measurement tool for the assessment of pain behaviour in real time. Physiotherapy 2004;90(1):12–8.
[77] Keefe FJ, Caldwell DS, Queen KT, et al. Pain coping strategies in osteoarthritis patients. J Consult Clin Psychol 1987;55(2):208–12.
[78] Weiner DK, Rudy TE. Attitudinal barriers to effective treatment of persistent pain in nursing home residents. J Am Geriatr Soc 2002;50:2035–40.
[79] Cook AKR, Niven CA, Downs MG. Assessing the pain of people with cognitive impairment. Int J Geriatr Psychiatry 1999;14(6):421–5.
[80] Shega J, Emanuel L, Vargish L, et al. Pain in persons with dementia: complex, common, and challenging. J Pain 2007;8(5):373–8.
[81] Zwakhalen SMG, Hamers JPH, Berger MPF. The psychometric quality and clinical usefulness of three pain assessment tools for elderly people with dementia. Pain 2006;126(1–3): 210–20.
[82] Fuchs-Lacelle S, Hadjistavropoulos HD. Development and preliminary validation of the pain assessment checklist for seniors with limited ability to communicate (PACSLAC). Pain Manag Nurs 2004;1(5):37–49.
[83] Wary B. Collectief Doloplus: Doloplus-2, une échelle pour évaluer la douleur. Soins Gérontologie 1999;19:25–7 [in French].
[84] Ferrell BA, Ferrell BR, Rivera L. Pain in cognitively impaired nursing home patients. J Pain Symptom Manage 1995;10(8):591–8.
[85] Parmelee PA, Smith B, Katz IR. Pain complaints and cognitive status among elderly institution residents. J Am Geriatr Soc 1993;41(5):517–22.
[86] Samanta J, Kendall J, Samanta A. 10-minute consultation: chronic low back pain. BMJ 2003;326(7388):535.
[87] Main CJ, Williams AC. ABC of psychological medicine: musculoskeletal pain. BMJ 2002; 325(7363):534–7.
[88] Jones AKP, Kulkarni B, Derbyshire SWG. Pain mechanisms and their disorders: imaging in clinical neuroscience. Br Med Bull 2003;65(1):83–93.
[89] Tolle TR, Kaufmann T, Siessmeier T, et al. Region-specific encoding of sensory and affective components of pain in the human brain: a positron emission tomography correlation analysis. Ann Neurol 1999;45(1):40–7.
[90] Kulkarni B, Bentley DE, Elliott R, et al. Arthritic pain is processed in brain areas concerned with emotions and fear. Arthritis Rheum 2007;56(4):1345–54.
[91] Kendall PC, Marrs-Garcia A, Nath SR, et al. Normative comparisons for the evaluation of clinical significance. J Consult Clin Psychol 1999;67(3):285–99.
[92] Kendall PC. Editorial. J Consult Clin Psychol 1997;65(1):3–5.
[93] Jacobson NS, Truax P. Clinical-significance—a statistical approach to defining meaningful change in psychotherapy-research. J Consult Clin Psychol 1991;59(1):12–9.
[94] Zigmond AS, Snaith RP. The hospital anxiety and depression scale. Acta Psychiatr Scand 1983;67(6):361–70.
[95] Rosenstiel AK, Keefe FJ. The use of coping strategies in chronic low-back-pain patients—relationship to patient characteristics and current adjustment. Pain 1983;17(1):33–44.
[96] Sullivan MJL, Bishop SR, Pivik J. The pain catastrophizing scale: development and validation. Psychol Assess 1995;7(4):524–32.
[97] Cleeland C, Ryan K. Pain assessment: global use of the brief pain inventory. Ann Acad Med Singapore 1994;23(2):129–38.

ELSEVIER
SAUNDERS

Rheum Dis Clin N Am
34 (2008) 331–349

RHEUMATIC
DISEASE CLINICS
OF NORTH AMERICA

Placebo Response: Relevance to the Rheumatic Diseases

Antonella Pollo, MD[a,b,*],
Fabrizio Benedetti, MD[b,c]

[a] *Department of Neuroscience, University of Turin, Faculty of Pharmacy, Corso Raffaello 30, I-10125 Turin, Italy*
[b] *National Institute of Neuroscience, Turin, Italy*
[c] *Department of Neuroscience, University of Turin Medical School, Corso Raffaello 30, I-10125 Turin, Italy*

Until recently, the word *placebo* carried the negative connotation of being a hindrance on the path of new treatment assessment and approval. A drug failing to show an effect stronger than that in the placebo arm of a clinical trial is appropriately dismissed as being ineffective, but in so doing, a strong link is established between the concepts of placebo and uselessness. In recent times, interest in the neurobiology of the placebo effect has brought about a new awareness of its potential exploitation for the patient's benefit, framing it as a positive context effect with the power to influence therapy outcome.

Placebo effects have been described in many different clinical and experimental settings, ranging from motor disorders like Parkinson's disease and neuropsychiatric conditions like depression and anxiety to endocrine and immune systems changes [1,2]. The field in which the most prominent effects have been observed and the largest number of studies has been conducted is that of placebo analgesia, that is, the lessening of pain experienced in response to a therapeutic act devoid of intrinsic analgesic activity. It is precisely this aspect that is most relevant to the rheumatologist, whose patients are often in a chronic pain state that negatively affects their quality of life. Pain is no longer considered the straightforward result of processing of nociceptive information but rather a multidimensional experience shaped

This work was supported by a grant from Istituto San Paolo di Torino and from Regione Piemonte.

* Corresponding author. Department of Neuroscience, University of Turin Medical School, Corso Raffaello 30, I-10125 Turin, Italy.

E-mail address: antonella.pollo@unito.it (A. Pollo).

doi:10.1016/j.rdc.2008.04.002

by attention, emotions, suggestions and expectations, mood, fear, and anxiety. Thus, the additional therapeutic opportunity offered by the modulation of psychologic factors must be eagerly taken, including nonpharmacologic approaches such as improvement of the patient–provider interaction, optimization of the psychosocial context surrounding the patient, and enhancement of those environmental factors eliciting expectation of pain relief. Moreover, knowledge of placebo mechanisms can be incorporated in the design of new clinical trials. When possible, the use of placebo groups can be limited to a minimum by employing the so-called "open/hidden" protocols, and simple measures such as the assessment of the patient's expectations about therapeutic outcomes can help in the interpretation of clinical trials results.

This article provides a short overview of neurochemical, pharmacologic, and neuroimaging studies that have contributed to our current view of placebo analgesia. Emphasis is placed on mechanisms of action, enlightening the role of expectation and conditioning in modulating the top-down control of pain during pharmacologic and procedural placebo administrations. The interested reader is referred to a number of specific reviews [1–7].

Placebo terminology

The definition of placebo still generates confusion in the scientific community, essentially because of the paradox intrinsic in the etymology of the word itself. The Latin *placēre* refers to the intent of pleasing the patient by administering an inert agent, which by definition cannot have any effect. How then can a "placebo effect" exist at all? The answer lies in the difference between the object—the substance without inherent properties—and the subject experiencing it, in whose brain sizable modifications are induced by its symbolic significance [8]. The proposed replacement of the term *placebo response* with *meaning response* underscores the importance of the patient's beliefs about the treatment and stresses what is present (something inducing the expectation of a benefit) rather than what is absent (the active principle of a drug or a manipulation of proven specific efficacy). Thus, the placebo can be reduced to the meaning that the patient attaches to it [9]. Proceeding along this line of reasoning, the concept of placebo may be extended to embrace all aspects of the therapeutic act. In fact, a healing meaning can be attached to virtually anything, and in the global perception of the cure, all factors are important, such as the physician's words, the sight and smell of the environment, and the memory of past experiences in similar situations [10,11]. Thus, the placebo effect can be expanded, becoming a context effect. The manipulation of the psychosocial context can result in the modulation of the placebo response, and the administration of a placebo can be broadened to the simulation of a complex therapeutic situation. At the limit, research protocols can even be applied whereby no placebo is given, but the context effect is elicited only by verbal suggestions or by other environmental clues inducing expectation of benefit. Strictly speaking, the effect resulting from such manipulations cannot be called a placebo response, but rather a placebolike or a placebo-related response. These protocols are useful, however, because they share with classic inert substance administration the generation of response anticipation (ie, one of the better-substantiated brain mechanisms of placebo action). Thus, in this review, many such studies are revised, taken especially among neuroimaging contributions.

It is common practice to use the terms *placebo effect* and *placebo response* as synonyms, but technically they refer to distinct phenomena. The placebo effect is the average effect observed in a group of subjects receiving a placebo, whereas the placebo response indicates the symptom improvement in a single individual given a sham treatment [12]. The difference is important because in the individual, the real psychobiologic phenomenon can best be studied, whereas the group effect (best exemplified by the placebo arm of randomized clinical trials) can be contaminated by other effects that have nothing to do with the placebo response but nonetheless induce symptom improvement (see later discussion). Even in the clinical or experimental setting in which placebo mechanisms are specifically investigated, average results are commonly reported because of the difficulty of evidencing placebo responses that are often small or absent in several subjects under study. This difficulty contributes to misinterpretation of placebo effects observed in clinical trials and placebo responses observed in experimental studies. For example, in a recent clinical trial meta-analysis, Hrobjartsson and Gotzsche [13] failed to show consistent placebo effects in a large number of diseases (with pain being a notable exception). Their work stimulated a lively debate on the appropriateness of protocols used to demonstrate placebo effects, which cannot always be revealed when the specific aim of the study is to assess the effectiveness of an active treatment, thus leaving important variables, such as psychologic factors, uncontrolled [14–16]. Therefore, knowledge of placebo neurobiology may best be acquired in clinical and experimental studies entirely targeted on placebo, as suggested by the larger placebo analgesic effects found in these studies compared with clinical trials [14].

Nonplacebo factors contributing to the placebo effect

When reporting placebo effects in clinical trials and experimental settings, care must be taken to dissect the real biologic phenomenon from bias and confounding factors that may add to the overall effect. These factors are often the cause of skepticism and disbelief in the placebo effect itself. The first and most important element is the natural history, that is, the time course of a symptom or disease in the absence of any external intervention. If the symptom (eg, pain) undergoes spontaneous fluctuations in time, simultaneous remission and placebo administration can result in wrong interpretation or, at best, overestimation of the placebo effect [17]. To obtain an accurate measurement, the effect in a group not receiving any treatment (the natural history group) must be subtracted from that in the placebo group. For ethical reasons (to limit the number of subjects not receiving therapy) or design reasons (eg, to limit the overall number of subjects), many clinical trials do not include a natural history group, thus making a precise quantification of the placebo effect impossible. Of note, the often-cited notion that, on average, 35% of subjects are adequately alleviated by a placebo derives from an early meta-analysis that included trials without an appropriate natural history group [18].

A second element to take into consideration is a statistical phenomenon called regression to the mean. When patients seek medical advice, their symptoms are likely to significantly deviate from normal values (eg, pain is strong rather than mild). In a second assessment, they have a higher probability of obtaining a lower pain score than a more elevated one (ie, the second value will move closer to the mean of its distribution) [19]. This improvement happens independently of any medical intervention, be it active or placebo and, again, has to be separated from placebo effects by means of a natural history group. In general, any selection of extreme physiologic parameters (eg, severe pain or very high values of blood glucose) produces a model of statistical regression to the mean.

Other possible confounding factors are biases, errors in the detection of relief (judgment errors), or concurrent actions of simultaneously intervening agents. An example of bias is the conscious or unconscious desire to please the clinician by providing the expected answer. A judgment error can occur when the symptom intensity change is small but has to be described in an all-or-none fashion such as "present/non present." In other words, it can be a false-positive error caused by the ambiguity of the signal, triggering the report of nonexistent relief. Finally, in a cointervention, two agents are acting at the same time—the placebo and an unidentified active principle (eg, a concomitant diet)—with the action of the latter mistakenly attributed to the placebo.

Pavlovian conditioning and cognitive mechanisms

The placebo effect was, at the beginning, considered only a demonstration of human suggestibility [20]; however, early scientific work emphasized the fact that comparable phenomena could be reproduced in animals [21,22]. Similar to the digestive reflexes of Pavlov's dogs (ie, salivation after presentation of food), which after proper training can also be elicited in response to stimuli not physiologically part of the reflex (ie, the sound of a bell), the placebo response can be viewed as an acquired reflex, resulting from the repeated pairing of the appropriate (ie, physiologic) stimulus with a new one devoid of the capability of eliciting the reflex. Thus, the repeated co-occurrence in the medical history of a patient of aspects of the clinical setting associated with drug assumption (such as taste, color, and shape of a tablet; white coats; or the peculiar hospital smell) and therapy outcome (eg, analgesia) can provoke what is called a *conditioned response*: the therapy outcome induced by the clinical setting alone in the absence of the pharmacologically active principle [23–26]. In the experimental setting, demonstration of the effectiveness of conditioning in mediating a placebo response comes from a series of studies by Voudouris and colleagues [27–29]. They applied a protocol whereby conditioning was achieved by pairing a placebo analgesic cream with a painful stimulation that was surreptitiously reduced with respect to a baseline condition to make the subjects believe that the cream was effective. In this way, a direct comparison could be made between a conditioned and an unconditioned group, with the former invariably showing a larger pain reduction.

Recently, a role for behavioral conditioning processes in the modulation of placebo responses was suggested for physiologic functions outside the conscious control, such as those involving the immune system or neuroendocrine secretions [30]. For example, in patients who have multiple sclerosis, decrements in peripheral leukocyte counts induced by cyclophosphamide can be conditioned by pairing the drug with a strongly flavored beverage [31]. In healthy subjects, a similar conditioning with cyclosporine A produced immunosuppression after placebo, as assessed by depressed mRNA expression of interleukin-2 and interferon-gamma and by lymphocyte proliferation [32]. Immunocompetent cells of healthy individuals subcutaneously injected with saline showed enhanced in vitro activation [33]. Likewise, placebo modulation of growth hormone and cortisol secretion could be obtained after conditioning with sumatriptan (a selective 5-HT$_{1B/1D}$ receptor agonist that stimulates growth hormone and inhibits cortisol secretion) [34]. The physiologic basis for these responses can conceivably be provided by autonomic nervous system activity and by the release of neuroendocrine substances from the pituitary gland induced by the psychosocial context through neural circuits including limbic and hypothalamic relays [30,35].

Conditioning alone, however, cannot completely account for placebo effects in all situations. Even more important, especially when the response falls in the conscious domain, are cognitive aspects such as expectations, motivations, and emotions [36]. These cognitive aspects are modulated by many factors, including anxiety, mood, credibility and dose of the cure, and likelihood of the response to occur. A large body of evidence points to their role in shaping the reaction to a sham treatment. For example, grading the degree of expectation produced graded responses, as showed in a study in which the same placebo cream applied to three contiguous skin areas induced a progressively stronger analgesia, according to the strength of the accompanying words ("it is a powerful/weak analgesic cream") [37]. In postoperative patients, changing the symbolic meaning of a basal saline infusion resulted in different analgesic requests. Although all patients received the same physiologic solution, the belief of receiving a painkiller prompted a higher analgesic demand than the belief of not receiving any drug. Moreover, the belief certainty also mattered: a group of patients who had uncertain expectations, warned that they could receive a painkiller or a placebo in a double-blind protocol, requested an intermediate dose of analgesics [38]. Prior experience is also important in determining the placebo response at a given time. In healthy volunteers undergoing electrical pain stimulation with different conditioning protocols, small, medium, or large effects were observed, depending on previous experience and time lag between conditioning and response assessment [39].

The two mechanisms of conditioning and expectation can overlap, at least to some extent. It has been argued that during the conditioning process, the subject learns what to expect [40–42]. In a conscious process such as analgesia, conditioning and expectation can be present simultaneously. In a study testing pain tolerance to arm ischemic pain with a conditioning protocol, with expectation induction, or with both, the placebo increase in pain tolerance was found in all cases, with additive effects [43]. An attempt to counteract one mechanism by means of the other (ie, to reverse placebo analgesia induced by conditioning with the generation of pain worsening expectation) was successful, but the same result could not be achieved with a protocol of hormonal modulation, an unconscious process in which suggestion does not play a role [34].

A different cognitive mechanism that has recently been proposed as a contributor to the genesis of placebo effects is the recruitment of the reward circuitry. It has been argued that placebos have reward properties. Rewards such as food and sex are usually directed to increase survival, but so are placebos with the beneficial outcome they provide. Until recently, only few active treatments existed, and the history of medicine largely matched that of placebo effects [44]. According to this view, the expected clinical benefit is a form of reward, which triggers the placebo response [45,46].

The next section provides data to support the involvement of specific neurochemicals associated with the onset of placebo effects induced by expectations and reward.

The neurochemical substrate of placebo analgesia

The science of placebo has come a long way since the days when psychologic effects were dismissed as unworthy of scientific enquiry or as phenomena devoid of any grounding in physiology. What brought the placebo back to the realm of biology and physiology was the neuropharmacologic approach.

Endogenous opioids

In 1978, Levine and colleagues [47] first proposed the involvement of endogenous opioids in placebo analgesia, based on a study of dental postoperative pain in which the opiate antagonist naloxone reduced the probability of a positive placebo response. Since then, placebo analgesia has been antagonized by naloxone in different models [17,48], and a model gradually emerged depicting the secretion of endogenous opioids in the brain as the central event of the pain modulation by a placebo, with activation of the descending antinociceptive pathway as its anatomic substrate (see later discussion). In the cerebrospinal fluid of placebo responders, the peak concentration of β-endorphin was found to be more than twice that of placebo nonresponders [49]. Opioids released by the central nervous system after a placebo procedure showed the same (naloxone-reversible) side-effects of exogenously administered narcotics, as measured by ventilation changes in thoracotomized patients conditioned with buprenorphine [50]. The endogenous opioid system was suggested to be somatotopically organized because the naloxone-sensitive effect showed a strict site specificity, being possible to reverse the placebo response of a cream applied on different body parts, together with locally circumscribed instructions as to where the cream would produce analgesia [51]. Finally, another naloxone-sensitive phenomenon was the inhibition of the β-adrenergic sympathetic system during placebo-induced expectation of analgesia, as measured by slowed heart rate and reduced β-adrenergic spectral component of heart rate variability. It is still unknown whether the heart effect is mediated by the pain reduction or caused by a direct action of endogenous opioids [52]. A different substance indirectly supporting the role of endogenous opioids is cholecystokinin (CCK), whose effects counteract those of opioids. Brain distribution of CCK and opioid peptides and their receptors largely overlap, suggesting interaction between the two systems [53]. The CCK antagonist proglumide has been showed to potentiate the placebo analgesic response in a model of experimental ischemic pain, suggesting an inhibitory role for CCK in placebo analgesia, which would thus appear to be under the opposing actions of promoting endogenous opioids and inhibiting endogenous CCK [54]. The opposing role of the two systems has also been extended to the emotional modulation of other external signals such as visual input [55].

The opioid antinociceptive system is certainly the best studied but not the only one implicated. Knowledge of other systems is scarce, but their existence emerges from the fact that in some situations, a placebo effect can still occur after blockade of opioid mechanisms by naloxone [56,57]. It seems that different agents can bring about different placebo effects. For example, with a morphine conditioning and/or expectation-inducing protocol, Amanzio and Benedetti [43] could, with naloxone, completely reverse placebo analgesia induced in experimental ischemic arm pain. With the use of ketorolac (a nonopioid analgesic) in the same protocol, however, only a partial blockade could be observed.

Dopamine

Drawing on studies in Parkinson's disease in which the motor placebo response is mediated by dopamine release in the dorsal striatum [58], it was proposed that the concomitant dopamine release in the ventral striatum (especially in the nucleus accumbens) also contributes to the generation of the placebo effect, thanks to the activation of the reward circuitry. The reward circuitry includes structures of the limbic system, such as the nucleus accumbens, the prefrontal cortex, and the amygdala [59]. Activation of electrodes implanted in these regions induces self-stimulation in humans [60], which is associated with dopamine release [61]. Although at present, neuropharmacologic evidence has not been presented and studies employing dopamine antagonists in protocols similar to those used with naloxone are still missing, support for the role of dopamine in shaping the placebo response comes from neuroimaging studies. Specific neurotransmission can be assessed with positron emission tomography (PET) using distinct radioactive tracers that bind to the neurotransmitter receptors in the absence of the endogenous substance but are displaced by its release (shown as a PET signal decrease). In a study combining placebo analgesia and a monetary reward task, it was demonstrated that the subjects who had stronger nucleus accumbens synaptic activation (as measured by functional MRI [fMRI]) during the monetary reward anticipation also showed more profound placebo responses and greater dopamine activity in the same nucleus (as measured with dopamine-agonist [^{11}C]raclopride PET) [62]. Moreover, in a subsequent PET study using the μ-opioid receptor-selective radiotracer [^{11}C]carfentanil and [^{11}C]raclopride, opioid and dopamine neurotransmission were assessed with a pain placebo procedure. It was found that they both were coupled with the placebo response, with changes of activity induced in several brain regions associated with the opioid and dopamine networks [63].

Imaging placebo analgesia in the brain

In the most recent literature on placebo analgesia, ample use is made of brain imaging and mapping techniques, such as PET, fMRI, magnetoelectroencephalography (MEG), and electroencephalography (EEG). Despite some technical limitations, their use is of crucial value to understand where and when placebo analgesia is generated in the central nervous system [64–66].

Placebo in action: evidence for the activation of the descending antinociceptive system

Following the discovery of endogenous enkephalins [67] and the autoradiographic mapping of opioid receptors throughout the brain, a complex pain control system has been delineated, the centers of which are largely coincident with those of nociceptive ascending pathways. Its best-characterized areas comprise the periaqueductal gray (PAG), the rostral ventromedial medulla, and the parabrachial nuclei at the brainstem level; and rostrally, the anterior cingulate cortex (ACC), the orbitofrontal cortex, the hypothalamus, and the central nucleus of the amygdala [68]. This top-down pain regulatory system has adaptive value, being called into action by fear or threat (as in stress-induced analgesia), depressing the incoming nociceptive signals [69]. The first neuroimaging study supporting the involvement of this network in placebo analgesia was a PET study measuring regional cerebral blood flow in healthy volunteers. This study showed overlapping of opioid-induced analgesia (by the μ-agonist remifentanil) and placebo-induced analgesia, with similar activation of the rostral ACC (rACC) and the orbitofrontal cortex, by a pharmacologic or a psychologic means [70]. In a subsequent fMRI study, the activity of different brain regions involved in pain transmission (thalamus, anterior insula, caudal rACC) was decreased in parallel with pain intensity reports following a placebo treatment, suggesting diminished transmission along the pain pathways [71]. In contrast to these findings, no decrease was found in pain regions in an fMRI study using sham acupuncture; however, the investigators confirmed rACC activation, with greater placebo analgesia corresponding to greater rACC activity [72]. Discrepancies in results could be explained by methodologic and procedural differences and by the employment of different placebos, highlighting the variability of the placebo response in distinct context and individual settings [46]. The first direct demonstration of endogenous opioid release was provided in another PET study measuring μ-opioid receptor availability [73]. In this study, [^{11}C]carfentanil was displaced by the activation of opioid neurotransmission, showing significant binding decrease after placebo in pregenual rACC, insula, nucleus accumbens, and dorsolateral prefrontal cortex (DLPFC). In all areas except DLPFC, this binding decrease was correlated with placebo reduction of pain intensity reports. In a subsequent study of the same group, the magnitude variability of the placebo response was showed by multiple regression analyses to be accounted for, at least in part, by the emotional state of the subject during pain and by the affective quality of experienced pain. Thus, individual variations in placebo response may depend on the underlying process for which relief is required; that is, on the individual experience of pain itself [74]. Further support for the role of descending inhibitory pain systems comes from an fMRI study that not only confirmed placebo-related activity in the rACC but also correlated rACC activity with activity in the PAG and bilateral amygdalae, suggesting that the rACC is a crucial cognitive control area, recruiting the subcortical antinociceptive network during placebo analgesia [75]. In an attempt to investigate what takes place at the spinal cord level, Matre and colleagues [76] measured skin areas of heat-induced mechanical hyperalgesia (thought to derive from central sensitization). These areas were smaller in placebo conditions relative to control. Also, expectations of reduced pain resulted in dampened spinal (withdrawal) reflexes and brain evoked-potentials after sural nerve stimulation [77]. Therefore, although no imaging placebo study has been performed so far at the level of the spinal cord, these studies suggest that placebos might modulate spinal activity.

It has been argued that the length of the painful stimulation may be critical for the measurement of placebo effects. Most studies used short heat or electric shock pain stimuli and recorded activity decreases during periods extending after stimulus offset, thus possibly including a later cognitive reappraisal of the significance of pain or late neural activity influenced by report bias (ie, compliance with the investigator's suggestions). Addressing this contention, Price and colleagues [78] examined whether placebo analgesia was accompanied by reductions in neural activity in pain-related areas of the brain during the time of stimulation in irritable bowel syndrome patients by long-duration rectal distension with a balloon barostat. These investigators found that placebo analgesia was accompanied by reductions in brain activity similar to those resulting from lowering the strength of stimulation (in the thalamus, somatosensory cortex, insula, and ACC) and that these reductions occurred during the stimulus presentation itself, not just when subjects reported pain. Of note, this study was conducted on a clinically relevant model of placebo analgesia and showed large placebo effects, consistent with the described discrepancy in magnitude between placebo responses in the experimental and clinical settings [79].

Imaging expectations

As mentioned earlier, expectation of benefit can induce a placebolike effect even without the physical administration of a placebo. Knowledge of placebo analgesia can therefore be gained by focusing on changes in brain activity that take place during pain anticipation. Anticipation alone, in the absence of noxious input, has been shown in fMRI studies to elicit signal intensity changes (increase or decrease) in primary somatosensory cortex, ACC, anterior insula, ventral medial prefrontal cortex, and PAG; that is, in brain areas associated with sensory and affective components of pain. These results have been interpreted as an indication of the influence of cognitive factors on cortical nociceptive networks [80–82].

In the study by Wager and colleagues [71], increased activity in DLPFC and other frontal regions in the anticipatory phase of the placebo analgesic response was found. This increase was negatively correlated with the signal reduction in pain regions and with reported pain intensity but was positively correlated with increase of activity in a midbrain region containing the PAG. Just before the onset of placebo analgesia, prefrontal cortical evaluation could drive the activation of the descending antinociceptive system. In an attempt to further isolate the modulatory effect of expectation on pain transmission, Keltner and colleagues [83] analyzed the regional activation produced by a strong painful stimulus following two different visual cues, one inducing expectation of strong pain and the other of mild pain. Areas showing significant differences included those already implicated in the control of the descending inhibitory pathway, including the ACC, the head of the caudate, the cerebellum, and the nucleus cuneiformis, with the nucleus cuneiformis postulated as the converging target of afferent nociceptive input and top-down modulatory regulation.

To discriminate whether expectancy exerts its psychophysical effect through changes of the perceptual sensitivity of early cortical processes (ie, in the primary and secondary somatosensory areas) or on later evaluative elaborations, such as stimulus identification and response selection (represented in the ACC), Lorenz and colleagues [84] used a combined application of the high temporal resolution techniques of EEG and MEG. They found that the amplitude of the laser-evoked MEG fields in secondary somatosensory areas was highly correlated to the expected stimulus intensity as signaled by an auditory cue, whereas the ensuing evoked responses with a source in the caudal ACC varied with stimulus intensity (requiring a varying level of task engagement) but failed to show any cue validity effects.

Taken together, these brain imaging studies help us understand the neural processes underlying the anticipatory phase before placebo administration and the response to the placebo itself. The involvement of a complex set of brain areas in placebo analgesia indicates that the placebo effect is a good model to help understand the intricate mechanisms linking mental activity (ie, expectation of a future outcome) to different neuronal systems.

Reversing the placebo: the nocebo effect

Because of its relevance in clinical practice as a phenomenon opposite to the placebo, the nocebo effect is worthy here of at least a brief mention. The term *nocebo* (from the Latin *nocēre*, to harm) was introduced to indicate the "toxic" placebo effects arising as sham-treatment side effects [85]. More recently, the concept has been expanded in parallel with that of placebo to include any harmful effect deriving from anticipation of a negative outcome. If the psychosocial context can act on the therapeutic outcome through positive conditioning and expectations, generating a beneficial result, just the reverse effect can be achieved by negative manipulations, leading to symptom worsening [86,87].

Although studies of this phenomenon are limited due to ethical constraints, current interest in nocebos is beginning to yield interesting results (for a review, see Ref. [88]). Experimental evidence in the field of pain suggests that the anticipatory anxiety about the impending pain, brought about by negative expectations, triggers the activation of CCK, which facilitates pain transmission and results in hyperalgesia. Consistently, CCK antagonists block nocebo hyperalgesia [89]. This block is related specifically to nocebo/anxiety-induced hyperalgesia rather than to the more general process of nocebo-induced anxiety, as demonstrated by the selective block by the CCK-antagonist proglumide of nocebo hyperalgesia but not of the concurrent stress-induced hypothalamic-pituitary-adrenal axis hyperactivity [90].

As for placebo analgesia, brain imaging techniques have helped shed light on the circuitry underlying nocebo hyperalgesia, centering in particular on nocebo-related effects. Thus, increased fMRI responses in the ACC and insula were found to be associated with the amplified unpleasantness of innocuous stimuli induced by negative expectation [91]. Likewise, in some of the placebo imaging studies, modulation of secondary somatosensory areas, ACC, and prefrontal cortex activity was bidirectional, showing sensitivity to decreased and increased pain expectation [83,84,92].

At least for pain, the placebo-nocebo phenomenon can best be viewed as a continuum, with opioid and CCK-ergic systems acting as the mediators of opposing effects. The close neuroanatomic distribution of CCK and opioid peptides in the ACC and other areas of the limbic system [53] suggests that they may favor or contrast pain perception, the first through the activation of descending pain inhibitory pathways and the second allegedly through descending pain facilitatory pathways.

Clinical implications

The relevance of placebo studies to clinical practice is manifold, and patients may greatly benefit from the application of research findings on placebo in general and on placebo analgesia in particular. An initial repercussion is on clinical trial design: here, the first recommendation is to control for patient expectations as an important variable influencing trial outcome. In acupuncture studies on osteoarthritis and other acute or chronic pain conditions, group assignment (to real or sham treatment) was unrelated to effects on pain, but regrouping the subjects according to perceived group assignment resulted in significant less pain for the subjects believing to be in the real treatment group [93,94]. A second recommendation is to exploit, whenever possible, the possibility of conducting a form of clinical trial whereby the placebo effect is indirectly measured as the difference between an "open" group receiving the treatment in full view, and a "hidden" group to which it is administered without the patient's knowledge. In the latter group, it is the psychosocial (placebo) component of the overall effect to be eliminated, rather than the active principle [95,96]. This open/hidden design has two advantages: to circumvent potential ethical limitations to the use of placebos in clinical trials and to check for potential direct interactions between the drug and the patient's expectations (ie, the potential activation of nonspecific brain pathways by the mere act of drug administration) [4].

Downstream to clinical trials, the skilful use of placebo in everyday clinical practice also has elevated therapeutic potential and has been knowingly or unknowingly exploited in medicine since ancient times. Despite ethical restrictions, even today, its practice is widespread, as demonstrated by the high percentage of physicians surveyed who reported the use of placebo usually to calm patients, avert requests for unnecessary medication, or as a supplemental treatment [97,98]. It can be argued that deception is not necessarily involved in the use of a placebo and that it can represent an effective treatment that would be unethical to withdraw [99]. Eventually, the appropriateness of placebo employment needs to be evaluated case by case, highlighting the importance of the clinician's awareness of its mechanisms of action. For example, to use a placebo as a diagnostic tool can be misleading, because its effectiveness does not necessarily imply malingering. As we have seen, it can, on the contrary, boost expectations and induce real symptom amelioration. Also, not all patients are placebo responders. Although the same inert pill may be given to many patients, it will induce unique health-related responses in different individuals. Despite attempts to characterize specific traits, behaviors, or neural activity of placebo responders [100], it has so far proved impossible to predict who will react positively to a placebo. Therefore, it is the physician's task to assess individual placebo usefulness.

Every real treatment administered in routine health care has two distinct components: the active constituent and the placebo (psychosocial) factor. Every effort should be made to enhance the latter to maximize the benefit of the therapeutic act. This behavior is perfectly acceptable and does not challenge ethical imperatives. A demonstration of the additive effect of the two components is offered by the lower analgesia obtained with hidden versus open administration of analgesics [95]. This difference disappears in cognitively impaired patients who are unable to communicate and purposefully interact with the caregiver [101]. Every aspect of the psychosocial context may be important, but certainly a central role is played by the patient/therapist relationship. Correct attitudes, skills of empathy, and appropriate words can positively impact on the patient's expectation and belief brain circuitry [11]. Nonverbal clues intentionally or unintentionally conveyed by the therapist are equally important. Deceiving clinicians as to the substance (placebo or drug) being administered to two groups of patients, when in fact both groups received a placebo, resulted in a bigger effect in the group believed by the clinicians to receive a drug [102]. Past experience, such as memory of previous treatments, is also likely to shape the placebo component of therapy outcome, as demonstrated for placebo analgesia in experimental pain [39]. The context influence has prompted Barrett and colleagues [103] to propose a list of eight specific clinical actions: speak positively about treatments, provide encouragement, develop trust, provide reassurance, support relationships, respect uniqueness, explore values, and create ceremony. It should be added that the reverse actions may act as nocebos, lessening the effectiveness of therapeutic agents, and should therefore be carefully avoided. Although the harmful effect of natural situations such as the impact of negative diagnoses or the patient's disbelief in a therapy are sometimes difficult to circumvent, care should be given at least to eliminate negligence and to minimize distrust. A nocebo suggestion can be very powerful. For example, the analgesic response induced by pharmacologic preconditioning with ketorolac together with placebo suggestions could be turned into a hyperalgesic response just by reversing the verbal instructions [34]. Even a seemingly innocuous act such as communicating to the patient that a therapy is going to be interrupted can have a negative impact, as showed by the faster and larger intensity relapse of pain after open versus hidden interruption of morphine analgesic therapy [104].

To sum up, design of clinical trials and placebo therapeutic use are the two main fields of application of the new notions derived from neurophysiologic and neurobiologic investigations on placebo effects. Therapeutic use includes administration of placebo per se (still open to ethical debate) and exploitation of the placebo component that is present in any treatment. Given the frequency of chronic pain complaints among their patients, rheumatologists will be particularly interested in findings on placebo analgesia, but it is hoped that the fallout of the acquisition of a "placebo-oriented" mentality will benefit all aspects of their patients' health.

Summary

The placebo effect is a phenomenon rooted in brain circuitry and biochemistry. Its mechanisms of actions are providing us with a holistic vision of mind–body interactions, enabling us to believe that we can influence our well-being, if not by sheer willpower, at least by employing means known to act on our central nervous system. Awareness of and feelings about treatments are able to influence patient responses psychologically and physiologically, two realms no longer segregated by Cartesian dualism.

Future directions for placebo research include investigation of the common and individual networks operating in different pathologic conditions, research into the mechanisms of action of cognitive factors, and elucidation of the different psychosocial variables interacting in the production of placebo effects. Today we are learning much about placebo effects in many medical conditions other than pain [1,2], although due to space limitations and a greater relevance of pain to the rheumatologist, the present review focuses on pain and analgesia. Nonetheless, it should be remembered that placebos have been found to induce the release of dopamine [58] and to affect the activity of subthalamic nucleus neurons [105] in Parkinson's disease, and they have been found to act on different brain regions in depressed patients [106]. Likewise, placebo treatments may affect a number of other conditions such as asthma [107] and apparatuses such as the immune system [30].

Most important, the knowledge gained in the laboratory must be applied in clinical practice, where the character of the clinician remains at the center of stage, confirming after more than half a century the assertion "the physician is a vastly more important institution than the drug store" [108].

References

[1] Benedetti F. Mechanisms of placebo and placebo-related effects across diseases and treatments. Annu Rev Pharmacol Toxicol 2008;48:33–60.

[2] Benedetti F. Placebo effects: understanding the mechanisms in health and disease. Oxford University Press; 2008. In press.
[3] Benedetti F, Mayberg HS, Wager TD, et al. Neurobiological mechanisms of the placebo effect. J Neurosci 2005;25:10390–402.
[4] Colloca L, Benedetti F. Placebos and painkillers: is mind as real as matter? Nat Rev Neurosci 2005;6:545–52.
[5] Finniss DG, Benedetti F. Mechanisms of the placebo response and their impact on clinical trials and clinical practice. Pain 2005;114:3–6.
[6] Benedetti F. Placebo and endogenous mechanisms of analgesia. Handb Exp Pharmacol 2007;177:393–413.
[7] Price DD, Finniss DG, Benedetti F. A comprehensive review of the placebo effects: recent advances and current thought. Annu Rev Psychol 2008;59:565–90.
[8] Brody H. The placebo response. New York: Harper Collins; 2000.
[9] Moerman DE. Meaning, medicine and the placebo effect. Cambridge (UK): Cambridge University Press; 2002.
[10] Di Blasi Z, Harkness E, Ernst E, et al. Influence of context effect on health outcomes: a systematic review. Lancet 2001;357:757–62.
[11] Benedetti F. How the doctor's words affect the patient's brain. Eval Health Prof 2002;25: 369–86.
[12] Hoffman GA, Harrington A, Fields HL. Pain and the placebo: what we have learned. Perspect Biol Med 2005;48:248–65.
[13] Hrobjartsson A, Gotzsche PC. Is the placebo powerless? An analysis of clinical trials comparing placebo with no treatment. N Engl J Med 2001;344:1594–602.
[14] Vase L, Riley JL 3rd, Price DD. A comparison of placebo effects in clinical analgesic trials versus studies of placebo analgesia. Pain 2002;99:443–52.
[15] Wampold BE, Minami T, Tierney SC, et al. The placebo is powerful: estimating placebo effects in medicine and psychotherapy from randomized clinical trials. J Clin Psychol 2005;61:835–54.
[16] Thorn B. Commentaries on the placebo concept in psychotherapy. J Clin Psychol 2007;63: 371–2.
[17] Fields HL, Levine JD. Placebo analgesia—a role for endorphins? Trends Neurosci 1984;7: 271–3.
[18] Beecher HK. The powerful placebo. JAMA 1955;159:1602–6.
[19] Davis CE. Regression to the mean or placebo effect? In: Guess HA, Kleinman A, Kusek JW, editors. The science of the placebo: toward an interdisciplinary research agenda. London: BMJ Books; 2002. p. 158–66.
[20] Tibbetts RW, Hawkings JR. The placebo response. J Ment Sci 1956;102:60–6.
[21] Herrnstein RJ. Placebo effect in the rat. Science 1962;138:677–8.
[22] Ader R, Cohen N. Behaviorally conditioned immunosuppression and murine systemic lupus erythematosus. Science 1982;215:1534–6.
[23] Wikramasekera I. A conditioned response model of the placebo effect: predictions of the model. In: White L, Tursky B, Schwartz GE, editors. Placebo: theory, research and mechanisms. New York: Guilford Press; 1985. p. 255–87.
[24] Siegel S. Drug anticipatory responses in animals. In: White L, Tursky B, Schwartz GE, editors. Placebo: theory, research and mechanisms. New York: Guilford Press; 1985. p. 288–305.
[25] Siegel S. Explanatory mechanisms for placebo effects: pavlovian conditioning. In: Guess HA, Kleinman A, Kusek JW, editors. The science of the placebo: toward an interdisciplinary research agenda. London: BMJ Books; 2002. p. 133–57.
[26] Ader R. The role of conditioning in pharmacotherapy. In: Harrington A, editor. The placebo effect: an interdisciplinary exploration. Cambridge (MA): Harvard University Press; 1997. p. 138–65.

[27] Voudouris NJ, Peck CL, Coleman G. Conditioned placebo responses. J Pers Soc Psychol 1985;48:47–53.
[28] Voudouris NJ, Peck CL, Coleman G. Conditioned response models of placebo phenomena: further support. Pain 1989;38:109–16.
[29] Voudouris NJ, Peck CL, Coleman G. The role of conditioning and verbal expectancy in the placebo response. Pain 1990;43:121–8.
[30] Pacheco-López G, Engler H, Niemi MB, et al. Expectations and associations that heal: immunomodulatory placebo effects and its neurobiology. Brain Behav Immun 2006;20: 430–46.
[31] Giang DW, Goodman AD, Schiffer RB, et al. Conditioning of cyclophosphamide-induced leukopenia in humans. J Neuropsychiatry Clin Neurosci 1996;8:194–201.
[32] Goebel MU, Trebst AE, Steiner J, et al. Behavioral conditioning of immunosuppression is possible in humans. FASEB J 2002;16:1869–73.
[33] Klein R, Buck S, Classen K, et al. Enhanced in vitro activation of immunocompetent cells in healthy individuals being subcutaneously 'vaccinated' with placebo (physiological saline). Clin Immunol 2008;126:322–31.
[34] Benedetti F, Pollo A, Lopiano L, et al. Conscious expectation and unconscious conditioning in analgesic, motor and hormonal placebo/nocebo responses. J Neurosci 2003;23: 4315–23.
[35] Ader R. Conditioned immunomodulation: research needs and directions. Brain Behav Immun 2003;17:S51–7.
[36] Kirsch I, Lynn SJ. Automaticity in clinical psychology. Am Psychol 1999;54:504–15.
[37] Price DD, Milling LS, Kirsch I, et al. An analysis of factors that contribute to the magnitude of placebo analgesia in an experimental paradigm. Pain 1999;83:147–56.
[38] Pollo A, Amanzio M, Arslanian A, et al. Response expectancies in placebo analgesia and their clinical relevance. Pain 2001;93:77–83.
[39] Colloca L, Benedetti F. How prior experience shapes placebo analgesia. Pain 2006;124: 126–33.
[40] Montgomery GH, Kirsch I. Classical conditioning and the placebo effect. Pain 1997;72: 107–13.
[41] Reiss S. Pavlovian conditioning and human fear: an expectancy model. Behav Ther 1980; 11:380–96.
[42] Rescorla RA. Pavlovian conditioning: it is not what you think it is. Am Psychol 1988;43: 151–60.
[43] Amanzio M, Benedetti F. Neuropharmacological dissection of placebo analgesia: expectation-activated opioid systems versus conditioning-activated specific sub-systems. J Neurosci 1999;19:484–94.
[44] de la Fuente-Fernández R, Schulzer M, Stoessl AJ. Placebo mechanisms and reward circuitry: clues from Parkinson's disease. Biol Psychiatry 2004;56:67–71.
[45] de la Fuente-Fernández R, Stoessl AJ. The placebo effect in Parkinson's disease. Trends Neurosci 2002;6:302–6.
[46] Lidstone SC, Stoessl AJ. Understanding the placebo effect: contributions from neuroimaging. Mol Imaging Biol 2007;9:176–85.
[47] Levine JD, Gordon NC, Fields HL. The mechanisms of placebo analgesia. Lancet 1978;2: 654–7.
[48] Benedetti F. The opposite effects of the opiate antagonist naloxone and the cholecystokinin antagonist proglumide on placebo analgesia. Pain 1996;64:535–43.
[49] Lipman JJ, Miller BE, Mays KS, et al. Peak B endorphin concentration in cerebrospinal fluid: reduced in chronic pain patients and increased during the placebo response. Psychopharmacology (Berl) 1990;102:112–6.
[50] Benedetti F, Amanzio M, Baldi S, et al. Inducing placebo respiratory depressant responses in humans via opioid receptors. Eur J Neurosci 1999;11:625–31.

[51] Benedetti F, Arduino C, Amanzio M. Somatotopic activation of opioid systems by target-directed expectations of analgesia. J Neurosci 1999;19:3639–48.
[52] Pollo A, Vighetti S, Rainero I, et al. Placebo analgesia and the heart. Pain 2003;102: 125–33.
[53] Noble F, Roques BP. The role of CCK2 receptors in the homeostasis of the opioid system. Drugs Today (Barc) 2003;39:897–908.
[54] Benedetti F, Amanzio M, Maggi G. Potentiation of placebo analgesia by proglumide. Lancet 1995;346:1231.
[55] Gospic K, Gunnarsson T, Fransson P, et al. Emotional perception modulated by an opioid and a cholecystokinin agonist. Psychopharmacology (Berl) 2008;197:295–307.
[56] Gracely RH, Dubner R, Wolskee PJ, et al. Placebo and naloxone can alter post-surgical pain by separate mechanisms. Nature 1983;306:264–5.
[57] Grevert P, Albert LH, Goldstein A. Partial antagonism of placebo analgesia by naloxone. Pain 1983;16:129–43.
[58] de la Fuente-Fernández R, Ruth TJ, Sossi V, et al. Expectation and dopamine release: mechanism of the placebo effect in Parkinson's disease. Science 2001;293:1164–6.
[59] Porrino LJ, Esposito RU, Seeger TF, et al. Metabolic mapping of the brain during rewarding self-stimulation. Science 1984;224:306–9.
[60] Bishop MP, Elder ST, Heath RG. Intracranial self-stimulation in man. Science 1963;140: 394–6.
[61] Wise RA, Rompre PP. Brain dopamine and reward. Annu Rev Psychol 1989;40:191–225.
[62] Scott DJ, Stoher CS, Egnatuk CM, et al. Individual differences in reward responding explains placebo-induced expectations and effects. Neuron 2007;55:325–36.
[63] Scott DJ, Stoher CS, Egnatuk CM, et al. Placebo and nocebo effects are defined by opposite opioid and dopaminergic responses. Arch Gen Psychiatry 2008;65:220–31.
[64] Rainville P, Duncan GH. Functional brain imaging of placebo analgesia: methodological challenges and recommendations. Pain 2006;121:177–80.
[65] Kong J, Kaptchuk TJ, Polich G, et al. Placebo analgesia: findings from brain imaging studies and emerging hypothesis. Rev Neurosci 2007;18:173–90.
[66] Colloca L, Benedetti F, Porro CA. Experimental designs and brain mapping approaches for studying the placebo analgesic effect. Eur J Appl Physiol 2008;102:371–80.
[67] Hughes J. Search for the endogenous ligand of the opiate receptor. Neurosci Res Program Bull 1975;13:55–8.
[68] Fields H. State-dependent opioid control of pain. Nat Rev Neurosci 2004;5:565–75.
[69] Millan MJ. Descending control of pain. Prog Neurobiol 2002;66:355–474.
[70] Petrovic P, Kalso E, Petersson KM, et al. Placebo and opioid analgesia-imaging: a shared neuronal network. Science 2002;295:1737–40.
[71] Wager TD, Rilling JK, Smith EE, et al. Placebo-induced changes in fMRI in the anticipation and experience of pain. Science 2004;303:1162–6.
[72] Kong J, Gollub RL, Rosman IS, et al. Brain activity associated with expectancy-enhanced placebo analgesia as measured by functional magnetic resonance imaging. J Neurosci 2006; 26:381–8.
[73] Zubieta JK, Bueller JA, Jackson LR, et al. Placebo effects mediated by endogenous opioid activity on μ-opioid receptors. J Neurosci 2005;25:7754–62.
[74] Zubieta JK, Yau WY, Scott DJ, et al. Belief or need? Accounting for individual variations in the neurochemistry of the placebo effect. Brain Behav Immun 2006;20:15–26.
[75] Bingel U, Lorenz J, Schoell E, et al. Mechanisms of placebo analgesia: rACC recruitment of a subcortical antinociceptive network. Pain 2006;120:8–15.
[76] Matre D, Casey KL, Knardahl S. Placebo-induced changes in spinal cord pain processing. J Neurosci 2006;26:559–63.
[77] Goffaux P, Redmond WJ, Rainville P, et al. Descending analgesia—when the spine echoes what the brain expects. Pain 2007;130:137–43.

[78] Price DD, Craggs J, Verne GN, et al. Placebo analgesia is accompanied by large reductions in pain-related brain activity in irritable bowel syndrome patients. Pain 2007;127:63–72.
[79] Charron J, Rainville P, Marchand S. Direct comparison of placebo effects on clinical and experimental pain. Clin J Pain 2006;22:204–11.
[80] Hsieh JC, Stone-Elander S, Ingvar M. Anticipatory coping of pain expressed in the human anterior cingulate cortex: a positron emission tomography study. Neurosci Lett 1999;262: 61–4.
[81] Ploghaus A, Tracey I, Gati JS, et al. Dissociating pain from its anticipation in the human brain. Science 1999;284:1979–81.
[82] Porro CA, Baraldi P, Pagnoni G, et al. Does anticipation of pain affect cortical nociceptive systems? J Neurosci 2002;22:3206–14.
[83] Keltner JR, Furst A, Fan C, et al. Isolating the modulatory effect of expectation on pain transmission: a functional magnetic resonance imaging study. J Neurosci 2006;26:4437–43.
[84] Lorenz J, Hauch M, Paur RC, et al. Cortical correlates of false expectations during pain intensity judgments—a possible manifestation of placebo/nocebo cognitions. Brain Behav Immun 2005;19:283–95.
[85] Pogge RC. The toxic placebo. Part I. Side and toxic effects reported during the administration of placebo medicine. Med Times 1963;91:773–8.
[86] Hahn RA. A sociocultural model of illness and healing. In: White L, Tursky B, Schwartz GE, editors. Placebo: theory, research and mechanisms. New York: Guilford Press; 1985. p. 167–95.
[87] Dworkin SF, Chen AC, LeResche L, et al. Cognitive reversal of expected nitrous oxide analgesia for acute pain. Anesth Analg 1983;62:1073–7.
[88] Benedetti F, Lanotte M, Lopiano L, et al. When words are painful: unraveling the mechanisms of the nocebo effect. Neuroscience 2007;147:260–71.
[89] Benedetti F, Amanzio M, Casadio C, et al. Blockade of nocebo hyperalgesia by the cholecystokinin antagonist proglumide. Pain 1997;71:135–40.
[90] Benedetti F, Amanzio M, Vighetti S, et al. The biochemical and neuroendocrine bases of the hyperalgesic nocebo effect. J Neurosci 2006;26:12014–22.
[91] Sawamoto N, Honda M, Okada T, et al. Expectation of pain enhances responses to nonpainful somatosensory stimulation in the anterior cingulated cortex and parietal operculum/posterior insula: an event-related functional magnetic resonance imaging study. J Neurosci 2000;20:7438–45.
[92] Koyama T, McHaffie JG, Laurienti PJ, et al. The subjective experience of pain: where expectations become reality. Proc Natl Acad Sci U S A 2005;102:12950–5.
[93] Bausell RB, Lao L, Bergman S, et al. Is acupuncture analgesia an expectancy effect? Eval Health Prof 2005;28:9–26.
[94] Linde K, Witt CM, Streng A, et al. The impact of patient expectations on outcomes in four randomized controlled trials of acupuncture in patients with chronic pain. Pain 2007;128: 264–71.
[95] Amanzio M, Pollo A, Maggi G, et al. Response variability to analgesics: a role for non-specific activation of endogenous opioids. Pain 2001;90:205–15.
[96] Colloca L, Lopiano L, Lanotte M, et al. Overt versus covert treatment for pain, anxiety, and Parkinson's disease. Lancet Neurol 2004;3:679–84.
[97] Sherman R, Hickner J. Academic physicians use placebos in clinical practice and believe in the mind-body connection. J Gen Intern Med 2007;23:7–10.
[98] Nitzan U, Lichtenberg P. Questionnaire survey on use of placebo. BMJ 2008;329:944–6.
[99] Lichtenberg P, Heresco-Levy U, Nitzan U. The ethics of the placebo in clinical practice. J Med Ethics 2004;30:551–4.
[100] Leuchter AF, Cook IA, Witte EA, et al. Changes in brain function of depressed subjects during treatment with placebo. Am J Psychiatry 2002;159:122–9.
[101] Benedetti F, Arduino C, Costa S, et al. Loss of expectation-related mechanisms in Alzheimer's disease makes analgesic therapies less effective. Pain 2006;121:133–44.

[102] Gracely RH, Dubner R, Deeter WD, et al. Clinician's expectations influence placebo analgesia. Lancet 1985;5:43.
[103] Barrett B, Muller D, Rakel D, et al. Placebo, meaning and health. Perspect Biol Med 2006; 49:178–98.
[104] Benedetti F, Maggi G, Lopiano L, et al. Open versus hidden medical treatments: the patient's knowledge about a therapy affects the therapy outcome. Prevention and Treatment 2003. Available at: http://journals.apa.org/prevention/volume6/toc-jun-03.html. Accessed May 16, 2008.
[105] Benedetti F, Colloca L, Torre E, et al. Placebo-responsive Parkinson patients show decreased activity in single neurons of subthalamic nucleus. Nat Neurosci 2004;7:587–8.
[106] Mayberg HS, Silva JA, Brannan SK, et al. The functional neuroanatomy of the placebo effect. Am J Psychiatry 2002;159:728–37.
[107] Kemeny ME, Rosenwasser LJ, Panettieri RA, et al. Placebo response in asthma: a robust and objective phenomenon. J Allergy Clin Immunol 2007;119:1375–81.
[108] Findley T. The placebo and the physician. Med Clin North Am 1953;37:1821–6.

ELSEVIER
SAUNDERS

Rheum Dis Clin N Am
34 (2008) 351–368

RHEUMATIC
DISEASE CLINICS
OF NORTH AMERICA

Psychologic Interventions and Lifestyle Modifications for Arthritis Pain Management

Francis J. Keefe, PhD[a,*], Tamara J. Somers, PhD[a], Lynn M. Martire, PhD[b]

[a]*Department of Psychiatry and Behavioral Sciences, Duke Medical Center, Duke Pain Prevention and Treatment Research Program, 2200 Main Street, Durham, NC 27705, USA*

[b]*Department of Psychiatry, University of Pittsburgh School of Medicine, 121 University Place, Room 508, University Center for Social and Urban Research, Pittsburgh, PA 15260, USA*

Over the past three decades there have been significant advances in medical and surgical approaches to treating patients suffering pain caused by rheumatic diseases. For example, early and more aggressive use of disease-modifying antirheumatic drugs has led to reductions in pain and pain-related disability for many patients suffering from rheumatoid arthritis (RA) [1]. Pain medication protocols developed, refined, and tested in other persistent disease-related pain conditions (eg, cancer pain) are now increasingly being applied to patients suffering from pain caused by osteoarthritis (OA) and RA [2]. Finally, surgical options, once held out as a last resort in the management of arthritis pain (eg, joint replacement surgery), are now being offered to arthritis patients earlier in their disease course [3].

Given these recent developments in the biomedical management of arthritis pain, one might expect that there is a diminishing emphasis in current practice on the role of patient self-management efforts in controlling arthritis pain. Yet, recent clinical guidelines for the management of arthritis [4–6] clearly recommend patient self-management interventions as part of a comprehensive approach to pain control. Among the recommendations

Preparation of this article was supported in part by National Institutes of Health (NIH) grants: R01 AG026469-01, R01 AG026010, AR47218, AR049059, AR050245, AR054626; T32 MH019109 and the Pittsburgh Mind-Body Center (NIH grants HL076852/076858).

* Corresponding author.
E-mail address: keefe003@mc.duke.edu (F.J. Keefe).

doi:10.1016/j.rdc.2008.03.001

offered by these guidelines are the increased use of protocols designed to enhance patients' pain coping skills and greater of involvement of significant others in pain management efforts.

Arthritis is a particularly appropriate target for interventions designed to enhance pain self-management. First, pain is one of the most common symptoms of arthritis patients and is a significant concern of both patients and the health care providers who treat them [7]. Second, there is growing evidence that the use of pain coping strategies and patients' confidence (self-efficacy) that they can use pain coping skills to control pain not only influences the experience of pain but also the impact of pain on psychologic distress and physical disability [2]. Third, recent randomized clinical trials have shown that psychosocial interventions for arthritis pain can produce significant improvements in pain and other outcomes (eg, pain coping, anxiety, joint swelling, and physical disability) [7]. Finally, training in self-management strategies for controlling pain may be especially important for those patients who have difficulty tolerating or have failed to respond to more traditional biomedical approaches to pain. This article provides an overview of self-management interventions currently being used to manage arthritis pain. The article is divided in two major sections. In the first section, the authors review psychologic interventions used to manage arthritis pain, including pain coping skills training and cognitive behavioral therapy for pain management, emotional disclosure interventions, and partner-assisted interventions. In the second section, the authors address lifestyle behavioral weight management interventions used to reduce arthritis pain. In each section the authors briefly describe the rationale and nature of the interventions, present data on their efficacy, and highlight potential future research directions.

Psychologic interventions

Pain coping skills training and cognitive behavioral therapy for pain management

The notion that training in cognitive and behavioral pain coping skills could alter disease-related pain grew out of developments in pain theory dating back to Melzack and Wall's gate control theory [8]. The gate control theory maintains that pain is not a simple sensory event (eg, a simple warning sign of tissue damage), but rather a complex experience that influences and can be influenced by brain processes related to sensation, cognition, emotion, and behavior. The gate control theory has two main tenets: (1) that a gating mechanism in the dorsal horn of the spinal cord can control the transmission of nociceptive signals from a peripheral site (eg, inflamed joint) to the brain and, (2) that the spinal gating of noxious signals is controlled not only by input from the periphery but also by input from higher brain centers responsible thoughts, feelings, and behaviors. The gate control theory provides an explanation for why some psychologic factors (eg, active coping, optimism, social support) can reduce pain, while others (eg, feelings of helplessness, depression) can increase pain. One important implication of the gate control theory is that systematic training in cognitive and behavioral coping skills for altering thoughts, feelings, and behaviors related to pain can reduce pain and help minimize the detrimental impact of pain on psychologic and physical functioning.

The neuromatrix theory of pain builds upon and extends the gate control theory [9] by highlighting the key role that stress and stress regulation systems play in persistent pain conditions. According to the neuromatrix theory, pain is a major stressor that, when it persists, can profoundly alter homeostatic mechanisms. Alterations in homeostasis that are caused by persistent pain can activate stress regulation processes to reinstate homeostasis (eg, release of cortisol, cytokines) that, in turn, can heighten pain. The neuromatrix theory's highlighting of the importance of stress dysregulation has led to an increased emphasis on teaching patients how to use pain coping skills to manage stress.

Pain coping skills training and cognitive behavioral therapy (CBT) for pain management typically consists of three components [7]. The first component involves providing an educational rationale (eg, the gate control theory) that helps patients better understand how their thoughts, feelings, and behaviors can influence pain and how, in turn, their own efforts to manage pain can influence the pain experience. The second component involves therapist-guided training in cognitive and behavioral coping strategies, such as progressive relaxation training, brief relaxation methods, goal setting, activity pacing, imagery, and strategies for altering overly negative thoughts related to pain (eg, cognitive restructuring). The third component involves extensive home practice with coping skills and learning how to apply those skills to challenging pain-related situations (eg, managing pain flares).

Bradley and colleagues [10] were among the first to conduct a methodologically rigorous trial to test the efficacy of a pain coping skills training and CBT intervention for patients having RA. A sample of 53 RA subjects was randomly assigned to receive either a 15-session protocol that provided extensive training in relaxation, biofeedback, goal setting, and self-rewards or to a control group that received 15 sessions of structured social support. When compared with the control condition, the pain coping skills training and CBT protocol produced significant reductions in pain behavior, disease activity, and trait anxiety.

An important focus of recent studies of pain coping skills training and CBT studies in RA patients has been on the effects of providing training early in the course of the disease. In a randomized, clinical trial of 53 subjects having a less than 2-year history of RA, Sharpe and colleagues [11] found that, when compared with a routine medical care control condition, a protocol that combined routine medical care with a comprehensive pain coping skills training and

CBT regimen led to significant improvements in joint stiffness, C-reactive protein levels, and depression. An 18-month follow-up study [12] reported that subjects who received the pain coping skills training and CBT regimen not only maintained their improvements in joint function and depression, but also showed additional benefits in terms of reductions in anxiety and disability. Taken together, these findings suggest that a pain coping skills training and CBT protocol may be a useful adjunct to routine care typically given to RA patients early in the course of their disease.

The authors' research group has conducted a number of clinical trials testing the efficacy of pain coping skills training and CBT protocols in patients having osteoarthritic knee pain. In the first study [13], the authors randomly assigned 99 subjects having OA of the knees to one of three conditions: pain coping skills training, arthritis education, or standard care control. Subjects in the pain coping skills training attended 10 weekly group sessions training them in cognitive and behavioral pain coping strategies, while those in the arthritis education condition attended 10 weekly group sessions providing educational information and lectures on arthritis. Data analyses showed that subjects in the pain coping skills training group had significant improvements in pain, psychologic disability, and physical disability when compared with those in the arthritis education and standard care control conditions. A 6-month follow-up study [14] revealed that subjects in the pain coping skills group maintained their gains in psychologic disability and showed a strong trend ($P = .051$) to show improvements in physical disability, compared with the arthritis education condition. In addition, those subjects who reported the greatest increases in their perceived efficacy of pain coping skills over the course of initial training had significantly lower levels of pain, physical disability, and pain behavior at 6-months follow-up. These findings suggest that pain coping skills training can benefit OA patients suffering from persistent knee pain and that changes in pain coping achieved with this training are related in meaningful ways to a number of long-term outcomes.

Pain coping skills training and CBT is one of the most widely used psychologic interventions for the control of arthritis pain. A recent meta-analysis of randomized psychosocial interventions found that, in fact, pain coping skills training and CBT, was the most frequently tested intervention (tested in 18 of 26 studies) [7]. As discussed above, controlled studies have shown that pain coping skills training and CBT can produce beneficial outcomes in patients suffering from either OA or RA pain. What makes the effects of this training impressive is that they are not restricted solely to pain, but also evident for other important indices of adjustment to persistent arthritis pain, including anxiety, depression, physical disability, and joint function. An important direction for future research on pain coping skills training and CBT interventions is to determine whether these interventions can be successfully disseminated into clinical practice. In a dual-site (SUNY-Stony Brook, Duke Medical Center) National Institutes of Health

(NIH)-supported study, the authors are currently testing the efficacy of nurse-practitioner delivered pain coping skills training protocol for patients with OA pain seen in a primary care practice. The authors are also working with investigators at Mt. Sinai to develop a Web-based platform for delivering pain coping skills training to OA patients being treated in primary care settings.

Emotional disclosure

Over the past 25 years, research by Pennebaker and other investigators has demonstrated that individuals who engage in the disclosure of emotionally difficult and stressful events (emotional disclosure) may experience significant benefits in their health status [15–19]. Typically, these studies require that participants write or talk privately in detail about their thoughts and feelings about a major life event they have not fully disclosed to others. Disclosure sessions are typically performed for 20 to 30 minutes daily for 4 days in a row. The effects of disclosure are usually compared with a control condition in which participants talk or write about a neutral topic. In these studies, all participants are followed up to examine long-term health benefits of the intervention. Studies have been performed in college students as well as a variety of other typically healthy populations. Although results vary, in general emotional disclosure has led to short-term increases in negative mood followed by longer term improvements in outcomes. Beneficial effects of emotional disclosure have included reductions in symptoms and health problems [16,17,19,20], decreases in the frequency of health care visits [19–21], and improvements in immune functioning [19].

There has been growing interest in testing the efficacy of emotional disclosure in patients suffering from pain caused by RA. RA is a good model in which to test emotional disclosure interventions for several reasons. First, there is evidence that RA patients experience high levels of stress [22,23] and are quite reactive to interpersonal stress [24–26]. Second, patients having RA often have high levels of negative emotions that are linked to increased pain [27]. Third, there is a body of literature that suggests that some patients with RA are particularly prone to inhibit their negative emotions and experience problems identifying and reporting their emotions [28].

Kelley and colleagues [29] were the first to systematically test the effects of emotional disclosure in persons with RA. In this study, 72 subjects having RA were randomly assigned to either an emotional disclosure condition (talking privately into a tape recorder about stressful life events for 4 consecutive days) or to a control condition (talking about neutral pictures for 4 consecutive days.) Results revealed that, while the emotional disclosure intervention produced significant, immediate increases in negative mood, at 3-months follow-up patients receiving this intervention reported significantly lower levels of affective disturbance and enhanced physical functioning. Interestingly, patients who experienced the largest initial increases in negative mood had the best outcomes at follow-up in terms of improvements in joint functioning. The results of this study attracted considerable attention, because they indicated that a brief emotional disclosure protocol can have lasting benefits for RA patients.

Subsequent studies of emotional disclosure in RA patients, however, have produced inconsistent results. In a study that involved both RA subjects and asthma subjects, Smyth and colleagues [30] reported that RA subjects who engaged in a written disclosure task for 3 days had significant improvements in physician ratings of their disease activity 4 months later. Broderick and colleagues [31] tested the effects of a standard 3-day home-based written emotional disclosure protocol in patients with RA. They found the disclosure intervention produced no significant effects on outcomes. Wetherell and colleagues [32] conducted a clinical trial comparing the effects of an emotional disclosure protocol to a control intervention in RA subjects and found that, when compared with the control condition, emotional disclosure was associated with reductions in disease activity and improvements in mood. Conclusions regarding the benefits of emotional disclosure, though, were tempered by the fact that the differences in outcome obtained mainly reflected the effects of the control getting worse.

Finally, the authors recently conducted a study to test whether the benefits of emotional disclosure in RA patients could be enhanced by having a trained nurse assist the patient in the disclosure process [33]. In this study, 98 subjects having RA were randomly assigned to one of four conditions: (a) private verbal emotional disclosure, (b) clinician-assisted verbal emotional disclosure, (c) arthritis information control, or (d) no-treatment, standard care only control group. Outcome measures of pain, disability, affect, and stress were collected at evaluation sessions conducted before treatment at 1-month, 3-months, and 12-months follow-ups. Data analyses revealed that there were no consistent benefits of either the clinician-assisted or private emotional disclosure protocols.

The application of emotional disclosure protocols to samples of RA patients is a relatively recent development. Prior studies have mainly been conducted in samples of healthy individuals. Meta analyses of the effects of emotional disclosure in healthy samples have shown this intervention produces moderate effect sizes [34,35]. Interestingly, the mixed findings obtained in emotional disclosure in RA patients are similar to those reported in other clinical populations. Indeed, meta-analyses of emotional disclosure in clinical populations [35,36] have shown that this intervention has a small effect size on average.

At this point it seems fair to conclude that emotional disclosure may be more effective in some RA patients than others. Future research is needed to identify those patients who are most likely to respond to emotional disclosure. For example, it could be that RA patients who are most likely to have difficulty identifying their emotions or who hold back on expressing negative emotions would benefit the most. Future research also needs to examine strategies for enhancing the effects of emotional disclosure in RA patients.

It is possible that having patients engage in an emotional disclosure task before training in pain coping skills and CBT for pain management could produce synergist effects that are stronger than what might be obtained with either intervention alone. With increased disclosure of life events and major stressors, patients may be more readily able to use learned coping skills to manage stressors that contribute to their pain.

Partner-assisted psychologic interventions

For many of the millions of adults who live with arthritis pain, the spouse or partner plays an important role in psychologic adjustment and illness management [37,38]. Therefore, patients may derive greater benefit from psychologic interventions for pain (eg, arthritis education, peer support, or CBTs) that incorporate their partner than from interventions that are solely patient-oriented [39]. In addition, because of the negative social impact of patient distress and pain expression for example [40], this treatment approach may benefit the partner as well. Specifically, the partner's emotional well-being, sense of mastery in providing support and assistance, and critical attitudes may improve as the result of being included in the patient's psychologic pain treatment [39].

Partner-assisted psychologic interventions for chronic illnesses such as arthritis vary in terms of whether or not they focus on interpersonal issues between patient and spouse. Some interventions provide education to both partners regarding etiology and treatment of the illness and may enlist the spouse or partner's help in changing patient health behaviors. In contrast, other interventions more directly address issues, such as the impact of such a painful illness on the spouse, communication between partners about pain and other symptoms, and need for support, or ways in which the spouse might be helpful or unhelpful [41]. Although the first approach may be beneficial to patients and partners, illness-related interactions between the patient and partner are more likely to improve with the latter, more interpersonally focused approach [39].

Several randomized, controlled studies have compared a couple-based intervention for OA that included such an interpersonal focus to a patient-based intervention using the same type of content (ie, cognitive-behavioral skills training, education, and support). In the first study, patients and their spouses were taught pain coping skills (eg, cognitive coping strategies) and couples skills (eg, communication, spouse reinforcement) [42,43]. In comparison to patients receiving pain coping skills training without spouse involvement for 10 weeks, patients in the 10-week couple-oriented intervention tended to experience better outcomes, such as decreased pain severity and pain behaviors.

More recent research tested an intervention that provided education and support to OA patients and spouses and also addressed issues, such as supportive and unsupportive communications and effective strategies for requesting and providing spousal assistance. Patients who received the

6-week couple-oriented intervention did not experience change in pain and physical function, but their spouses reported greater reductions in stress and tended to have less critical attitudes than spouses of patients who received the 6-week patient-oriented intervention [44]. Moderators of patient treatment outcomes also were identified. Wives who received the couples intervention reported decreased stress, whereas husbands who received the couples intervention became more stressed, consistent with the finding that female family caregivers benefit more from psychosocial treatment than male caregivers [45]. In addition, only spouses who were highly satisfied in their marriage experienced decreased depressive symptoms and increased caregiver mastery from the couples intervention, suggesting that future partner-assisted interventions addressing problematic relationship issues may enhance the effects of these interventions for spouses who are in unhappy marriages.

An analysis of secondary outcomes from the same study showed that patients in the couple-oriented intervention experienced greater improvements in spousal support and punishing responses to pain than those who received education and support without spouse involvement [46]. Specifically, patients in the couple-oriented intervention reported a greater decrease in their spouses' punishing responses to pain (eg, anger, irritation) than patients in the patient-oriented intervention. A trend effect was observed in regard to the advantage of couple-oriented intervention for increasing spouses' attempts to distract patients from their pain. In addition, patients in the couple-oriented intervention reported greater increased spouse support than those in the patient-oriented intervention.

There are several possible explanations for the seemingly discrepant findings regarding enhanced quality of pain-related interactions with the spouse on the one hand [46] but no effects on patients' pain or physical function on the other hand [44]. One explanation is that changes in pain-related interactions may have been too small to affect patients' pain and function. Findings from post-hoc analyses focused on patients in the dyadic intervention were consistent with this explanation, in that changes in spousal support, distracting responses, or punishing responses were not significantly associated with changes in patient pain or physical function. A second explanation is that the largest effects observed in this study were for positive spouse behaviors and these factors may have less impact on patient pain and function than negative spouse behaviors.

Partner-assisted psychologic interventions also have been developed and tested for individuals with RA. In a study by Radojevic and colleagues [47], RA patients who received 6 weeks of behavior therapy alone showed greater decreased joint swelling than those who received a 6-week educational intervention with a family member. A study by Riemsma and colleagues [48] on RA patients and their partners (88% spouses) found that, contrary to prediction, a 5-week educational program attended by both partners resulted in decreased self-efficacy and increased fatigue, whereas patients who attended a 5-week patient-oriented educational program experienced increased self-efficacy and decreased fatigue. A third study of RA patients incorporated the spouse in a 4-week educational intervention that also used cognitive-behavioral techniques (ie, rational emotive therapy to restructure disease-related cognitions and teach effective coping) and resulted in patients' improved disease-related communication with the spouse. However, there was no advantage of the partner-assisted intervention over a similar patient-oriented intervention. Of these three studies focused on RA, only the study conducted by van Lankveld and colleagues [49] examined effects of intervention on the spouse, reporting no differences in these outcomes.

Several tentative conclusions can be drawn regarding the efficacy of partner-assisted psychologic interventions for arthritis pain. First, the advantage of patient-oriented pain coping skills and cognitive-behavioral intervention over partner-assisted educational intervention [42,43,47] may reflect that patients with pain conditions typically respond best to psychosocial treatments that use a cognitive-behavioral approach, regardless of whether a spouse or partner is involved or not. Second, the efficacy of educational interventions that focus on providing information is not clear, especially in interventions that may not fully address the partner's concerns or interpersonal issues between patient and partner, for example [48]. Third, future interventions may have greater impact if they are more intensive (ie, more weeks or sessions) and also target spousal social control strategies that have been linked to health behaviors [50,51]. For example, given the importance of physical activity for promoting long-term function in many arthritis conditions, it may be useful to enhance positive social control strategies that encourage physical activity (eg, encouragement to stay active, modeling an active lifestyle) and reduce negative social control strategies that may evoke resentment and lead to less activity (eg, nagging the patient to exercise more often). Finally, in future research testing partner-assisted treatment approaches it will be especially important to include outcome measures that enable researchers to evaluate the benefits of interventions for both patients and partners.

Lifestyle behavioral weight management for arthritis pain management

Lifestyle behavioral weight management programs are designed to help overweight and obese individuals with arthritis minimize the impact of pain on their day-to-day life. Lifestyle behavioral weight management programs encourage arthritis patients to gradually lose weight through permanent lifestyle changes. Small weight losses (5% to 10% of initial body weight) can improve obesity-related complications [52–59] and maintenance of small weight losses through changes in diet and exercise or activity patterns can sustain improvements in health [60,61]. Lifestyle behavioral weight management programs typically focus on altering one or more behavioral factors (eg, eating habits, dietary patterns, activity or exercise) and one or more psychosocial factors (eg, cognitions, feelings, attitudes, relationships) known to impact weight management. Meta-analysis and systematic reviews of the obesity literature have shown that lifestyle behavioral weight management programs can reduce weight in obese persons [62,63]. There is evidence that lifestyle behavioral weight management programs not only reduce weight in OA patients, but also decrease pain levels, improve body mechanics, and positively impact adjustment to OA [64–68]. There is also increasing interest in the possibility that some of the strategies offered by lifestyle behavioral weight management may be beneficial in reducing pain and disability in patients having RA.

Osteoarthritis

Obesity and OA commonly co-occur [69], making lifestyle behavioral weight management programs particularly relevant for many individuals with OA. Research has shown that increased weight contributes to the development and progression of OA and negatively impacts adjustment to OA pain and disability [70]. A recent meta-analysis concluded that weight-loss is a significant predictor of reductions in disability in persons with OA [71]. Messier and colleagues [72] found that for each pound of weight loss in obese OA patients there is a fourfold reduction in the load exerted on the knee per step during daily activities, which has significant clinical implications. Research has shown that increased weight contributes to the development and progression of OA and negatively impacts adjustment to OA pain and disability [70].

It is expected that the incidence of both obesity and obesity-related OA will increase in the coming years [73,74]. Given this, the application of lifestyle behavioral weight management programs to overweight and obese OA patients will become increasingly important. To date, there have been a number of clinical trials testing the effects of lifestyle behavioral weight management protocols in overweight and obese OA patients. Although the content of these protocols varies somewhat across studies, the results obtained generally support the notion that lifestyle behavioral weight management can have beneficial effects in OA patients.

Studies examining the impact of lifestyle behavioral weight management programs have largely focused on older adults with knee OA ($\geq$ 60 years; body mass index $\geq$ 28). In an early study, Messier and colleagues [64] randomly assigned 24 overweight and obese knee OA subjects to either a weight management program that included diet therapy and exercise training or to an exercise only control group. The exercise component consisted of aerobic and strength training exercises for 1 hour, 3 days a week, for 6 months. In addition to exercise, participants in dietary therapy received 1 hour of nutrition class that included instruction on how to modify caloric intake and cognitive-behavioral strategies to promote behavioral change. Both groups showed improvements in pain and physical disability at 6-months follow-up. However, participants in the combined group (eg, exercise and diet) lost significantly more weight (M = 18.8 lb [8.5 kg] versus M = 4 lb [1.8 kg]) and demonstrated greater loading weight rate and maximum breaking force with biomechanical testing than patients in the exercise-only group.

Based on preliminary evidence from their early work, Messier and colleagues [65] conducted a second, larger and more rigorous clinical trial that incorporated a longer follow-up. This trial compared the separate and combined effects of exercise and dietary weight loss in improving pain, physical function, and mobility in older overweight and obese OA subjects ($n = 252$). Participants were randomized to exercise intervention, diet intervention, exercise and diet intervention, or a control group (eg, attention, social interaction, health education). Consistent with their earlier findings, Messier and colleagues found that the exercise plus diet intervention produced the greatest benefit in knee pain and physical function (eg, self-reported physical function, 6-minute walk distance, and stair climb time). All three treatment groups maintained treatment gains for at least 18 months, while the control group (eg, healthy lifestyle training) regressed toward baseline values.

Encouraging substantial weight loss in older populations has been controversial because of the potentially harmful effects of weight loss in accelerating loss of lean tissue. To examine how intense weight-loss impacts outcomes in older adults with OA, Miller and colleagues [66] tested a lifestyle behavioral weight-loss program in older OA patients that incorporated severe calorie restriction (daily energy deficit of 1,000 kcal). Study outcomes included self-report and performance task measures of physical function and body composition. The weight-loss intervention (eg, partial meal replacements, nutrition education, lifestyle behavioral modifications, three weekly exercise sessions) was compared with a weight stable intervention (eg, newsletters and bimonthly session health sessions). The weight-loss intervention group obtained a mean weight loss of 8.5%, compared with no change in the weight-stable group, and reported less pain, stiffness, and higher physical functioning than the weight-stable condition. Importantly, despite loss of lean body mass, the weight-loss intervention group reported less pain, stiffness, and higher physical function and did significantly better on performance tasks (eg, 6-minute walk, stair climb time) than the weight-stable group. This study demonstrated important benefits and no detrimental effect of weight loss for older OA patients.

Although diet and exercise are the two most common components of lifestyle behavioral weight management programs, additional components have also been investigated. One study compared the impact of a weight-loss program that included diet, exercise, and acupuncture to electrotherapy for pain in obese OA patients, for example [75]. Subjects who received the weight-loss program reported significantly greater pain reduction, better ambulation, and decreases in disability, compared with subjects treated with only electrotherapy. This study demonstrated that a lifestyle behavioral weight-loss program may have greater benefits than traditional medical approaches.

Lifestyle behavioral weight management programs for OA patients not only impact OA pain and disability, but have been shown to have other positive benefits for overweight and obese patients with OA. Rejeski and colleagues [67] reported that a lifestyle behavioral weight management program applied to overweight and obese OA patients had positive effects on self-report measures of physical role functioning, general health, social functioning, satisfaction with physical functioning, and satisfaction with physical appearance when compared with a control group. Another study found that a lifestyle behavioral weight management program had a positive impact on mobility related self-efficacy in older, obese OA patients [68]. This is particularly important, as self-efficacy has emerged as an important psychologic predictor of adjustment to OA pain [76,77].

Rheumatoid arthritis

Patients with RA suffer from pain, restricted mobility, reduced muscle strength, and low endurance [78]. There is emerging evidence that increased exercise and modified diet, both components of lifestyle behavioral weight management, may have positive benefits for RA patients. Traditionally, it has been thought that exercise would worsen RA symptoms and cause additional joint damage. However, newer work has lead to the realization that exercise and general physical activity plays an essential role in managing disability [79] and can increase aerobic capacity and muscle strength in RA [80]. Physical inactivity in RA has been associated with increased pain, obesity, comorbid health problems, low functional capacity, and higher levels of disease activity and fatigue [81]. A recent study found that RA patients who self-initiated long-term regular exercise (eg, $\geq$ 20 minutes, $\geq$ 3 times a week) reported less fatigue and disability than RA patients who do not exercise [82]. Another study found that RA subjects assigned to aerobic exercise had less pain, fatigue, and depression and improved grip strength and walk time than a control group [83].

There is epidemiologic evidence to suggest that a lifelong diet of certain foods (eg, fish, olive oil, cooked vegetables) may decrease the incidence and severity of RA [84,85]. There is some data suggesting that implementing a modified diet may lead to decreases in RA symptoms. In a randomized, controlled trial of RA subjects, Skoldstam and colleagues [86] found that diet modification decreased physiologic markers of RA activity, improved physical functioning, and improved self-report quality of life. Other research has found that RA patients who modified their diet though a 6-week cooking course intervention with an emphasis on a Mediterranean-type diet reported decreased pain, stiffness, and increased quality of life at a 6-month follow-up when compared with a control group [87].

Although patients with RA who are obese are more likely to experience impaired physical and mental quality of life than normal weight RA patients [88], evidence supporting weight loss per se in this population is not available. However, there is evidence that important components of lifestyle behavioral weight-loss interventions (eg, exercise and diet modification) may have significant physical benefits and other quality of life benefits for patients with RA. To date, there are no studies examining the application of a comprehensive lifestyle behavior modification (eg, exercise and diet) in patients with RA, but emerging lines of evidence suggest that this is an important area to explore and better understand. Furthermore, although obesity appears to be associated with negative outcomes in RA, there is limited empiric evidence to that support weight loss in obese RA patients. This is a critical empiric question that needs to be answered.

Comment

Lifestyle behavioral weight management interventions confer clear benefits for overweight and obese patients with OA. Evidence also suggests that the exercise and diet modification components of lifestyle behavioral weight management programs may have important benefits for patients with RA. Although exercise and diet alone provide some benefit, compared with control groups in both OA and RA studies, it appears that combining these two elements of lifestyle behavioral weight management provide the greatest effect.

The majority of patients with OA are older [89]; however, OA is not limited to older populations. Reasons that individuals may have symptoms of OA at earlier ages include joint injury and overweight or obesity [90]. Obesity has been rising across all age groups during the past two decades [91] and it is expected that obesity-related OA will also increase [73,74]. It will be important that future work in this area is not limited to only older adults, but also includes younger individuals. The authors are currently conducting an NIH-supported clinical trial that is examining lifestyle behavioral weight loss in radiographically confirmed OA patients. Over 50% of the authors' sample is under the age of 60; this study will yield data for us to examine the benefits of lifestyle behavioral weight loss among younger overweight and obese OA samples. As mentioned above, future research is also need to determine how much patients with RA might benefit from combined components of lifestyle behavioral. To date, studies of RA patients have tested separate components of lifestyle behavioral modification strategies, usually exercise or diet. The results of OA trials strongly suggest that combining such strategies may be most beneficial.

Most approaches to arthritis pain are based on a traditional biomedical model that emphasizes pharmacologic or surgical interventions (eg, joint replacement, knee replacement). However, there is evidence that these approaches do not eliminate pain and disability faced by patients with OA and RA. Lifestyle behavioral weight management programs are not often prescribed to OA and RA patients and are not widely available in clinical settings. It is important that health care professionals understand the benefits of lifestyle behavioral weight management programs for OA and RA and insist on the availability of such programs for their patients. It will be important that training in lifestyle behavioral change strategies be available to health care professionals and that there are appropriate facilities available to support these interventions.

References

[1] O'Dell JR. Therapeutic strategies for RA. N Engl J Med 2004;350:2167–79.
[2] Keefe FJ, Abernethy AP, Campbell LC. Psychological approaches to understanding and treating disease-related pain. Annu Rev Psychol 2005;56:601–30.
[3] Ranawat AS, Ranawat CS. Pain management and accelerated rehabilitation for total hip and total knee arthroplasty. J Arthroplasty 2007;22:12–5.
[4] American College of Rheumatology Subcommittee on Rheumatoid Arthritis Guidelines. Guidelines for the management of rheumatoid arthritis: update. Arthritis Rheum 2002;46: 328–46.
[5] American College of Rheumatology Subcommittee on Osteoarthritis Guidelines. Guidelines for the medical management of osteoarthritis of the hip and knee. Arthritis Rheum 2000;43: 1905–15.
[6] American Pain Society. Guidelines for the management of pain in osteoarthritis, rheumatoid arthritis, and juvenile chronic arthritis. Glenview (IL): American Pain Society; 2002.
[7] Dixon KE, Keefe FJ, Scipio CD, et al. Psychological interventions for arthritis pain management in adults: a meta-analysis. Health Psychol 2007;26:241–50.
[8] Melzack R, Wall PD. Pain mechanisms: a new theory. Science 1965;150(3699):971–9.
[9] Melzack R. Pain and the neuromatrix in the brain. J Dent Educ 2001;65(12):1378–82.
[10] Bradley LA, Young LD, Anderson KO, et al. Effects of psychological therapy on pain behavior of rheumatoid arthritis patients. Treatment outcome and six-month follow-up. Arthritis Rheum 1987;30(10):1105–14.
[11] Sharpe L, Sensky T, Timberlake N, et al. A blind, randomized, controlled trial of cognitive-behavioral intervention for patients with recent onset rheumatoid arthritis: preventing psychological and physiological morbidity. Pain 2001;89(2–3):275–83.
[12] Sharpe L, Sensky T, Timberlake N, et al. Long-term efficacy of a cognitive-behavioral treatment from a randomized controlled trial for patients recently diagnosed with rheumatoid arthritis. Rheumatology 2003;42:435–41.
[13] Keefe FJ, Caldwell DS, Williams DA, et al. Pain coping skills training in the management of osteoarthritis knee pain: a comparative study. Behav Ther 1990;21(1):49–62.
[14] Keefe FJ, Caldwell DS, Williams DA, et al. Pain coping skills training in the management of osteoarthritic knee pain: II. Follow-up results. Behav Ther 1990;21(4):435–47.
[15] Pennebaker JW. Putting stress into words: the impact of writing on psychological, absentee and self-reported emotional well being measures. Am J Health Promot 1992;6:280–7.
[16] Greenberg MA, Stone AA. Emotional disclosure about traumas and its relation to health: effects of previous disclosure and trauma severity. J Pers Soc Psychol 1992;63:75–84.
[17] Pennebaker JW, Beall SK. Confronting a traumatic event: toward an understanding of inhibition and disease. J Abnorm Psychol 1986;95:274–81.
[18] Petrie KJ, Booth RJ, Pennebaker JW, et al. Disclosure of trauma and immune response to a hepatitis B vaccination program. J Consult Clin Psychol 1995;67:787–92.
[19] Esterling BA, Antoni MH, Fletcher MA, et al. Emotional disclosure through writing or speaking modulates latent Epstein-Barr Virus antibody titers. J Consult Clin Psychol 1994;62:130–40.

[20] Greenberg MA, Wortman CB, Stone AA. Emotional expression and physical health: revising traumatic memories or fostering self-regulation? J Pers Soc Psychol 1996;71:588–602.
[21] Pennebaker JW, Colder M, Sharp LK. Accelerating the coping process. J Pers Soc Psychol 1990;58:528–37.
[22] Koehler T. Stress and rheumatoid arthritis: a survey of empirical evidence in human and animal studies. J Psychosom Res 1985;29:655–63.
[23] Rimon R, Laakso RL. Life stress and rheumatoid arthritis. Psychother Psychosom 1985;43: 38–43.
[24] Thomason BT, Brantley PJ, Jones GN, et al. The relation between stress and disease activity in rheumatoid arthritis. J Behav Med 1992;15:215–20.
[25] Zautra AJ, Burleson MH, Matt KS, et al. Interpersonal stress, depression, and disease activity in rheumatoid arthritis and osteoarthritis patients. Health Psychol 1994;13:139–48.
[26] Potter PT, Zautra AJ. Stressful life events' effects on rheumatoid arthritis disease activity. J Consult Clin Psychol 1997;65:319–23.
[27] Affleck G, Tennen H, Urrows S, et al. Person and contextual features of daily stress reactivity: individual differences in relations of undesirable daily events with mood disturbance and chronic pain intensity. J Pers Soc Psycho 1994;66:329–40.
[28] Fernandez A, Sriram TG, Rajkumar S, et al. Alexithymic characteristics in rheumatoid arthritis: a controlled study. Psychother Psychosom 1989;51:45–50.
[29] Kelley JE, Lumley MA, Leisen JCC. Health effects of emotional disclosure in rheumatoid arthritis patients. Health Psychol 1997;16:331–40.
[30] Smyth JM, Stone AA, Hurewitz A, et al. Effects of writing about stressful experiences on symptom reduction in patients with asthma or rheumatoid arthritis: a randomized trial. JAMA 1999;281:1304–9.
[31] Broderick JE, Stone AA, Smyth JM, et al. The feasibility and effectiveness of an expressive writing intervention for rheumatoid arthritis via home-based videotaped instructions. Ann Behav Med 2004;27:50–9.
[32] Wetherell MA, Byrne-Davis L, Dieppe P, et al. Effects of emotional disclosure on psychological and physiological outcomes in patients with rheumatoid arthritis: an exploratory home-based study. J Health Psychol 2005;10:277–85.
[33] Keefe FJ, Anderson T, Lumley M, et al. A randomized, controlled trial of emotional disclosure in rheumatoid arthritis: can clinician assistance enhance the effects? Pain, in press.
[34] Smyth JM. Written emotional expression: effect sizes, outcome types, and moderating variables. J Consult Clin Psychol 1998;66:174–84.
[35] Harris AH. Does expressive writing reduce health care utilization? A meta-analysis of randomized trials. J Consult Clin Psychol 2006;74:243–52.
[36] Frisina PG, Borod JC, Lepore SJ. A meta-analysis of the effects of written emotional disclosure on the health outcomes of clinical populations. J Nerv Ment Dis 2004;192: 629–34.
[37] Kiecolt-Glaser JK, Newton TL. Marriage and health: his and hers. Psychol Bull 2001;127: 472–503.
[38] Schmaling KB, Sher TG. The psychology of couples and illness: theory, research, practice. Washington, DC: Am Psychol Assoc.; 2000.
[39] Martire LM, Lustig AP, Schulz R, et al. Is it beneficial to involve a family member? A meta-analytic review of psychosocial interventions for chronic illness. Health Psychol 2004;23: 599–611.
[40] Stephens MAP, Martire LM, Cremeans-Smith JK, et al. Older women with osteoarthritis and their caregiving husbands: effects of patients' pain and pain expression. Rehabil Psychol 2006;51:3–12.
[41] Baucom DH, Shoham V, Mueser KT, et al. Empirically supported couple and family interventions for marital distress and adult mental health problems. J Consult Clin Psychol 1998; 66:53–88.

[42] Keefe FJ, Caldwell DS, Baucom D, et al. Spouse-assisted coping skills training in the management of osteoarthritic knee pain. Arthritis Care Res 1996;9:279–91.
[43] Keefe FJ, Caldwell DS, Baucom D, et al. Spouse-assisted coping skills training in the management of knee pain in osteoarthritis: long-term follow up results. Arthritis Care Res 1999;12:101–11.
[44] Martire LM, Schulz R, Keefe FJ, et al. Couple-oriented education and support intervention: effects on individuals with osteoarthritis and their spouses. Rehabil Psychol 2007;52: 121–32.
[45] Sorenson S, Pinquart M, Duberstein P. How effective are interventions with caregivers? An updated meta-analysis. Gerontologist 2002;42:356–72.
[46] Martire LM, Schulz R, Keefe FJ, et al. Couple-oriented education and support intervention for osteoarthritis: effects on spouses' support and responses to patient pain. Families, Systems & Health, in press.
[47] Radojevic V, Nicassio PM, Weisman MH. Behavioral intervention with and without family support for rheumatoid arthritis. Behav Ther 1992;23:13–30.
[48] Riemsma RP, Taal E, Rasker JJ. Group education for patients with rheumatoid arthritis and their partners. Arthritis Rheum 2003;49:556–66.
[49] van Lankveld W, van Helmond T, Naring G, et al. Partner participation in cognitive-behavioral self-management group treatment for patients with rheumatoid arthritis. J Rheumatol 2004;31:1738–45.
[50] Fekete EM, Stephens MA, Druley JA, et al. Effects of spousal control and support on older adults' recovery from knee surgery. J Fam Psychol 2006;20(2):302–10.
[51] Lewis MA, Rook KS. Social control in personal relationships: impact on health behaviors and psychological distress. Health Psychol 1999;18(1):63–71.
[52] Williams RA, Foulsham BM. Weight reduction in osteoarthritis using phentermine. Practitioner 1981;225:231–2.
[53] NHLBI obesity education initiative expert panel on the identification, evaluation, and treatment of overweight and obesity in adults. Clinical guidelines on the identification, evaluation, and treatment of overweight and obesity in adults: the evidence report 1998. Bethesda (MD): National Heart Lung and Blood Institute; 1998.
[54] Wolf AM, Colotz GA. Current estimates of the economic cost of obesity in the United States. Obes Res 1998;8:97–106.
[55] Flegal KM, Carroll MD, Kuczmarski RJ, et al. Overweight and obesity in the United States: prevalence and trends 1990–1994. Int J Obes Relat Metab Disord 1999;22:39–47.
[56] Willett WC, Dietz WH, Colotz GA. Guidelines for health weight. N Engl J Med 1999;341: 427–34.
[57] Wadden TA, Anderson DA, Foster GD. Two year changes in lipids and lipoproteins associated with maintenance of a 5% to 10% reduction in initial weight: some findings and some questions. Obes Res 1999;7:170–8.
[58] Huang Z, Willett WC, Manson JE, et al. Body weight, weight change, and risk for hypertension in women. Ann Intern Med 1998;128:81–9.
[59] Colotz GA, Willett WC, Rotnitzky A, et al. Weight gain as a risk factor for clinical diabetes mellitus in women. Ann Intern Med 1995;122:481–6.
[60] Goldstein DJ. Beneficial health effects of modest weight loss. Int J Obes Relat Metab Disord 1992;16:397–418.
[61] Institute of Medicine. Weighing the options: criteria for evaluating weight management programs. Washington, DC: Institute of Medicine; 1995.
[62] Blackburn GL. Effect of degree of weight loss on health benefits. Obes Res 1995;3(Suppl 2): 211s–8s.
[63] Glenny AM, O'Meara S, Melville A, et al. The treatment and prevention of obesity: a systematic review of the literature. Int J Obes Relat Metab Disord 1997;21:715–37.
[64] Messier SP, Loeser RF, Mitchell MN, et al. Exercise and weight loss in obese older adults with knee osteoarthritis: a preliminary study. J Am Geriatr Soc 2000;48:1062–72.

[65] Messier SP, Loeser RF, Miller GD, et al. Exercise and dietary weight loss in overweight and obese older adults with knee osteoarthritis. Arthritis Rheum 2004;50(5):1501–10.
[66] Miller GD, Nicklas BJ, Davis C, et al. Intensive weight loss program improves physical function in older obese adults with knee osteoarthritis. Obesity(Silver Spring) 2006;14(7):1219–30.
[67] Rejeski WJ, Focht BC, Messier SP, et al. Obese, older adults with knee osteoarthritis: weight loss, exercise, and quality of life. Health Psych 2002;21(5):419–26.
[68] Focht BC, Rejeski WJ, Ambrosius WT, et al. Exercise, self-efficacy, and mobility performance in overweight and obese older adults with knee osteoarthritis. Arthritis Rheum 2005;53(5):659–65.
[69] Marks R. Obesity profiles with knee osteoarthritis: correlation with pain, disability, disease progression. Obesity (Silver Spring) 2007;15(7):1867–74.
[70] Hartz AJ, Fischer ME, Bril G, et al. The association of obesity with joint pain and osteoarthritis in the HANES data. J Chronic Dis 1986;39(4):311–9.
[71] Christensen R, Bartels EM, Astrup A, et al. Effect of weight reduction in obese patients diagnosed with knee osteoarthritis: a systematic review and meta-analysis. Ann Rheum Dis 2006;66:433–9.
[72] Messier SP, Gutekunst DJ, Davis C, et al. Weight loss reduces knee-joint loads in overweight and obese adults with knee osteoarthritis. Arthritis Rheum 2005;52(7):2026–32.
[73] Flegal KM, Carrol MD, Ogden CL, et al. Prevalence and trends in obesity among US adults, 1999–2000. JAMA 2002;288(14):1772–3.
[74] World Health Organization. Diet, nutrition and the prevention of chronic diseases. World Health Organ Tech Rep Ser 2003;916:1–149.
[75] Huang MH, Chen CH, Chen TW, et al. The effects of weight reduction on the rehabilitation of patients with knee osteoarthritis and obesity. Arthritis Care Res 2000;13(6):398–405.
[76] Keefe FJ, Blumenthal J, Baucom D, et al. Effects of spouse-assisted coping skills training and exercise training in patients with osteoarthritic knee pain: a randomized controlled study. Pain 2004;110(3):539–49.
[77] Pells JJ, Shelby RA, Keefe FJ, et al. Arthritis self-efficacy and self-efficacy for resisting eating: relationship to pain, disability, and eating behavior in overweight and obese individuals with osteoarthritic knee pain. Pain 2007; [epub ahead of print].
[78] Wolfe F, Allaire S, Michaud K. The prevalence and incidence of work disability in rheumatoid arthritis, and the effect of anti-tumor necrosis factor on work disability. J Rheumatol 2007;34(11):2126–68.
[79] Plasqui G. The role of physical activity in rheumatoid arthritis. Physiol Behav 2008; [epub ahead of print].
[80] Gaudin P, Leguen-Guegan S, Allenet B, et al. Is dynamic exercise beneficial in patients with rheumatoid arthritis? Joint Bone Spine 2008;75(1):11–7.
[81] Sokka T, Hakkinen A, Kautiainen H, et al. Physical inactivity in patients with rheumatoid arthritis: data from twenty-one countries in a cross-sectional, international study. Arthritis Rheum 2008;59(1):42–50.
[82] Lee EO, Kim JI, Davis HT, et al. Effects of regular exercise on pain, fatigue, and disability in patients with rheumatoid arthritis. Fam Community Health 2006;29(4):320–7.
[83] Neuberger GB, Aaronson LS, Gajewski B, et al. Predictors of exercise and effects of exercise on symptoms, function, aerobic fitness, and disease outcomes of rheumatoid arthritis. Arthritis Rheum 2007;57(6):943–52.
[84] Linos A, Kaklamani VG, Kaklamani E, et al. Dietary factors in relation to rheumatoid arthritis: a role for olive oil and cooked vegetables? Am J Clin Nutr 2000;70:1077–82.
[85] Shapiro JA, Koepsell TD, Voigt LF, et al. Diet and rheumatoid arthritis in women: a possible protective effect of fish consumption. Epidemiology 1996;7:256–63.
[86] Skoldstam L, Brudin L, Hagfors L, et al. Weight reduction is not a major reason for improvement in rheumatoid arthritis from lacto-vegetarian, vegan, or Mediterranean diets. Nutr J 2005;4(15):1–6.

[87] McKellar G, Morrison E, McEntegart A, et al. A pilot study of a Mediterranean-type diet intervention in female patients with rheumatoid arthritis living in areas of social deprivation in Glasgow. Ann Rheum Dis 2007;66(9):1239–43.
[88] Garcia-Poma A, Segami MI, Mora CS, et al. Obesity is independently associated with impaired quality of life in patients with rheumatoid arthritis. Clin Rheumatol 2007;26: 1831–5.
[89] Anderson JJ, Felson DT. Factors associated with osteoarthritis of the knee in the first national health and nutrition examination survey (HANES I). Evidence for an association with overweight, race, and physical demands of work. Am J Epidemiol 1988;28(1):179–89.
[90] Englund M, Lohmander LS. Risk factors for symptomatic knee osteoarthritis fifteen to twenty two years after meniscectomy. Arthritis Rheum 2004;50(9):2811–9.
[91] Nelson DE, Bland S, Powell-Griner E, et al. State trends in health risk factors and receipt of clinical preventive services among US adults during the 1990s. JAMA 2002;287(20):2659–67.

ELSEVIER
SAUNDERS

Rheum Dis Clin N Am
34 (2008) 369–385

RHEUMATIC
DISEASE CLINICS
OF NORTH AMERICA

The Pharmacotherapy of Chronic Pain

Mary E. Lynch, MD

Pain Management Unit, Queen Elizabeth II Health Sciences Centre, Department of Anesthesiology, Psychiatry, and Pharmacology, Dalhousie University, 4th Floor Dickson Centre, Room 4086, Halifax, NS B3H 1V7, Canada

In spite of significant advances over the past 2 decades in the treatment of rheumatic and inflammatory conditions, chronic pain remains a significant clinical problem for a majority of patients with these conditions. As with many chronic diseases, one must consider treatment along more than one axis. That is, one must consider both axis 1 treatment, which involves appropriate disease-modifying agents for the condition underlying the pain, and axis II treatment, which involves additional measures needed to control the pain. This article focuses on axis II.

Significant advances in the field of pain have expanded our understanding of the underlying mechanisms causing chronic pain (see article by Fitzcharles and Shir in this issue), along with an appreciation of the complexity of the pain modulatory system. In assisting the patient suffering with chronic pain, it is important to consider the whole person, starting with the patient's narrative [1]. After hearing the patient's story, the clinician is in a better position to engage with the patient in his or her understanding of the causes of the pain and what the patient can do about it. Pharmacotherapy should take place within an overall active participatory approach toward assisting patients with managing their own pain.

Overview

The agents for which there is well-established evidence of analgesic efficacy include the acetaminophen and nonsteroidal anti-inflammatory drugs (NSAIDs), the tricyclic antidepressants, specific anticonvulsants, and the opioids. There is support for cannabinoids as a second- or third-line treatment. Specific topically delivered analgesics may also be used as a sole agent or in combination with systemic therapy [2].

E-mail address: mary.lynch@dal.ca

doi:10.1016/j.rdc.2008.04.001 ***rheumatic.theclinics.com***

Once the physician has established the working diagnosis and has identified that analgesic medication is appropriate, the usual approach for mild to moderate pain is to start with a nonopioid analgesic, such as an NSAID or acetaminophen (Fig. 1). If this is inadequate or poorly tolerated, and if there is an element of sleep loss, it is then reasonable to add an antidepressant with analgesic qualities (see the article by Perrot and colleagues in this issue). If there is a component of neuropathic pain or fibromyalgia, then a trial of one of the gabapentinoids is appropriate. If these steps are inadequate, then an opioid analgesic may be added. For moderate to severe pain, one would initiate a trial of chronic opioid earlier. Cannabinoids and topicals may also be appropriate as single agents or in combination. The above assumes that the clinician has also addressed appropriate therapy targeting the specific disease.

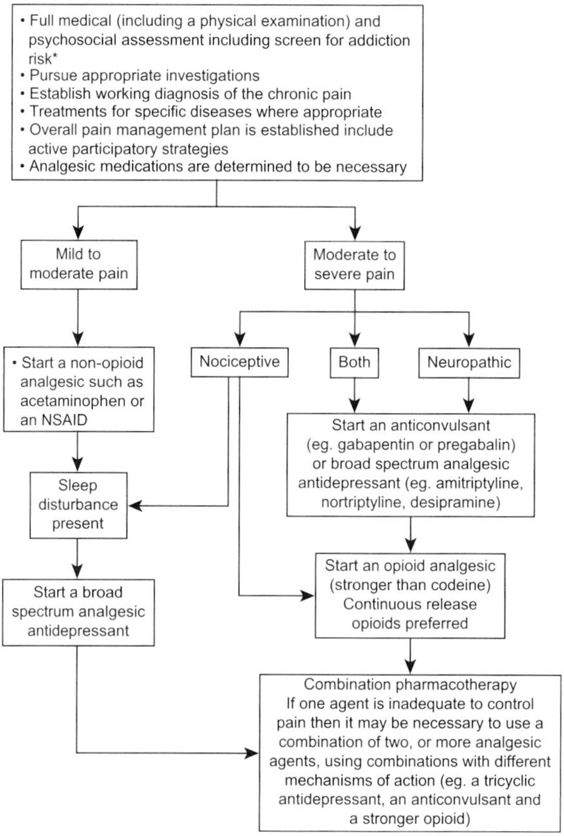

Fig. 1. Treatment algorithm for pharmacotherapy of chronic noncancer pain. In general, if one agent in a class of medications does not provide adequate analgesia or causes limiting side effects, it is worth pursuing serial trials of one or two others from the class. Topicals may be introduced at any point as sole agent or in combination. Cannabinoids may be introduced as second- or third-line agents.

In rheumatological conditions, one or several mechanisms for each an individual patient may be at play in the etiology of the pain, and more than one pharmacotherapeutic agent may be necessary for pain control. It is appropriate to use a combination of agents with different mechanisms of action for adequate pain control. This combination approach has been supported by a randomized, double-blind, active placebo-controlled trial in neuropathic pain, which found that gabapentin and morphine combined achieved better analgesia at lower doses than when the agents were used alone [3].

Specific agents

Nonsteroidal anti-inflammatory drugs and acetaminophen

Acetylsalicyclic acid (ASA), ibuprofen, and acetaminophen are available over-the-counter in North America and are widely used for pain control. ASA and ibuprofen, members of the NSAID group, exhibit analgesic, antipyretic, and anti-inflammatory effects. Acetaminophen is a different agent and does not exhibit significant anti-inflammatory effects, but does act as a good analgesic and antipyretic [2].

There are at least 10 different drug classes represented within the NSAID group. The analgesic action has been established for some time. Most NSAIDs exhibit analgesic efficacy comparable with ASA, and a few exhibit superior efficacy. There is poor correlation between anti-inflammatory activity and analgesic efficacy, so the relief of pain involves additional mechanisms, both central and peripheral [2]. Unfortunately these agents generally provide only mild relief and are associated with potentially serious adverse effects, including hypertension, gastric ulceration, and bleeding. An increased risk of cardiovascular events, such as myocardial infarction and stroke has been identified with the cyclooxygenase-inhibiting class. For these reasons, drugs in this class have limited usefulness in assisting patients with moderate to severe chronic pain.

Acetaminophen is equi-analgesic with ASA in most types of pain except that related to inflammatory arthritis. In head-to-head patient preference studies comparing acetaminophen with NSAIDs, over twice as many patients preferred NSAIDs. However, given its safety profile, acetaminophen is still considered a first-line drug for patients with osteoarthritis [4]. As noted, acetaminophen does not possess a significant anti-inflammatory effect. The mechanism of action is unknown but there is growing evidence supporting a central serotonergic mechanism [2] and a possible cannabinoid/vanilloid-receptor connection [5].

In recommended doses, acetaminophen is well tolerated and side effects are mild. The gastrointestinal profile of this agent is usually benign. On occasion, patients may experience abdominal pain or diarrhea, which may improve with decrease in the dose of acetaminophen or discontinuation of the drug. There is no effect on platelet function. The main concern is hepatotoxicity in patients who are alcoholic or who have liver disease. In acute overdose, hepatic necrosis, a potentially fatal adverse effect, may result. The conventional oral or rectal adult dose of acetaminophen is 500 to 1000 mg every 4 to 6 hours. There is a shallow dose-response curve, so increasing the dose further does not confer additional analgesia. The total daily dose should not exceed 4000 mg and, for chronic long-term use, the dose should be limited to 2500 mg/d [2].

Antidepressants

Tricyclic antidepressants

Several systematic reviews and meta-analyses have concluded that the tricyclic antidepressants (TCAs) exhibit clear analgesic efficacy in a number of chronic pain conditions [2,6–8]. The number needed to treat (NNT)[1] is generally in the range of 2.1 to 2.6. Specifically, TCAs have demonstrated efficacy in pain caused by diabetic neuropathy, postherpetic neuralgia, tension headache, migraine, atypical facial pain, fibromyalgia, and low back pain. TCAs relieve various qualities of pain, including brief lancinating pain, constant dysesthetic pain, allodynia, and spontaneous pain. The pain relief from TCAs is generally moderate and is accompanied by side effects, such as sedation, postural hypotension, and anticholinergic side effects, including dry mouth and constipation. The analgesic effect is independent of the effect on mood. TCAs with a balanced inhibition of serotonin (5-hydroxytryptamine) and noradrenaline reuptake, such as amitriptyline, imipramine, and clomipramine, as well as agents with greater noradrenaline reuptake inhibition, such as desipramine and nortriptyline, appear to be effective analgesics. The mechanism of action is unknown but probably multifactorial as these agents are capable of multiple actions relevant to pain transmission [2].

Other antidepressants

Venlafaxine. There are several other chemical groups of antidepressants. However, to date, only the serotonin noradrenaline reuptake inhibitors have exhibited potential as analgesics in randomized controlled trials. The two antidepressants available from this group include venlafaxine and duloxetine. Both are effective antidepressants with strong inhibition of 5-hydroxytryptamine and noradrenaline reuptake. This balanced neurotransmitter profile is similar to that found with the TCAs.

There are seven randomized controlled trials examining the analgesic effects of venlafaxine [9–15]. An analgesic effect was demonstrated in studies of 29 patients with polyneuropathy [10] and 244 patients with diabetic neuropathy [11]. In a third study involving neuropathic pain, there was

[1] Number needed to treat refers to the number of patients who must be exposed to the treatment to experience a significant reduction in pain. In this case, that means a 50% or more reduction in pain.

a significant decrease in hyperalgesia, but not in pain [13]. In postsurgical neuropathic pain, there was a significant improvement in average pain relief and maximum pain intensity, but not in average pain intensity [9]. In addition, administration of vanlafaxine for 2 weeks starting the night before surgery led to a 25% to 30% decrease in the incidence of postmastectomy pain syndrome at 6 months [15]. A study examining venlafaxine in migraine prophylaxis reported a decrease in the number of headaches and analgesic consumption along with an improvement in daily activities [14]. There was no analgesic effect found in a study of 20 patients with atypical facial pain [12]. The NNT is generally higher than that found with the TCAs and is reported in the range of 4.5 to 5.2 [10,11].

In summary, there is initial evidence indicating that venlafaxine in a dose range of 150 to 225 mg/d may exhibit some analgesic effect. However, the NNT to obtain an analgesic effect is higher than with the TCA group. Further controlled trials are necessary. One potential advantage is the different and nonanticholinergic side effect profile compared with TCAs.

Duloxetine. There are several randomized controlled trials examining efficacy of duloxetine in the treatment of pain. Four trials examined duloxetine in treatment of diabetic neuropathy and two in fibromyalgia. Others have examined painful symptoms associated with depression.

Four trials involving a total of 1139 patients with diabetic neuropathy found duloxetine 60 and 120 mg/d significantly reduced pain severity as compared with placebo [16–19]. In fibromyalgia, there are two randomized controlled trials involving 561 patients [20,21]. In the first trial, there was no significant difference in the Fibromyalgia Impact Questionnaire (FIQ) pain score. However, in both trials, duloxetine led to a significant decrease in Brief Pain Inventory pain scores and the total score on the FIQ as compared with placebo in females with or without major depression [20,21]. A randomized controlled trial examined duloxetine 60 mg once daily in treatment of painful physical symptoms in patients with major depressive disorder [22]. According to the Brief Pain Inventory Average Pain Score, which was the primary outcome measure for pain, results indicated that duloxetine was significantly better than placebo at early and intermediate visits (1, 2, and 5 weeks), but the difference was not significant at the end of the study (7 weeks). Additional publications have pooled data from studies examining duloxetine in treatment of depression and have identified in post hoc analyses that painful physical symptoms in depressed patients exhibited greater improvement than those in placebo-treated patients. However, one cannot conclude an analgesic effect for duloxetine from these studies [23,24]. Thus, preliminary evidence suggests that duloxetine may be helpful in painful diabetic neuropathy. There is some initial support that it may benefit patients with fibromyalgia according to the FIQ. Further randomized controlled trials in nondepressed patients with pain are required. Details on the clinical use of the antidepressant agents appear in Chapter 10.

Anticonvulsants

Good evidence indicates that certain anticonvulsants exhibit analgesic action in neuropathic pain. This is on the basis of their ability to reduce neuronal excitability, a mechanism that may also be important in certain rheumatological conditions. Supporting this is the fact that recent randomized controlled trials have demonstrated that gabapentin [25] and pregabalin [26] are effective in treatment of pain in fibromyalgia. There are no controlled trials regarding the other anticonvulsant agents in rheumatological conditions. Therefore this discussion focuses on the gabapentinoids (Table 1).

Gabapentin

Gabapentin was originally developed as a structural analog of γ-aminobutyric acid (GABA) but does not actually bind to GABA or affect GABA reuptake or metabolites [27]. Gabapentin binds with high affinity

Table 1
Anticonvulsants with documented analgesic effects in neuropathic pain and fibromyalgia

Agent	Dose range (mg/d)	Mechanism of action	Indications supported by at least one RCT[a]	Side effects	Comments
Gabapentin (Neurontin)	1200–3600	α_2-δ protein of voltage-gated Ca^{2+} channels	PHN, DN, mixed neuropathic pain, fibromyalgia	Sedation, dizziness, ataxia, confusion	Does not require metabolism in liver, so is a better choice in liver dysfunction; clearance will be diminished in renal dysfunction
Pregabalin (Lyrica)	150–600	α_2-δ protein of voltage-gated Ca^{2+} channels	PHN, DN, fibromyalgia	Dizziness, somnolence	Analgesic effect is seen within first 3 days; does not require liver metabolism; renal excretion primary route of elimination

Abbreviations: DN, diabetic neuropathy; PHN, postherpetic neuralgia; RCT, randomized placebo-controlled trial; TN, trigeminal neuralgia.

[a] For details, see section relating to the specific agent in the text.

to the α_2-δ subunit of voltage-dependent Ca^{2+} channels and it is thought that inhibition of high voltage activated Ca^{2+} currents is a potential mechanism of action in analgesia [28]. However, this remains to be determined.

Several large randomized controlled trials have provided evidence that gabapentin is significantly more analgesic than placebo in postherpetic neuralgia [29,30], diabetic neuropathy [31–33], mixed diagnoses of neuropathic pain [34], and fibromyalgia [20]. There is also support for an analgesic effect in spinal cord injury [35], trigeminal neuralgia [34], pain of Guillain-Barre [36], phantom limb pain [37], and in prophylaxis of chronic daily headache [38]. Overall, gabapentin was well tolerated and the most common adverse events were mild to moderate dizziness and somnolence, most of which occurred in the initiation phase. Additional side effects include ataxia and confusion. Dosing usually starts with 300 mg by mouth once daily. This can be increased by 300 mg every 5 days until adequate analgesia is accomplished or until limiting side effects are encountered. The large trials used doses of 1200 mg and 2400 mg per day. In the trial using two doses, there did not appear to be a significant difference between the two doses with regards to efficacy as compared with placebo, but the trial was not designed to look at dose response. Most investigators recommend a dose range of 1800 to 3600 mg/d. There are only two comparative trials comparing gabapentin with other analgesics: one head-to-head trial with amitriptyline [32], which found both agents to exhibit similar efficacy but with different side effects; and one placebo-controlled trial examining gabapentin alone and in combination with morphine, which demonstrated the combination to be superior than either agent alone [3]. Table 1 presents further detail regarding dosing and side effects.

Pregabalin

Pregabalin exhibits the same mechanism of action as gabapentin. Large randomized controlled trials have indicated that pregabalin exhibits significant analgesic efficacy in postherpetic neuralgia [39–42], painful diabetic peripheral neuropathy [43–45], and fibromyalgia [26]. There is also support for efficacy in spinal cord injury pain [46]. Pregabalin is generally well tolerated. The most common side effects are dizziness and somnolence. Renal excretion is the primary route of elimination, with 98% of the administered drug eliminated unchanged in the urine. Pregabalin has been studied in individuals with varying degrees of renal function and was effectively cleared in patients with end-stage renal failure undergoing dialysis. It has also been determined that the analgesic effect of pregabalin is evident within the first week of treatment. The effective dose range is from 150 to 600 mg/d orally and is given in two or three divided doses per day. In some patients, 150 mg/d may be inadequate. In subjects who received start doses of 300 mg/d, significant analgesia was identified within 1 to 3 days. An initial dose of 150 mg/d may be increased to 300 mg after 3 to 7 days based on response and tolerability. If necessary, the dose may be increased to 600 mg/d after an additional 7 days. In cases of renal impairment, the lower dose range should be used.

The overall benefit of pregabalin is that it seems to offer approximately a 30% advantage over placebo. This benefit is similar to that of gabapentin. To date, there are no head-to-head trials comparing pregabalin with gabapentin.

Opioids

The endogenous opioid system is a part of the body's natural defense network allowing the modulation of pain-related transmission. The endogenous opioid peptides (β-endorphin, enkephalins, dynorphins) inhibit synaptic transmission and are released at several central nervous system sites in response to noxious stimuli. Opioid receptors fall into three classes designated μ, κ, and δ. Opioid receptors are found in several areas of the brain and brainstem, throughout the spinal cord, and in the peripheral nervous system. In the brain, opioids alter mood and reaction to pain. In the brainstem, opioids increase the activity of cells involved in descending inhibition of pain. At the spinal and peripheral level, opioids have an inhibitory effect on transmission in nociceptive systems. At the molecular level, opioid receptors are linked to G proteins and are able to affect ion channel gating. On the presynaptic nerve terminal, agonists of all three receptor types result in closure of voltage-gated Ca^{2+} channels, leading to decreased Ca^{2+} influx and a decrease in neurotransmitter release. μ-Opioid receptor agonists also hyperpolarize second-order primary afferents by increasing K^+ conductance, resulting in decreased neuronal excitability and inhibition of postsynaptic neurons [27,47]. Previously, it was thought that opioid analgesia was mediated via central effects only. It is now known that opioids exhibit a peripheral action as well [48].

Most available opioids are μ-opioid receptor agonists or drugs with direct affinity for μ-opioid receptors. When an opioid is administered exogenously, it is essentially augmenting the endogenous system in place. The pure agonists have no apparent ceiling effect for analgesia. The exception is meperidine (Demerol) limited by an active metabolite, nor-meperidine, which is associated with excitatory side effects with risk of seizures. Meperidine is not recommended for treatment of chronic pain. For the remaining agents, the analgesic effect increases as the dose is raised, until analgesia is achieved or dose-limiting adverse effects occur. Antagonists, such as naloxone, interfere with the action of agonists blocking their effects. Clinically, the antagonists are used to treat overdoses of opioids. It is important to be aware that agents with mixed agonist-antagonist and partial-agonist action are available (eg, pentazocine [Talwin], buprenorphine). However, these mixed agents are generally not indicated for treatment of chronic pain.

There is a growing body of evidence that controlled-release opioid analgesics have a role to play in a subset of patients with chronic pain. A recent meta-analysis of 41 randomized controlled trials involving 6019 patients found that opioids were more effective than placebo for both pain and functional outcomes in both nociceptive and neuropathic pain [49]. Guidelines for the use of opioid analgesics in chronic noncancer pain have been established by the Canadian Pain Society [50], and details regarding treatment using opioids for chronic noncancer pain are presented in a recent review [2]. The main message is that the evidence supports the assertion that opioids are a reasonable and efficacious treatment for people with chronic pain [2]. The average duration of trials was only 5 weeks (range 1–16 weeks) and there is a need for longer-term trials examining efficacy and safety parameters. Recommended front-line agents include hydromorphone, morphine, oxycodone, and tramadol used orally on a time-contingent basis. Additional options include the fentanyl patch, in cases where the oral route is not a reasonable option (malabsorption, vomiting) or has failed, and methadone, if the previous conventional opioids have failed [51]. Details regarding clinical use appear in article by Katz in this issue.

Cannabinoids

The potent antinociceptive and antihyperalgesic effects of cannabinoid agonists in animal models of acute and chronic pain; the presence of cannabinoid receptors in pain-processing areas of the brain, spinal cord and periphery; and evidence supporting endogenous modulation of pain systems by cannabinoids support the premise that cannabinoids exhibit significant potential as analgesics [52–56].

Fifteen of 18 randomized controlled trials examining cannabinoids in the treatment of pain have demonstrated a significant analgesic effect [57]. Cannabinoid agents tested included synthetic analogs as well as cannabis and cannabis-based extracts. These agents were tested in a number of pain conditions. Smoked cannabis was demonstrated to exhibit a significant analgesic effect in a randomized controlled trial of 50 patients with HIV neuropathy [58]. Five published randomized controlled trials have examined a cannabis-based buccal spray: Three were positive [59–61], one was negative [62], and one exhibited a statistically significant reduction but the reduction in pain was not to the full 2-point reduction required for a clinically significant effect [63]. An oral cannabis-based extract led to significant reductions in pain of multiple sclerosis in a large multisite trial at 14 weeks [64] and at 52 weeks [65]. Regarding the oral synthetic analogs, two recent trials examining nabilone found a significant decrease in pain in multiple sclerosis [66] and in chronic spinal pain and headache [67]. Dronabinol also led to significant but modest (1-point reduction on a 0- to 10-point scale) reductions in multiple sclerosis pain [68]; and CT-3, a synthetic analog of THC-11-oic acid, led to significant reduction of neuropathic pain associated with hyperalgesia or allodynia [69]. In n-of-1 trials, oral tetrahydorcannabinol (THC) was found to reduce painful spastic paraparesis [70] and led to a significant reduction in the amount of morphine required for management of the pain associated with familial Mediterranean fever [71]. Four trials examined THC or analogs available in the 1970s in cancer pain. Three of these demonstrated significant reduction in pain. Sedation was noted to be a problem [72–74]. A study examining a THC cogener (benzopyranoperidine) did not demonstrate an analgesic effect [75].

The weight of evidence indicates that cannabinoids exhibit a moderate analgesic effect in neuropathic and cancer pain with preliminary evidence for action in other types of pain, such as spinal pain and headache. In Canada, four cannabinoid agents are available (Table 2). These include the naturally occurring agent (cannabis) available under the Medical Marihuana Access Regulations (MMAR), a cannabis buccal spray (Sativex), nabilone (Cesamet), and dronabinol (synthetic δ-9-THC in sesame oil sold under the trade name Marinol). Guidelines for the use of cannabinoids available in Canada in chronic pain management have been established [76] and recently updated [77]. Based on current evidence showing that cannabinoids are analgesic and safe, it is reasonable to use a cannabinoid as

Table 2
Indications and dosing guidelines for cannabinoids available for clinical use in Canada

Agent	"On label" indications	Dose supplied	Start dose	Dose titration and maximum dose[a]
Nabilone (Cesamet)	Nausea and vomiting pain	0.5 mg, 1 mg capsule	0.25–0.5 mg	Increase dose by 0.25–0.5 mg every 2–3 d to maximum 3 mg bid
Δ-9-THC (Marinol)	Nausea and vomiting	2.5 mg, 5 mg, 10 mg capsules	2.5 mg	Increase dose by 2.5 mg every 2–3 days to a maximum dose of 10 mg tid
Sublingual extract of cannabis (Sativex)	Pain in multiple sclerosis; pain in cancer	1:1 ratio THC/CBD bucchal spray	1 buccal spray once or twice daily	Increase dose by 1–2 buccal sprays every 2–3 d to a maximum dose of 16 sprays per d
Cannabis under the MMAR program		14% THC in cannabis supplied by the program		3–5 gm/d smoked or oral route

Abbreviations: CBD, cannabidiol; MMAR, Medical Marihuana Access Regulations.

[a] Route is oral unless otherwise indicated.

Data from Clark AJ, Lynch ME, Ware M, et al. Guidelines for the use of cannabinoid compounds in chronic pain. Pain Res Manage, 2005;10:44A–46A; and Clark AJ, Lynch ME, Ware M, et al. Updated guidelines for the use of cannabinoid compounds available in Canada for the treatment of chronic pain [abstract]. ICRS Annual Meeting Abstracts; 2007. p. 126.

a second- or third-line agent either as a single agent or in combination with other agents exhibiting a different mechanism of action. In patients exhibiting a constellation of symptoms, including nausea, anorexia, or spasticity, one might consider introducing a cannabinoid earlier as there is evidence cannabinoids exhibit antiemetic and antispasticity action [78].

The guidelines for the use of cannabinoids [76] are similar to those used for opioids [50]. To summarize the key points, one must do a full assessment to establish a working diagnosis; assess psychosocial issues, including screening for risk of addiction; ensure that traditional approaches have been tried or considered; discuss potential for adverse effects (Box 1); and monitor and document treatment. Once the decision is made to use a cannabinoid agent, it is best to try one of the agents available by prescription before proceeding to the MMAR program if the patient is able to afford the medication.

Medical marihuana access program

Since July 2001, the MMAR regulations have been established allowing Canadians to apply to possess cannabis (marihuana) for medicinal purposes. This program involves an application process initiated by the patient. The patient requires the support of a physician, who also completes a form. The patient sends the forms, along with two passport photos, to the Office of Cannabis Medical Access, Health Canada, where the application is reviewed. If all requirements are met, a license to possess is granted. Patients may also apply for a license to produce or may purchase cannabis from Health Canada. Further information regarding this program is available at www.hc-sc.gc.ca/hecs-sesc/ocma/index.htm. As of October 5, 2007, there were 2261 Canadians authorized to possess marihuana for medical purposes and 1256 physicians in Canada who supported these applications. Updated statistics are available at the Web site indicated above.

Further study regarding marihuana as a therapeutic agent is needed regarding both efficacy and safety, neither of which has been established in controlled trials. Studies are underway. In the meantime, physicians in Canada should be aware that 10% to 16% of patients presenting to pain and multiple sclerosis clinics are using cannabis for symptom control [79,80], and that pain is one of the top symptoms for which people in the general population are using cannabis for medical purposes [81]. Physicians should always ask about the use of cannabis and any other herbal or complementary therapies as a routine part of the history.

Muscle relaxants

For most muscle relaxants, the indication is for management of acute pain. However, in practice, many patients who suffer with chronic pain are using muscle relaxants to find relief. A recent systematic review of controlled trials examining the use of muscle relaxants in nonspecific low back

Box 1. Common and important side effects of cannabinoids

Central nervous system
Euphoria
Anxiety
Panic
Paranoia
Psychosis
Sedation
Dizziness
Somnolence
Depression
Ataxia
Visual or hearing disturbances
Asthenia
Cognitive effects

Cardiovascular
Tachycardia
Postural hypotension
Palpitations
Vasodilation (flushing, red eyes)
Increased risk of myocardial infarction within 1 hour of use[b]

Respiratory (if smoked)
Bronchitis, chronic obstructive pulmonary disease
Lung infection
Increased risk for upper airways cancer[a]

Other
Dry mouth
Headache
Abdominal pain or bloating

[a] A recent large case control trial found no evidence to support an association between use of marihuana and an increased risk of lung or upper aerodigestive tract cancers, even in long-term heavy use [83].
[b] Only with marihuana that is smoked.

pain identified 30 studies that met inclusion criteria [82]. Four trials studied benzodiazepines, 11 nonbenzodiazepines, and 2 antispasticity muscle relaxants in comparison with placebo. Results showed that muscle relaxants are effective for short-term symptomatic relief in patients with acute and chronic low back pain. However, the incidence of drowsiness, dizziness, and other side effects is high. Caution was recommended and it was left to the discretion of the physician to review the risk/benefit analysis. It was acknowledged that large high-quality trials are necessary.

Topical analgesics

The involvement of peripheral mechanisms in the generation of chronic pain suggests the use of topical agents in management. There is considerable interest in this area with the probability that new agents will become available. Controlled trials have demonstrated efficacy for topical NSAIDs, capsaicin, local anesthetics, and doxepin. There is preliminary evidence that a topical combination of amitriptyline and ketamine is analgesic in neuropathic pain [2]. Details are presented in Chapter 8.

Summary

Although there have been significant advances in disease-modifying agents for rheumatic diseases, the majority of patients with these conditions experience difficulties with chronic pain. For this reason, it is important to address the pain directly. To assist clinicians in this task, this clinically focused article has presented a treatment approach and algorithm (see Fig. 1) based on best evidence.

References

[1] Carr DB, Loeser JD, Morris DB. Why narrative? In: Carr DB, Loeser JD, Morris DB, editors. Narrative, pain, and suffering. Seattle (WA): IASP Press; 2005. p. 1–13.
[2] Lynch ME, Watson CP. The pharmacotherapy of chronic pain, a review. Pain Res Manag 2006;11:11–38.
[3] Gilron I, Bailey JM, Dongsheng T, et al. Morphine, gabapentin, or their combination for neuropathic pain. N Engl J Med 2005;352:1324–34.
[4] Tannenbaum H, Bombardier C, Davis P, et al. An evidence based approach to prescribing NSAIDs. The Third Canadian Consensus Conference. J Rheumatol 2006;33:140–57.
[5] Hogestatt ED, Jonsson BAG, Ermund A, et al. Conversion of acetaminophen to bioactive N-acylphenolamine AM404 via fatty acid amide hydrolase-dependent arachidonic acid conjugation in the nervous system. J Biol Chem 2005;280:31405–12.
[6] Lynch ME. Antidepressants as analgesics. A review of random controlled trials examining analgesic effects of antidepressant agents. J Psychiatry Neurosci 2001;26:30–6.
[7] McQuay HJ, Moore RA. Antidepressants and chronic pain. BMJ 1997;314:763–4.
[8] McQuay HJ, Tramer M, Nye BA, et al. A systematic review of antidepressants in neuropathic pain. Pain 1996;68:217–27.
[9] Tasmuth T, Hartel B, Kalso E. Venlafaxine in neuropathic pain following treatment of breast cancer. Eur J Pain 2002;6:17–24.
[10] Sindrup SH, Bach FW, Madsen C, et al. Venalfaxine versus imipramine in painful polyneuropathy: a randomized, controlled trial. Neurology 2003;60:1284–9.
[11] Rowbotham M, Goli V, Kunz NR, et al. Venlafaxine extended release in the treatment of painful diabetic neuropathy: a double-blind, placebo-controlled study. Pain 2004;110: 697–706.

[12] Forssell H, Tasmuth T, Tenovuo O, et al. Venlafaxine in the treatment of atypical facial pain: a randomized controlled trial. J Orofac Pain 2004;18:131–7.
[13] Yucel A, Ozyalcin S, Koknel Talu G, et al. The effect of venlafaxine on ongoing and experimentally induced pain in neuropathic pain patients: a double blind, placebo controlled study. Eur J Pain 2005;9:406–16.
[14] Ozyalcin SN, Koknel Talu G, Kiziltan E, et al. The efficacy and safety of venlafaxine in the prophylaxis of migraine. Headache 2005;45:144–52.
[15] Reuben SS, Makari-Judson G, Lurie SD. Evaluation of efficacy of the perioperative administration of venlafaxine XR in the prevention of postmastectomy pain syndrome. J Pain Symptom Manage 2004;27:133–9.
[16] Goldstein DJ, Lu Y, Detke MJ, et al. Duloxetine vs. placebo in patients with painful diabetic neuropathy. Pain 2005;116:109–18.
[17] Wernicke JF. Duloxetine in treatment of diabetic neuropathic pain. Pharmacotherapy 2004; 24:1422, abstract 17.
[18] Raskin J, Pritchett YL, Wang F, et al. A double blind, randomized multicenter trial comparing duloxetine with placebo in management of diabetic peripheral pain. Pain Med 2005;5: 346–56.
[19] Wernicke JF, Pritchett YL, D'Souza DN, et al. A randomized controlled trial of duloxetine in diabetic peripheral neuropathic pain. Neurology 2006;67:1411–20.
[20] Arnold LM, Lu Y, Crofford IJ, et al. A double-blind, multicenter trial comparing duloxetine with placebo in treatment of fibromyalgia patients with or without major depressive disorder. Arthritis Rheum 2004;50:2974–84.
[21] Arnold LM, Rosen A, Pritchett YL, et al. A randomized double blind, placebo-controlled trial of duloxetine in the treatment of women with fibyalgia with and without major depressive disorder. Pain 2005;119:5–15.
[22] Brannan SK, Mallinckrodt CH, Brown EB, et al. Duloxetine 60 mg once-daily in the treatment of painful physical symptoms in patients with major depressive disorder. J Psychiatr Res 2005;39:43–53.
[23] Fava M, Mallinckrodt CH, Detke MJ, et al. The effect of duloxetine on painful physical symptoms in depressed patients: Do improvements in these symptoms result in higher remission rates? J Clin Psychiatry 2004;65:521–30.
[24] Goldstein DJ, Detke MJ, Iyengar S. Effects of duloxetine on painful physical symptoms associated with depression. Psychosomatics 2004;45:17–28.
[25] Arnold LM, Goldenberg DL, Stanford SB, et al. Gabapentin in the treatment of fibromyalgia: a randomized, double-blind, placebo-controlled, multicenter trial. Arthritis Rheum 2007;56:1336–44.
[26] Crofford LJ, Rowbotham MC, Mease PJ, et al. Pregabalin for treatment of fibromyalgia syndrome: results of a randomized, double-blind, placebo-controlled trial. Arthritis Rheum 2005;52:1264–73.
[27] Griffin RS, Woolf CJ. Pharmacology of analgesia. In: Principles of pharmacology: the pathophysiologic basis of drug therapy. Philadelphia: Lippincott, Williams and Wilkins; 2005. p. 229–43.
[28] Rogawski MA, Loscher W. The neurobiology of antiepileptic drugs for the treatment of nonepileptic conditions. Nat Med 2004;10:685–92.
[29] Rice ASC, Maton S, PNS Group. Gabapentin in postherpetic neuralgia: a randomised, double blind, placebo controlled study. Pain 2001;94:215–24.
[30] Rowbotham M, Harden N, Stacey B, et al. Gabapentin for the treatment of postherpetic neuralgia. JAMA 1998;280:1837–42.
[31] Morello CM, Leckband SG, Stoner CP, et al. Randomized double blind study comparing efficacy of gabapentin with amitriptyline on diabetic peripheral neuropathy pain. Arch Intern Med 1999;159:1931–7.
[32] Backonja M, Baydoun A, Edwards KR, et al. Gabapentin for the symptomatic treatment of painful neuropathy in patients with diabetes mellitus. JAMA 1998;280:1831–6.

[33] Gorson KC, Schott C, Herman RM, et al. Gabapentin in the treatment of painful diabetic neuropathy: a placebo controlled trial. J Neurol Neurosurg Psychiatry 1999;66:251–2.
[34] Serpell MG, NPS Group. Gabapentin in neuropathic pain syndromes: a randomised, double blind, placebo-controlled trial. Pain 2002;99:557–66.
[35] Levendoglu F, Ogun CO, Ozerbil O, et al. Gabapentin is a first line drug for the treatment of neuropathic pain in spinal cord injury. Spine 2004;29:743–51.
[36] Pandey CK, Bose N, Garg G, et al. Gabapentin for the treatment of pain in Guillain-Barre syndrome: a double-blinded, placebo-controlled, crossover study. Anesth Analg 2002;95: 1719–23.
[37] Bone M, Critchley P, Buggy DJ. Gabapentin in postamputation phantom limb pain: a randomized, double-blind, placebo-controlled, cross-over study. Reg Anesth Pain Med 2002;27:481–6.
[38] Spira PJ, Beran RG, AGCDH Group. Gabapentin in the prophylaxis of chronic daily headache: a randomized, placebo-controlled study. Neurology 2003;61:1753–9.
[39] Dworkin RH, Corbin AE, Young JP, et al. Pregabalin for treatment of postherpetic neuralgia, a randomized, placebo-controlled trial. Neurology 2003;60:1274–83.
[40] Sabatowski R, Galvez R, Cherry DA, et al. Pregabalin reduces pain and improves sleep and mood disturbances in patients with post-herpetic neuralgia: results of a randomized, placebo-controlled clinical trial. Pain 2004;109:26–35.
[41] Freynhagen R, Strojek K, Griesing T, et al. Efficacy of pregabalin in neuropathic pain evaluated in a 12-week, randomised, double-blind, multicenter, placebo-controlled trial of flexible- and fixed-dose regimens. Pain 2005;115:254–63.
[42] van Seventer R, Feister HA, Young JPJ, et al. Efficacy and tolerability of twice-daily pregabalin for treating pain and related sleep interference in postherpetic neuralgia: a 13 week, randomized trial. Curr Med Res Opin 2006;22:375–84.
[43] Richter RW, Portenoy RK, Sharma U, et al. Relief of painful diabetic peripheral neuropathy with pregabalin: a randomized, placebo controlled trial. J Pain 2005;6:253–60.
[44] Lesser H, Sharma U, LaMoreaux L, et al. Pregabalin relieves symptoms of painful diabetic neuropathy. Neurology 2004;63:2104–10.
[45] Rosenstock J, Tuchman M, LaMoreaux L, et al. Pregabalin for the treatment of painful diabetic peripheral neuropathy: a double-blind, placebo-controlled trial. Pain 2004;110: 628–38.
[46] Siddall PJ, Cousins MJ, Otte A, et al. Pregabalin in central neuropathic pain associated with spinal cord injury, a placebo-controlled trial. Neurology 2006;67:1792–800.
[47] Schumacher HE, Basbaum AI, Way WL. Opioid analgesics and antagonists. In: Katzung BG, editor. Basic and clinical pharmacology. 9th edition. New York: Lange Medical Books, McGraw-Hill; 2004. p. 497–518.
[48] Stein C. The control of pain in peripheral tissue by opioids. N Engl J Med 1995;332:1685–90.
[49] Furlan AD, Sandoval JA, Mailis-Gagnon A, et al. Opioids for chronic noncancer pain: meta-analysis of effectiveness and side effects. CMAJ 2006;174:1589–94.
[50] Jovey RD, Ennis J, Gardner-Nix J, et al. Use of opioid analgesics for the treatment of chronic noncancer pain—a consensus statement and guidelines from the Canadian Pain Society, 2002. Pain Res Manag 2003;8:3A–28A.
[51] Lynch ME. A review of the use of methadone for treatment of chronic non-cancer pain. Pain Res Manage 2005;10:133–44.
[52] Rice ASC. Cannabinoids and pain. Curr Opin Investig Drugs 2001;2:399–413.
[53] Lynch ME. Preclinical science regarding cannabinoids as analgesics: an overview. Pain Res Manage 2005;10:7A–14A.
[54] Pertwee RG. Cannabinoid receptors and pain. Prog Neurobiol 2001;63:569–609.
[55] Walker JM, Strangman NM, Huang SM. Cannabinoids and pain. Pain Res Manage 2001;6: 74–9.
[56] Rice ASC. Cannabinoids. In: McMahon S, Koltzenburg M, editors. Wall and Melzack's textbook of pain. Online edition. Philadelphia: Elsevier; 2008. p. 521–40.

[57] Lynch ME. Pharmacotherapy of chronic pain. In: Taenzer P, Rashiq S, Schopflocher D, editors. Health policy perspectives on chronic pain. Institute of Health Economics: Edmonton (Canada), in press.
[58] Abrams D, Jay CA, Shade SB, et al. Cannabis in painful HIV-associated sensory neuropathy: a randomized controlled trial. Neurology 2007;68:515–21.
[59] Rog DJ, Nurmikko TJ, Friede T, et al. Randomized controlled trial of cannabis based medicine in central pain due to multiple sclerosis. Neurology 2005;65:812–9.
[60] Notcutt W, Price M, Miller RD, et al. Initial experiences with medicinal extracts of cannabis for chronic pain: results from 34 'N of 1' studies. Anesthesia 2004;59:440–52.
[61] Wade DT, Robson P, House H, et al. A preliminary controlled study to determine whether whole-plant cannabis extracts can improve intractable neurogenic symptoms. Clin Rehabil 2003;17:21–9.
[62] Wade DT, Makela P, Robson P, et al. Do cannabis based medicinal extracts have general or specific effects on symptoms in multiple sclerosis? A double-blind, randomized, placebo-controlled study on 160 patients. Mult Scler 2004;10:434–41.
[63] Berman JS, Symonds C, Birch R. Efficacy of two cannabis based medicinal extracts for relief of central neuropathic pain from brachial plexus avulsion: results of a randomized controlled trial. Pain 2004;112:299–306.
[64] Zajicek J, Fox P, Sanders H, et al. Cannabinoids for treatment of spasticity and other symptoms related to multiple sclerosis (CAMS study): multicentre randomised placebo-controlled trial. Lancet 2003;362(9395):1517–26.
[65] Zajicek JP, Sanders HP, Wright DE, et al. Cannabinoids in multiple sclerosis (CAMS) study: safety and efficacy data for 12 months follow-up. J Neurol Neurosurg Psychiatry 2005;76:1664–9.
[66] Wissell J, Haydn T, Muller JE, et al. Low dose treatment with the synthetic cannabinoid nabilone significantly reduces spasticity-related pain. J Neurol 2006;253:1337–41.
[67] Pinsger M, Schimetta W, volc D, et al. Benefits of an add-on treatment with the synthetic cannabinomimetic nabilone on patients with chronic pain—a randomized controlled trial. Wein Klin Wochenschr 2006;118:327–35.
[68] Svendsen KB, Jensen TS, Bach FW. Does the cannabinoid dronabinol reduce central pain in multiple sclerosis? Randomised double blind placebo controlled crossover trial. BMJ 2004;329(7460):253.
[69] Karst M, Salim K, Burstein S, et al. Analgesic effect of the synthetic cannabinoid CT-3 on chronic neuropathic pain. JAMA 2003;290:1757–62.
[70] Maurer M, Henn V, Dittrich A, et al. Delta-9-tetrahydrocannabinol shows antispastic and analgesic effects in a single case double-blind trial. Eur Arch Psychiatry Clin Neurosci 1990;240:1–4.
[71] Holdcroft A, Smith M, Jacklin A, et al. Pain relief with oral cannabinoids in familial Mediterranean fever. Anesthesia 1997;52:483–8.
[72] Noyes RJ, Smith M, Jacklin A, et al. Analgesic effect of delta-9-tetrahydrocannabinol. J Clin Pharmacol 1975;1:139–43.
[73] Noyes RJ, Brunk SF, Avery DH, et al. The analgesic properties of delta-9-tetrahydrocannabinol and codeine. Clin Pharmacol Ther 1975;18:84–9.
[74] Staquet M, Gantt C, Machin D. Effect of a nitrogen analog of tetrahydrocannabinol on cancer pain. Clin Pharmacol Ther 1978;23:397–401.
[75] Jochimsen PR, Lawton RL, VerSteeg K, et al. Effect of benzopyranopyridine a delta-9-THC cogener on pain. Clin Pharmacol Ther 1978;24:223–7.
[76] Clark AJ, Lawton RL, VerSteeg K, et al. Guidelines for the use of cannabinoid compounds in chronic pain. Pain Res Manage 2005;10:44A–46A.
[77] Clark AJ, Lynch ME, Ware M, et al. Updated guidelines for the use of cannabinoid compounds available in Canada for the treatment of chronic pain [abstract]. ICRS Annual Meeting Abstracts; 2007. p. 126.

[78] Watson SJ, Benson AJ Jr, Joy JE. Marijuana and medicine: assessing the science base: a summary of the 1999 Institute of Medicine Report. Arch Gen Psychiatry 2000;57(6): 547–52.

[79] Clark AJ, Ware MA, Yazer E, et al. Patterns of cannabis use among patients with multiple sclerosis. Neurology 2004;62:2098–100.

[80] Ware MA, Doyle CR, Woods R, et al. Cannabis use for chronic non-cancer pain: results of a prospective survey. Pain 2003;102(1–2):211–6.

[81] Ogborne AC, Smart RG, Adlaf EM. Self-reported medical use of marijuana: a survey of the general population. CMAJ 2000;162:1685–6.

[82] Van Tulder MW, Touray T, Furlan AD, et al. Muscle relaxants for nonspecific low back pain. Cochrane Database Syst Rev 2003;(4):CD004252, 10.1002/14651858.

[83] Hashibe M, Morgenstern H, Cui Y, et al. Marihuana use and the risk of lung and upper aerodigestive tract cancers: results of a population-based case-control study. Cancer Epidemiol Biomarkers Prev 2006;15:1829–34.

ELSEVIER
SAUNDERS

Rheum Dis Clin N Am
34 (2008) 387–413

RHEUMATIC
DISEASE CLINICS
OF NORTH AMERICA

Opioids for Nonmalignant Pain

Warren A. Katz, MD[a,b,c,*]

[a]*University of Pennsylvania School of Medicine, Philadelphia, PA, USA*
[b]*Rheumatology Division, Penn-Presbyterian Medical Center, Philadelphia, PA, USA*
[c]*Rothman Institute, Philadelphia, PA, USA*

Pain is the most common symptom in the world for which patients seek professional help. In the United States, 9 out of 10 Americans older than age 18 report suffering pain at least once a month, whereas 42% experience pain every day [1]. Most have reported that pain lasts for at least 5 years [2].

Chronic pain is defined as pain that continues beyond the time normally associated with healing for a specific illness or initial injury, usually 3 months [3,4]. Because of its great impact, chronic pain represents a major health problem, resulting in personal suffering, reduced productivity, and substantial health care costs [5,6]. According to the 1999 National Pain Survey [7], chronic pain prevented 42% of subjects surveyed from working and 63% of subjects from performing their desired daily activities. Of those who were able to work, 24% reported that chronic pain decreased the time they were able to work by an average of 26 hours per week [8].

The National Institutes of Health reported that pain costs more than $100 billion per year in medical expenses, lost wages, and lost productivity [9]. Episodic migraine headaches, arthritis, back pain, and other musculoskeletal conditions, the most common non-cancer-related painful conditions, result in a 13% loss in United States workforce productivity and a $61.2 billion per year loss in productive work time. Migraine headaches alone account for $13 billion annually in lost worker productivity, of which $8 billion results from lost work days [10]. Similarly, osteoarthritis pain is a leading cause of disability in the United States, with an estimated annual cost of $7.11 billion in lost productive work time; 65.7% of the cost results from chronic pain [11]. An estimated 30 million Americans report chronic back pain, usually in the lower back, thus making this syndrome the leading cause of inactivity in young adults and the cause of $28 billion losses in worker productivity each year [12]. Depression is common in primary

* 790 Newtown Yardley Road, Suite 424, Newtown, PA 18940.
E-mail address: wakatzmd@aol.com

doi:10.1016/j.rdc.2008.04.004

care, and its recognition has important management implications in the elderly [13].

Definition of pain

Pain is an uncomfortable symptom that varies greatly from one patient to another; it is often difficult for them to explain and clearly has different meaning to each patient. How a person perceives and responds to pain and how each describes it is highly variable. What one patient describes as very painful, another might not even notice. For many, reaction to pain may reflect the sum substance of the patient's upbringing and personality. Pain has been defined as "an unpleasant sensory and emotional experience associated with actual or potential tissue damage, or described in terms of such damage" [14]. Interpatient inconsistency and the subjective nature of pain require the clinician to objectively treat pain based on the patient's perceptions.

General causes of rheumatic pain

Simplistically, there are two types of pain: nociceptive and neuropathic. Pain caused by injury, malignancy, infection, inflammation, or tissue degeneration is generally referred to as nociceptive pain: that is, it has a fairly specific, identifiable source. Neuropathic pain is usually less recognizable and, therefore, tends to be undertreated. The International Association for the Study of Pain [15] describes neuropathic pain as being "initiated or caused by a primary lesion or dysfunction in the nervous system." Depending on where the nervous system lesion or dysfunction occurs, neuropathic pain can be classified as either peripheral or central. This article will be limited to pain caused by rheumatic diseases.

Types of pain

Both nociceptive and neuropathic pain may be acute, chronic, or breakthrough (that is, chronic pain that intensifies periodically). Breakthrough pain sometimes is related to a specific cause, such as a decrease in medication, or may occur spontaneously without cause. Persistent pain is more difficult to treat than acute pain because of its complex biologic, psychologic, and social dimensions. Acute pain is usually nociceptive (transmitted by normal pain pathways), but persistent pain is often neuropathic (because of peripheral or central nervous system dysfunction) or it may be mixed. It makes intuitive sense that if pain is managed early, then persistent pain is less likely, but there is little hard evidence for this.

Overview of rheumatic pain management

Simple mandates in both acute and chronic pain management call for the patient's complaints to be recognized, validated, and respected. Obviously, patients explain their pain in different ways, some with just a few words or gestures, other with a flourish, verbosity, and intricate body language. Regardless, listening and observing are not only diagnostic attributes of a good health care provider, but they have therapeutic value as well. Not all pain, for example that which is mild or intermittent, needs to be specifically treated, but if a health care provider and the patient both make a mutual decision to treat, early aggressive treatment is advisable. Mild symptoms not causing disability can often be managed with monotherapy; however, polypharmacy, often integral to a multidisciplinary approach, is best. Pharmacotherapy may be used to facilitate a rehabilitation plan with the aim of improving function; it should involve clear goals, with plans for steady progress toward them. All health care professionals who manage persistent pain should address fear and behaviors that increase disability. As an overview, effective, minimally abusive, and safe analgesic medicines are essential. The need of patients with all types of pain is great, but the expertise of most health care providers trusted to help relieve the agony of pain is often lacking, and many continue to demonstrate reluctance to use drugs in truly analgesic doses. Nonpharmacologic management helps increase functionality in many painful disorders, and enhances the net effectiveness of pharmacologic therapy. As an example of the high regard for comprehensive management of pain, the American College of Rheumatology's *Recommendations for the Medical Management of Osteoarthritis of the Hip and Knee* [16] calls for nonpharmacologic management foremost, but in conjunction with appropriate drug management. However, the two approaches really are complementary [17]. The more severe the osteoarthritis, the more nonpharmacologic therapy is needed [18].

Consequence of inadequately treated pain

Inadequately treated pain can lead to other serious comorbidities, including depression, anxiety, fatigue, impaired ambulation, dementia, aphasia, sexual activities, and decreased socialization [19–21]. Inadequately treated pain unquestionably contributes to the poor quality of life. However, there are some interesting data that link widespread body pain with excess mortality from cancer [22]. The association with death directly related to unremitting pain is unclear, but, in one study, symptoms of depression were associated with an adverse prognosis in patients who had heart failure, which could provide an indirect connection [23]. It stands to reason that sedentary patients with chronic pain are more prone to deconditioning, congestive heart failure, and pulmonary emboli, which might eventually prove fatal.

Therapeutic options

The major analgesic options for treating pain pharmacologically are limited to the following classes: acetaminophen, nonsteroidal anti-inflammatory drugs (NSAIDs), which include cyclooxygenase (COX)-2 selective inhibitors, opioids, and weak opioid tramadol preparations [24]. Certain other drugs, such as antidepressants, anticonvulsants, and muscle relaxants give adjunctive relief to persons with certain painful conditions [25–27]. Generally, they are used to enhance the effects of analgesics. Of course, there are numerous drugs that may afford relief of pain by suppressing or eliminating the underlying cause of pain, such as corticosteroids for polymyalgia rheumatica or antibiotics for infection, respectively.

Opioids

Background

Opioids are among the oldest of the analgesic agents, dating back centuries; however, only over the past 50 years have we been able to used evidence-based medicine to understand the pharmacokinetics of this class of drug, it's clinical use, and in particular, how these drugs can best be employed by health care providers to treat nonmalignant sources of pain, especially those caused by rheumatic disease. Short- and long-acting opioids of all types are widely used worldwide. In most instances, they are predictably effective and safe; however, both physician and patient misperceptions and concerns about legal ramifications of opioids, addiction, side effects, and the stigma of abuse and diversion may pose barriers to their more extensive usage [28].

The World Health Organization [29] analgesic ladder promoted acceptance that adequate, regular doses of opioids, such as morphine, are needed for moderate or severe cancer pain. The use of long-term, strong opioids, such as oxycodone or morphine, has been shown to be superior to certain NSAIDs and antidepressants for non-cancer pain relief but not for improving function [30]. Yet their use has been met with less enthusiasm [31–33].

Since the 1980s, worldwide opinion proposes that in certain such patients, opioids can provide analgesia and improve quality of life, without necessarily escalating recommended doses or precipitating problem drug use [34]. Clinical anecdotes and published case series support this notion; there are few adequate randomized, controlled trials to provide truly credible documentation. The several studies that show that opioids relieve persistent musculoskeletal or neuropathic pains still fail to answer questions about how they should be use effectively [30]. For example, the use of opioids even as a first-line drug for a patient with osteoporosis who presents acutely with excruciating vertebral fracture-related back pain is easy to accept, especially with the basic science recognition that inadequately treated pain may lead to chronicity [35]. The pathology is well defined, and historically we know that most patients will need short-term opioids for relief. Patients with persistent pain, though, are more challenging, because frequently the pathology is less defined and the chronicity of their symptoms may cause behavioral and social problems. Furthermore, clinical research studies tend to be of short duration and exclude patients with significant psychologic problems. Thus, there is a knowledge gap in the evidence-based long-term benefits and safety of opioids in this population. The use of opioids must be carefully considered so that patients in need are not undertreated, yet indiscriminate prescribing must not be encouraged.

Lack of opioid acceptance

Many health care providers are reluctant to prescribe opioids for patients who have non-cancer related pain [36]. In one survey of multidisciplinary pain clinics and centers, beliefs in what kind of chronic pain for which they were likely to use opioids varied; they were most consistently accepted for pain associated with sickle cell anemia and least commonly endorsed for headaches, myofascial pain, and fibromyalgia [37]. Many patients are hesitant about taking them, when they are prescribed, for a variety of reasons. Both physicians and patients may fear perceived inevitable or substantial side effects. Other general reasons include concern for addiction, the specter of medicolegal retribution, social stigmatization, or annoyance and time burden of administering this class of drugs when compared with most others. For example, documentation of opioid prescriptions and the requisite education is essential but burdensome. Unless dealt with early, these misconceptions may be hard to overcome. Attitudes of 72 internal medicine and medicine-pediatrics residents who completed a survey questionnaire about opioid prescribing were assessed. Residents were far more concerned about using opioids to treat chronic low back pain than cancer-related pain [38].

The overall prevention and management of opioid-related issues may pose barriers to their use. An effective reassuring response to concerns of a long-standing complaining patient ultimately may reduce office visits, hospitalizations, and frequent telephone calls. Then there is the problem of patient anxiety, created as they run low on their prescriptions, particularly before a weekend. Health care providers may have concerns about undertreating or overtreating their patients who need opioids for pain relief. Yet, these matters must be discussed with patients before starting treatment and managed promptly if they occur; otherwise, undertreatment with needed opioids may ensue [39]. The consequences of overtreatment may be more realistic. Excessive sedation may have safety, social, and economic consequences for the patient.

Another reason for reluctance to prescribe opioids is the concern for drug diversion. Diverters try to obtain opioids under false pretenses for the illicit purpose of reselling or giving the drugs to others. Diverters may use an oral drug formulation for an intravenous quick "high." Providers can prevent medication diversion with patient agreements and prescription safety, among other things. Although all health care professionals should be concerned about this, even though there may be a time burden attached, the prevention of diversion is part of effective management of pain with opioid use. This requires the use of tamperproof medications and close communication with the dispensing pharmacy if there is a suspicion cast.

Pharmacology of opioids

Opioids are defined as any natural or synthetic compound, which pharmacologically produces morphine-like properties. Opioid analgesics inhibit pain pathways by binding to opioid receptors in the nervous system. Because most opioid analgesics are structurally related to morphine, morphine is considered to be the prototype. That morphine exerts its analgesic properties by directly acting on nervous system receptors was suspected in the 1960s, but research over the last half century has documented that opioids affect both central and peripheral specific mu, kappa, and delta receptors that inhibit the transmission and perception of nociceptive input. Opioids may have an affinity for one or more of three receptors: mu (μ1, μ2), kappa (κ), or delta (δ). However, most opioids used clinically are relatively selective for mu receptors.

Opiod action at various receptors has provided a classification of opioids as full agonist, partial agonist, mixed agonist-antiagonist, and antagonist. Most of the opioids used in clinical practice are full agonists, which are drugs that can interact with receptors to stimulate drug actions or effects that are evoked by naturally occurring opioids (Table 1). Morphine, methadone, oxycodone, hydrocodone, heroin, codeine, meperidine, propoxyphene, and fentanyl are examples of full agonist opioids. Buprenorphine is a partial agonist opioid, which is a drug that can both activate and block opioid receptors. Thus, partial agonists can produce effects similar to those of either agonists or antagonists depending on the clinical situation. An antagonist is a drug that prevents molecules of other drugs from binding to a receptor (eg, an opioid receptor). Antagonists can displace other opioids, precipitate withdrawal, or block the effects of other opioids, an example being naloxone and naltrexone. Pentazocine, butorphanol, and nalbuphine are examples of mixed agonist-antagonist opioids that have different effects on various opioid receptors. They have a ceiling effect, whereas full agonists do not [38,40–44]. Tramadol is a weak mu opioid agonist that also has inhibitory effects on norepinephrine and serotonin reuptake [41].

The analgesic effects of opioids go beyond their effect on receptors and are multidimensional because they have both sensory and affective components. Their nociceptive action is mediated at multiple sites of pain mechanisms, including spinal transmission to the brain.

Opioid selections for rheumatic diseases

Opioids significantly decrease pain intensity compared with placebo in patients who have osteoarthritis [45]. Many considerations will influence the choice of drug, particularly as first-line therapy. These include: (1) etiology of rheumatic pain, (2) pain intensity, (3) dose forms and route of

Table 1
Oral and transcutaneous opioid analgesics for nonmalignant pain in adults

Drug	Mechanism of action	Duration of action	Starting dose	Frequency	DEA scheduled	Comment
Codeine	Single[a]	SA	30 mg–60 mg	q3–4 h	ii/iii	iii with APAP; ineffective at low doses
Hydrocodone	Single[a]	SA	5 mg–10 mg	q3–4 h	ii/iii	iii at 5-mg dose with APAP or NSAIDs
Oxycodone	Single[a]	SA	5 mg–10 mg	q3–4 h	ii	Often used with APAP or ASA
Oxycodone	Single[a]	LA	10 mg	q12 h	ii	High abuse and diversion potential
Morphine	Single[a]	SA	10 mg–30 mg	q3–4 h	ii	
Morphine	Single[a]	LA (CR)	15 mg	q24 h	ii	
Morphine	Single[a]	LA (CR)	15 mg–20 mg	q12/24 h	ii	
Morphine	Single[a]	LA (ER)	30 mg	q24 h	ii	
Hydromorphone	Single[a]	SA	2 mg	q4–6 h	ii	
Oxymorphone	Single[a]	SA	5 mg–10 mg	q4–6 h	ii	
Oxymorphone	Single[a]	LA (ER)	5 mg–10 mg	q12 h	ii	High abuse and diversion potential; caution in elderly
Levorphanol	Single[a]	LA	2 mg	q6–8 h	ii	Every 8 h after steady state
Methadone	Single[a]	LA	2.5 mg–5 mg	q6–8 h	ii	Decrease frequency after steady state
Fentanyl	Single[a]	LA	25 mg m/h	q72 h	ii	
Tramadol	Dual[a]	SA	25 mg–50mg	q6 h	Not scheduled	Often used with APAP
Tramadol	Dual[a]	LA (ER)	100 mg–300 mg	q24 h	Not scheduled	

Guidelines for dosing and frequency vary. A patient's responses to opioid analgesics can be highly variable, so it is important to individualize treatment, taking into account pain severity, analgesic needs, and previous history of efficacy and safety responses.

Abbreviations: APAP, acetaminophen; ASA, acetylsalicylic acid; CR, continued release; DEA, Drug Enforcement Administration; ER, extended release; LA, long acting; SA, short acting; SR, sustained release.

[a] All opioids block mu opioid receptors to varying degrees.

Data from Refs. [109–111].

administration, (4) comorbid conditions, (5) prior patient compliance, (6) history of substance abuse, and (7) previous adverse effects. Adverse events, although reversible and usually not life threatening, may cause patients to stop opioids and could limit their usefulness. The ability to improve one's activities of daily living would be an additional reason for selection, but, as will be noted, they may have small benefits on function [45]. Overall, there is a trend to use more opioids in the treatment of resistant rheumatic diseases, using osteoarthritis as the chronic arthritis pain model, but the long-term efficacy and safety of opioids in this setting has not yet been determined because of the short mean trial duration in patients that were studied [45].

Etiology and onset of rheumatic pain

The approach to prescribing opioids for rheumatic disease varies according to the onset of the specific rheumatic disease. The scientific evidence or consensus for using opioids in this setting is presented below. Acute, severe musculoskeletal problems, such as trauma, are indications for opioids, often as a first-line choice [46]. The use of opioids in chronic rheumatic disease like osteoarthritis, which has been controversial, especially when it is recommended as first-line therapy, is becoming more acceptable when all other options, such as NSAIDs and weaker pure analgesics like tramadol have failed [45,47]. Rheumatoid arthritis and inflammatory rheumatic diseases are generally treated initially with anti-inflammatories, whether NSAIDs or corticosteroids. Exceptions are most likely at either spectrum of the disease: that is, early for the first day or two when the initial inflammation causes intense pain or after unremitting painful secondary degenerative changes have set in. In that the selective COX-2 inhibitors have been associated with renal and cardiovascular adverse effects that may limit their use in the elderly with renal or cardiovascular disease, opioids provide an additional treatment option. However, various therapeutic difficulties are encountered in the heterogeneous elderly population, such as increased risk of adverse effects, multimorbidity, and polypharmacy [48]. Considering the above-stated objections, it is hard to justify the use of opioids early in the course of disease, yet mild opioids, such as codeine with acetaminophen, are often prescribed. Patient and prescriber acceptance would seem to be better after other pharmacologic and nonpharmacologic options have failed.

The effectiveness of opioids for fibromyalgia has been questioned, yet for some individual patients both short- and long-term opioids could mean the difference between function and disability [49]. A problem of using potent long-acting opioids, such as long-acting oxycodone in fibromyalgia, even when reported pain is severe, is that there are no more pharmacologic options if the drug fails.

The use of opioids in patients with low back pain is variable, with one study indicating relatively low use compared with other rheumatic diseases

[50]. Two other articles indicate that opioids are commonly prescribed for chronic low back pain and also may be efficacious for short-term use [51,52].

Pain intensity

Examples of opioid analgesics used to treat moderate, acute, or chronic pain include codeine, oxycodone, dihydrocodeine, propoxyphene, and tramadol. Codeine, dihydrocodeine, hydrocodone, oxycodone, and propoxyphene are opioid analgesics with a short half-life, used alone or in combination with aspirin, acetaminophen, or ibuprofen for mild to moderately severe pain. Opioid analgesics with a short half-life used to treat severe, acute, or chronic pain include morphine, oxymorphone, fentanyl, hydromorphone, and oxycodone as a single agent in higher doses (see Table 1).

An examination of national trends in outpatient analgesic treatment for musculoskeletal pain in the office setting compared data from 1980 and 2000 [46]. During this time, opioid use increased for acute pain (8% versus 11%) and doubled for chronic pain (8% versus 16%). The use of more potent opioids (hydrocodone, oxycodone, morphine) for chronic musculoskeletal pain increased from 2% to 9% of visits, indicating that the threshold for both the general use of opioids and choice of more potent ones has dropped [46].

Opioid analgesics with a long half-life usually reserved for more intense persistent pain include methadone and levorphanol [53]. The analgesia of methadone is short (6 hours). Both propoxyphene and methadone are to be used with caution, if at all, because of cardiac events, arrhythmia, and pulmonary toxic events [47]. Reviews of propoxyphene and methadone discourage their use in chronic diseases [54,55]. In addition, the accumulation of the parent compound and metabolites of certain opioids, such as codeine, hydrocodone, dihydrocodeine, and methadone may occur in patients with renal impairment; therefore, patients with insufficient renal function should not use these agents. In a variety of chronic painful conditions, the average daily dose of tramadol alone (> 250 mg) was comparable to five doses of acetaminophen 300 mg with codeine phosphate 30 mg, five doses of aspirin 325 mg with codeine phosphate 30 mg, or two to three doses of acetaminophen 500 mg with oxycodone hydrochloride 5 mg [41].

Dose forms and route of administration

Available dosage forms (eg, transdermal, extended-release tablet, short-acting tablet, injectable, transmucosal, intranasal) and the required dosing interval will determine choice. For example, agonist drugs may be short or long acting; therefore, morphine, a short-acting drug, requires frequent dosing to maintain analgesia. However, extended-release oral (eg, morphine, oxycodone, oxymorphone) and transdermal (eg, fentanyl) formulations, and oral opioids with long half-lives (eg, methadone, levorphanol) are alternatives to short-acting opioids that are preferred for the management of persistent pain.

Comorbid conditions

The presence of chronic obstructive pulmonary disease (respiratory depression), sleep apnea, severe neuromuscular diseases (increased rigidity), and tendency to fall (light-headedness) are examples of diseases that could alter the drug choice of opioids [56]. These issues might be more concerning in the elderly, as they are sensitive to opioids because clearance and respiratory function are altered. Coexisting neurologic disease may make it more difficult to assess sedation and pain control. Pharmacotherapy for coexisting disease may prove difficult because of interactions.

Advantages of opioids for rheumatic diseases

There is little question that opioids are effective for most acute and chronic painful conditions because they are powerful, centrally acting analgesic agents, which also have peripheral effects. Some exceptions may be incomplete analgesia, even at high doses, for musculoskeletal pain when the involved body part is moved or in certain neuropathic diseases. In a recent Canadian meta-analysis, 41 randomized trials involving 6,019 subjects were evaluated for the effectiveness of opioids: 80% of the subjects had nociceptive pain, including osteoarthritis, rheumatoid arthritis, or back pain; 12% had neuropathic pain (post-herpetic neuralgia, diabetic neuropathy, or phantom limb pain); 7% had fibromyalgia; and 1% had "mixed pain." The average duration of treatment was 5 (range 1–16) weeks. "Dropout rates averaged 33% in the opioid groups and 38% in the placebo groups. Opioids were more effective than placebo for both pain and functional outcomes in patients with nociceptive or neuropathic pain or fibromyalgia. Strong, but not weak, opioids were significantly superior to naproxen and nortriptyline, and only for pain relief. Among the side effects of opioids, only constipation and nausea were clinically and statistically significant" [30].

Benefits of opioids in specific rheumatic diseases

Osteoarthritis

Several review articles and guidelines support the use of opioids for appropriate patients unresponsive to other first- or second-line treatments. The Osteoarthritis Research Society International [57] most recently has issued 25 evidence-based, expert consensus recommendations for the management of osteoarthritis of the hip and knee, including weak opioids and stronger "narcotics" for intractable pain. These are not too dissimilar to the European League Against Rheumatism (EULAR) guidelines of 2005, which state: "Opioid analgesics, with or without paracetamol, are useful alternatives in patients in whom NSAIDs including COX-2 selective inhibitors (coxibs) are contraindicated, ineffective, and/or poorly tolerated" [58]. All guidelines suggest that NSAIDs be tried first, but because of concomitant illness in the usual osteoarthritis populations, NSAIDs may not be safe. Some recommend the same World Health Organization analgesic ladder used for decision making for cancer pain, in which nonscheduled opioids be tried before scheduled opioids [59]. Furthermore, there are no published studies showing that NSAIDS alleviate pain by reducing inflammation in osteoarthritis. Because they appear to have a pure analgesic effect, there is no mandate to use them in this condition except for their pain relieving properties.

Ironically, recent studies have shown that the endogenous opioid endomorphin-1 (EM-1) plays an anti-inflammatory role in osteoarthritis. EM-1 assays show their presence in inflamed synovial linings [60]. The number of randomized clinical trials is limited. In that indications for total joint replacement for osteoarthritis require intractable pain, one can argue that intractability cannot be declared until a patient has had a course of opioids, recognized to be the most potent analgesic. Patterns of opioid analgesic prescriptions during a 1-year period were studied in 3,061 patients with osteoarthritis at a federal Veterans Affairs Medical Center. Specific prescription variables included: any opioid, number of specific opioid drugs prescribed, total number of opioid prescriptions, total number of days supply of opioids, and daily opioid doses. Results revealed that 41% of patients received at least one opioid prescription, opioids were prescribed significantly less frequently among African Americans than Caucasians, the number of opioid prescriptions declined with increasing age, and daily opioid doses averaged below recommended daily doses for the treatment of osteoarthritis. This 2004 study concluded that opioids may be gaining acceptability for the treatment of chronic musculoskeletal pain [61]. The author of an article on the short-term efficacy of pharmacotherapeutic interventions in osteoarthritic knee pain involving a meta-analysis of over 14,000 patients cautions that the efficacy of opioids may be inflated because of high drop-out rates in controlled studies, and the "best case " scenarios reported in intention-to-treat analysis [62].

A few scheduled opioids have been studied specifically in osteoarthritis, the knee and hip being the major target joints. Randomized placebo-controlled studies showed reduction in pain and improvement in function over a few weeks to a month [63–66]. No long-term studies reflecting benefit for more than a year have been reported. Most commonly, side effects of nausea, vomiting, and somnolence were reported [63–66]. Atypical non-scheduled opioids in the form of tramadol preparations, both short and long acting, have also been shown to show efficacy and tolerance in diverse populations. Benefits included pain relief, tolerance, and improved sleep. Side effects mirrored other scheduled opioids, with less nausea and constipation in some studies. A Cochrane meta-analysis of 1,019 subjects in 11 randomized clinical trials of tramadol alone or combined with acetaminophen revealed decreased pain intensity and improved function, but the investigators concluded that the benefits were small [67]. Once-daily long-acting tramadol was at least as effective and well tolerated as normal release in the treatment of osteoarthritic knee pain [68,69]. A pivotal study of an extended-release form of tramadol administered for 84 days and compared with placebo showed less pain, improved function, and better sleep [70].

Rheumatoid arthritis

Data supporting the use of opioids in inflammatory arthropathies is limited. A study of Medicare beneficiaries in Pennsylvania included selected patients who had a diagnosis of rheumatoid arthritis, osteoarthritis, chronic low back pain, or ischemic heart disease since 1995. Chronic opioid use, defined as at least six 30-day prescriptions in a year, was found in 4% of those with rheumatoid arthritis, and less than 1% in each of the other diagnostic groups [50]. In a 28-day treatment study of subjects with rheumatoid arthritis ($n = 104$) and osteoarthritis ($n = 159$), fentanyl patches increased pain control from 4% to 29% of subjects, while the number of subjects reaching adequate pain control in the first treatment week was increased to 75%, increased further to 88% on day 28, and to 80% at endpoint. Nausea and vomiting were the most common adverse events, mainly occurring at treatment initiation [71]. A similar study of 104 subjects, specifically for the treatment of pain from rheumatoid arthritis inadequately controlled by nonopioid analgesics or weak opioids, indicated that treatment was assessed favorably: greater than or equal to 78% would recommend it. In both studies, 25 micrograms was the initial dose, with an option for increase [72]. Tramadol or acetaminophen, when added to regular therapy for rheumatoid arthritis, offered pain relief but no change in function compared with placebo. It was suggested as another option for symptomatic control [73].

Several studies demonstrate that opioids modulate the immune response via opioid receptors expressed directly on the immune cells themselves. Reduction of lipopolysaccharide-induced interleukin-6 production by the κ-opioid U50,488 was shown in a mouse monocyte-like cell line [74]. An Australian group found κ-opioid drugs to be powerfully anti-inflammatory, reducing disease severity by as much as 80%, attenuating arthritis in a dose-dependent, stereoselective, antagonist-reversible manner [75]. As noted above for osteoarthritis, a recent study revealed that endogenous endomorphins (EM-1) had anti-inflammatory effects in patients with rheumatoid arthritis and in a model of adjuvant-induced polyarthritis. The research suggested that local enhancement of EM-1 might be a therapeutic option in different forms of arthritis [60]. These findings suggest a role for opioids in the treatment of chronic inflammatory diseases such as rheumatoid arthritis and connective tissue disorders.

Low back pain

Acute low back pain usually resolves spontaneously if the red flags of diagnosis—fracture, malignancy, infection, cauda equina syndrome—are not present. Even though fracture management is generally in the purview of the orthopedist, rheumatologists and other osteoporosis specialists are often the first to manage patients with the sudden onset of severe back pain when they sustain a fracture of one or more vertebrae. Patients with various other causes of low back pain frequently present to rheumatologists. Many with mild to moderate acute pain respond to acetaminophen or NSAIDs, but if idiopathic low back pain or any of the painful red flag conditions are severe, then short-term unscheduled or scheduled opioids may be required.

Employment of long-acting opioids for chronic low back pain, which could be a lifetime problem, is more speculative. Long-acting opioids, if used, need to be part of a multidisciplinary approach. The question is, when are opioids appropriate and how onerous is the responsible monitoring? In addition, health care providers need to weigh any negative public perception about opioids, varying from one community to another, with the true benefit in resolving the unmet analgesic needs of the patient. A major advantage, as noted above, is that the most commonly prescribed agonist opioids have no ceiling effect, whereas all other analgesics used for rheumatic diseases have dosage limits. Although there may be some unease in using them in older populations, opioids may be safer in those at risk for NSAID complications, such as bleeding peptic ulcers, coronary artery disease, congestive heart failure, edema, hypertension, or renal failure. Furthermore, the distinctive pain-relieving attribute, which differentiates the opioids from other antirheumatic medications, is their apparent psychotropic component. Several modes of opioid actions are responsible for this effect, viewed as a disadvantage by some, the most important one being that the emotional, negative affective pain response in the limbic system is reduced. Therefore, opioids may render a sense of contentment and euphoria. Anxiety aggravates pain, whereas opioids allay anxiety. Generic concerns about opioid dosage-creep—lost prescriptions and renewals of scheduled drugs not withstanding—can be addressed by the fact that most patients at any age are able to take opioids at stable doses as prescribed, even for long periods if appropriate.

The results of an expert panel studying the use of strong opioids in chronic low back pain were reported at the EULAR 2005 meeting. The consensus was that patients taking the maximum tolerated dose of nonopioid analgesics, who continue to experience moderate or severe pain that limits activity, are usually good candidates for strong opioids [76]. The report emphasized that "Strong opioids should be prescribed as part of a multimodal and ideally interdisciplinary treatment plan. As a general rule, opioids should not be used as a substitute for treating specific causes of pain unless pain is severe." Recommendations for treatment include:

Predicted duration at the starting dose;

Speed of titration based on clinical judgment;

Clear patient instructions about dosing, which should not be too low;

Treating side effects while maintaining dose;

Switching opioids if necessary;

Concomitant treatments, such as anticonvulsants, which should not be started during an initial opioid test period of 1 to 3 months;
The use of sustained-release formulations;
The use of short-acting, nonopioids, or weak opioids over immediate-release strong opioids for breakthrough pain; and
Referral to a specialist pain clinic if needed.

Most studies of opioid treatments are directed toward short-term use. A recent Cochrane review of four studies, three including tramadol, showed that opioids are commonly prescribed for chronic back pain but may be more efficacious for short-term pain relief [77]. Another investigation indicated that fentanyl buccal tablets were efficacious and well tolerated in the treatment of patients with chronic low back pain [78]. Efficacy has also been demonstrated in chronic low back pain with oxymorphone, hydromorphone, and tramadol [79–81]. Substance abuses and aberrant medication-taking behaviors are common in patients taking opioids for back pain (24%). Long-term (> 16 weeks) efficacy is unclear [52].

Fibromyalgia

There is currently no clear evidence that opioids help fibromyalgia, with the exception of tramadol. In fact, there is some substantiation that opioids might be ineffective in fibromyalgia. The underlying neurophysiology of acute pain is fairly well characterized, whereas the central mechanisms operative in chronic pain states are less well understood. In that fibromyalgia is thought to originate largely from altered central neurotransmission, investigators at the University of Michigan Medical School compared a sample of 17 fibromyalgia patients with 17 age- and sex-matched healthy controls, using μ-opioid receptor positron emission tomography. Their findings of altered endogenous opioid analgesic activity in fibromyalgia suggest a possible reason for why exogenous opiates appear to have reduced efficacy [82].

Yet opioids continue to be used. A survey of academic medical centers in the United States indicated that about 14% of fibromyalgia patients were treated with opiates [83]. A recent, 4-year, nonrandomized study revealed that patients with fibromyalgia did not experience significant improvement from opioids at the end of follow-up, compared with baseline. Furthermore, participants reported increased depression in the last 2 years of the study [84]. In addition, there is emerging evidence that opioid-induced hyperalgesia might limit the usefulness of opioids in controlling chronic pain [85].

However, two controlled studies have evaluated the efficacy of oral tramadol products in fibromyalgia. One was a 3-week, open-label phase of tramadol 50-mg to 400-mg per day, followed by a 6-week double-blind phase in which only subjects who tolerated tramadol and perceived benefit were enrolled [86]. Another was a multicenter, double-blind, randomized, placebo-controlled, 91-day study, which examined the efficacy of the combination of tramadol (37.5 mg) and acetaminophen (325 mg) in 315 subjects with fibromyalgia. In both there were improvements in pain and physical functioning [87].

Perhaps the dual mechanism of action, blockage of μ-opioid receptors, and inhibition of serotonin and norepinephrine, account for this apparently beneficial response when compared with traditional opioids.

Sample case history

A 43-year-old accountant lifted his 35-pound daughter and swung her around simultaneously. He immediately fell to a carpeted floor because of an initial "searing" severe pain in the right lower back. The child landed on top of him. The patient, after lying still for 10 minutes while waiting for the pain to subside, was so profoundly stiff that his wife had to call "fire rescue" to lift him into his bed. Severe (Visual Analog Scale 9/10) pain with any type of motion was present for 2 to 3 days. There was no radiation, and a physician friend could not find any neurologic involvement. Neither acetaminophen nor ibuprofen in high doses alleviated his symptoms. Oxycodone with acetaminophen (7.5/750) and local heat periodically made the pain "bearable." By the fourth day he required the medication every 6 hours, but was more functional and eager to return to work. His physician switched him to a fentanyl patch of 25 micrograms every 72 hours and recommend physical therapy. He was able to return to work, which was sedentary. No breakthrough analgesics were required. He was weaned from the patch 2 weeks later.

Side effects and disadvantages of opioids for rheumatic diseases

Of course, the adverse events associated with opioids used in rheumatic disease reflect those of any type of pain, including cancer. There is no widely accepted documented evidence to the contrary. Among these are nausea and vomiting, which often resolve within days of commencing treatment, and constipation, which tends to persist and many need active management. Sedation, dizziness, myoclonus, and urinary retention all depend upon patient sensitivity and dose [88–90]. Also reported are dose-related respiratory depression, sometimes leading to accumulation of secretions in the tracheobronchial tree, thus predisposing the patient to a variety of pulmonary complications. Peripherally acting opioid antagonists may be useful for dealing with this distressing side effect. Opioid-induced histamine liberation may lead to pruritus that necessitates discontinuation of the drug. True allergic reactions to opioids are rare, but some patients inaccurately refer to recurring gastrointestinal reactions to opioids as an "allergic reaction." Tramadol side effects include nausea, vomiting, constipation, abdominal pain, and lightheadedness. Known side effects are usually controlled by gradual titration of the drug [41]. The neurotoxicity of tramadol may manifest as generalized tonic-clonic seizures, occurring most frequently within 24 hours after tramadol intake. In research studies, seizures were more common in younger abusers who took high doses of the drug combined with alcohol [91].

Cognitive effects are common when opioid treatment is started or with dose changes. This phenomenon may be distressing and particularly difficult to manage in the elderly; however, the cognitive effects of long-term opioids are less clear. Several studies suggest that stable opioid treatment does not adversely affect driving, but patients are warned not to drive or use dangerous machinery until they do not have the adverse effects of the drug [92,93]. Patients should be reminded about their social responsibilities when taking opioids and to not use alcohol concomitantly. Long-term opioid treatment has endocrine and immunologic effects; the clinical significance of these is not certain [94]. As with the use of all drugs, adverse effects need to be put into context; opioids are less organ-toxic than many drugs, for example nonsteroidal anti-inflammatory agents administered to elderly patients with renal failure.

Effect of opioids on sleep

Many patients suffering from chronic pain have disturbed sleep; approximately 65% complain of sleep disruptions or nonrestorative sleep [95]. The effects of opioids on sleep are unclear. The issue is important because sleep difficulties are often associated with untreated painful rheumatic diseases. Yet, there is consistent evidence that self-report sleep improvement occurs in patients who benefit from the analgesic benefits of opioids [70]. However, the relationship between opioids and sleep architecture remain unresolved [56]. Opioids increase nonrapid-eye movement (REM) light sleep and decrease slow-wave sleep in stages 3 and 4. REM sleep is also decreased, but how does it translate clinically [96,97]? The level of pain intensity that would interfere with sleep and the degree of pain relief from opioids is not known. What is clear is that patients with known obstructive sleep apnea have prolonged apnea and hypoxia during non-REM sleep [56].

Discontinuation of opioids

Few patients in pain are started on opioids with the intent of continuing them prescribed forever, so it is wise, if possible, to have an exit plan from the start. Although opioids may be considered by some as last resort therapy, they may not be as effective as desired, tolerated, or safe for all users. Certainly, there is no need to continue therapy if there is a low likelihood of benefit or high risk of side effects, thus leading to a poor risk:benefit ratio. Obviously, opioids are discontinued if they have been ineffective for either acute or chronic painful conditions. Whether or not the opioid efficacy trial is successful, when opioids are discontinued, patients are monitored to minimize physiologic withdrawal symptoms. However, some patients must remain on long-term therapy.

Opioid withdrawal

Supervising opioid withdrawal in an office setting can pose some problems. The probability of exacerbating the original pain varies among patients. How patients respond to the withdrawal is often a reflection of factors that affected the initial response to pain, such as personality, anxiety, depression, stress, and concomitant illness. Patients undergoing opioid withdrawal usually need a great deal of empathy, understanding, positive coaching, and reassurance. A reliance on other elements of nonpharmacologic interventions, such as exercise, is psychologically boosting and likely to release analgesic endogenous endorphins. Several nonopioid adjunctive agents may provide additional relief from withdrawal symptoms. These include clonidine, an alpha-2-adrenergic agonist, which can help relieve many of the autonomic symptoms of opioid withdrawal. Other concomitant agents include acetaminophen, NSAIDs, muscle relaxants, hypnotics, and anxiolytics as well as nonpharmacologic measures may help.

Gradual tapering of the dose is the key to successful opioid withdrawal. Unless there are intolerable side effects, there is no need to rush. Even with slow tapers, it might be necessary to return to the previous dose for a few days until there is apparent equilibrium. The process must weigh the risk of drug toxicity with the severity of the withdrawal reaction. It is wise to warn the patient that tapering opioids might be uncomfortable and distressing, not only to the patients but to those with whom they are in contact.

Opioid misuse and abuse terminology

Many drug prescriptions for a variety of conditions are renewed for a lifetime, and patients, perhaps reluctantly, accept them. For example, the use of digitalis for chronic congestive heart failure is not likely to raise eyebrows. Whereas because opioids tend to give patients in pain a satisfying sense of well-being, their continued use often causes suspicions about whether the drugs are no longer used for their intended purpose. Perhaps the difference lies in the total subjectivity of pain compared with pathophysiologic changes that can be objectively measured in disorders like congestive heart failure. Many of the definitions dealing with opioid misuse and abuse were developed in the context of drug use in the absence of pain. Only an overview of the use of opioids in rheumatic diseases is presented in this article, but excellent sources of additional information on opioid prescribing, withdrawal, switching, and abuse may be found in other sources [42,98–102].

Most specialists in pain medicine and addiction medicine agree that patients treated with prolonged opioid therapy usually do develop some degree of physical dependence and sometimes tolerance, but do not usually develop addictive disorders (Table 2). Addiction, unlike tolerance and physical dependence, is not a predictable drug effect, but represents an idiosyncratic reaction in genetically predisposed and psychosocially susceptible individuals. Adverse consequences of addictive use of medications may include persistent sedation or intoxication because of overuse; increasing functional impairment and other medical complications; psychologic manifestations, such as irritability, apathy, anxiety, or depression; or adverse personal legal,

Table 2
Some features of opioid dependence and diversion

Signs of dependence	Behavioral changes
Irritability	Opioid dose escalation
Nausea, vomiting	Lost prescriptions
Hot flashes	Missed appointments
Chills	Prescription tampering
Arthralgias	Calls from several pharmacists
Lacrimation	Poor drug compliance
Sleep disorder	Concomitant psychoactive drugs

economic, or social consequences. Common and expected side effects of the medications, such as constipation or sedation because of use of prescribed doses, are not viewed as allergic or even true adverse responses in this setting (Table 3).

Pseudo-addiction is a term that has been used to describe patient behaviors that may occur when pain is undertreated and the patient is seeking more medication for pain relief. Patients with unrelieved pain may become focused on obtaining medications, so it seems that they are exhibiting inappropriate drug-seeking behavior. Even such behaviors as illicit drug use and deception can occur in the patient's desperate efforts to obtain relief. Importantly, pseudo-addiction can be distinguished from true addiction in that the behaviors resolve when pain is effectively treated. Distinguishing true addiction or other abuse from pseudo-addiction can be time-consuming and frustrating for some practitioners; therefore, referral to a pain specialist is often recommended.

Medicolegal and social issues

Despite the established need for effective opioids in the treatment of any type of pain, many physicians, other health care providers, and patients still express concern about underuse or overuse of these drugs. The regulatory and legal environment continues to be in a state of flux without uniform, clear-cut direction. As a consequence, clinicians are forced to consider the risk-benefit legal-social ratios. Some doctors avoid prescribing opioids in adequate doses for fear of "addicting" their patients, who in turn are dissatisfied with their treatment [103,104]. Other patients refuse to take opioids at

Table 3
Frequent side effects of opioids

Gastrointestinal	Central nervous system	Miscellaneous
Nausea	Sedation	Urinary retention
Vomiting	Dizziness	Respiratory depression
Constipation	Myoclonus	Pruritis
Abdominal pain	Cognitive dysfunction	Acute opioid toxicity
Ileus	Sleep disorder	

all because they believe they will be socially stigmatized. Several studies have described the underuse of analgesic treatment (oligoanalgesia) in emergency departments, despite patients so often seeking help there for pain [105,106]. Until medicolegal guidelines are more clarified, health care providers need to weigh the upside of adequate opioid relief with the downside of inadequate therapy, leading to pain, disability, and morbidity. In so doing, a diligent history, patient education, informed consent, documentation, patient adherence, and monitoring remain important. It is wise for prescribers to have a comprehensive therapeutic armamentarium that includes opioids among other choices. All involved parties must try to find the "...right balance between promoting adequate pain management and protecting against opioid diversion and abuse" [107].

Positioning opioid therapy in rheumatic diseases

Pain management is rheumatic diseases is best accomplished through the skillful application of one or multiple therapeutic modalities. In some cases, particularly early in the treatment of acute pain, a single modality, such as an analgesic drug or a local corticosteroid injection is appropriate. In other cases, when pain is persistent, intense, resistant to analgesic trials in the past, or physically or psychologically disabling, the best approach is a multimodality strategy. Clinicians should carefully consider the broad range of options in these categories when developing the plan of care for a patient with pain. In so doing, one should consider when to treat and when to refer.

When to treat

The primary outcome of treatment of rheumatic disease is pain relief, using both pharmacologic and non-pharmacologic modalities. Some initial plans, however simple, are initiated on a triage basis. Acetaminophen or NSAIDs are preferred for mild to moderate pain. Opioid analgesics are reserved for severe acute pain; they can also be used in a primary care setting for moderate to severe persistent pain often caused by arthritis, musculoskeletal trauma, or low back pain, or for breakthrough pain in patients on milder drugs. The role of long-term opioid therapy for persistent nonmalignant pain continues to be controversial. It is reasonable to consider these opioids in patients with moderate to severe persistent pain, but also to weigh the answers to some questions before deciding whether to prescribe:

Is the diagnosis as clear as possible?
How severe is the pain (Visual Analog Scale of 1–10)?
Is pain disabling, particularly from the personal and occupation activities of daily living?
Does the pain or intended opioid treatment pose any imminent dangers, such as driving or using machinery?

Does the patient have a history of effectiveness or safety problems with previous prescriptions for opioids?
Are there comorbidities, such as chronic obstructive pulmonary disease?
Is there a history of drug misuse or abuse?
How quickly and safely has the patient responded to intended treatment in the past?
Is there a history of drug intolerance or side effects?

Primary health care providers and specialists need to recognize that opioids do have a place in the humane, successful, safe treatment of rheumatic diseases. Yet, determining the degree of pain and proximate disability so that appropriate medication can be prescribed is challenging. More than a dozen opioids are readily available in the United States. The American Medical Association [102] has published guidelines in a comprehensive series of modules on pain. Under any circumstances, effective communication is needed among treating health care providers, their patients, and pharmacies. Some states require that a physician should write the initial prescription of strong opioids for persistent non-cancer pain, but other health care professionals may assist with monitoring and maintaining opioid therapy. Psychologic comorbidity, social problems, or a history of alcohol or misuse of drugs does not necessarily preclude the use of opioids but raises concerns and highlights the need for closer monitoring. Health care professionals who prescribe or maintain opioid treatment for persistent rheumatic pain should consider an individualized treatment plan. It is sometimes difficult to make patients aware of the limitations and side effects of opioids, and, importantly, of their own responsibilities for their treatment plan.

Besides treatment or modification of the underlying disease, demonstrable improvements in physical, psychologic, and social function are important secondary aims. Sustained release or transdermal opioids are preferable to immediate release formulations for chronic pain, even though the latter are more affordable alternatives. Parenteral opioids are not usually appropriate in the management of persistent non-cancer rheumatic pain. Patients who are prescribed opioids for persistent rheumatic pain are assessed regularly at intervals determined by clinical need. The assessment should include documented evaluation of pain relief; physical, psychologic and social function; adequacy of sleep; drug side effects; and signs of problem drug use. Several of the national and international pain societies have developed recommendations for the use of opioids in persistent non-cancer pain (available at www.painsociety.org).

Although opioids can be sedating, they should not be used as primary anxiolytics or sedatives. As noted previously, all opioids are not the same, and individuals may vary in their response to the same opioids. Therefore, if one opioid is not effective or safe, an alternative may be tried. Opioid switching is standard in the management of cancer pain, but is equally applicable in patients who do not have malignancy. A Cochrane review of the practice concluded that: "For patients with inadequate pain relief and intolerable opioid-related toxicity/adverse effects, a switch to an alternative opioid may be the only option for symptomatic relief. However, the evidence to support the practice of opioid switching is largely anecdotal or based on observational and uncontrolled studies" [108].

For the management of moderate to severe pain in opioid-naïve patients who can use oral medications, such as those with acute trauma or those who have undergone ambulatory surgery, the usual opioids selected include tramadol or one of a group of full agonist short-acting drugs conventionally selected for pain of this type. These drugs include codeine, hydrocodone, and oxycodone, which are available as combination products with acetaminophen, aspirin, or ibuprofen. Full mu agonists—morphine, hydromorphone, oxymorphone, methadone, levorphanol, and fentanyl—do not exhibit a ceiling effect with increasing dose. In practice, the "ceiling" relates either to the safe maximum dose of the nonopioid constituent (eg, 4,000-mg acetaminophen daily) or to the occurrence of opioid-related side effects as the dose is increased. Most patients experience satisfactory analgesia before this treatment-limiting toxicity occurs. Codeine is a commonly used mu agonist, especially combined with acetaminophen and often referred to as "T3." It is usually a poor choice as an analgesic because codeine appears to produce more constipation and nausea at equianalgesic doses than other pure mu agonists. Meperidine and propoxyphene are mu agonists that are metabolized to metabolites (normeperidine and norpropoxyphene, respectively), thus posing a potential for neurotoxicity (eg, tremulousness and seizures) and cardiotoxicity with overdose.

When to refer

A subset of patients requiring comprehensive care presumably would be optimally managed through consultation with an interdisciplinary team of pain specialists. Referral to a program with expertise in managing these patients (eg, multidisciplinary pain center or addiction service) is recommended. These sources can provide advice for opioid withdrawal or switching. A history of drug-seeking behavior or even pseudo-addiction (see above) can be a red flag for transfer to specialty care.

Summary

The pharmacologic armamentarium for treating nonmalignant pain, notably that caused by rheumatic diseases, is limited to a just a few classes of drugs. Ideally, clinicians try to suppress or eliminate the underlying disease, such as by using corticosteroids or biologic agents in rheumatoid arthritis. Acetaminophen is often the safest option for mild rheumatic pain. Although NSAIDs have been used for pain control for more than 35 years, there is growing concern about the long-term safety of both selective and nonselective COX-2 drugs, particularly in older populations who are at risk for heart disease, hypertension, and peptic ulcer disease. Opioids offer an appropriate and safe treatment for some but not all patients with nonmalignant chronic pain. Potential risks, including drug abuse and intolerable side effects, appear to be manageable or even preventable in most cases. Patients with persistent rheumatic pain who have failed traditional treatments should be considered for long-acting opioids. A recommended approach is "start low and slow as you go," gradually increasing the dose to the endpoint of efficacy or intolerable side effects. Opioids are best administered in the framework of weighing the good against the bad in each patient, recognizing the potential morbidity and sometimes mortality in untreated patients who have daily, severe, disabling pain.

References

[1] American Pain Society. Chronic pain in America: roadblocks to relief. Available at: http://www.ampainsoc.org/whatsnew/forward_road.htm. Accessed March 1, 2008.
[2] Becker W, Bondegaard N, Thomsen A, et al. Pain epidemiology and health related quality of life in chronic non-malignant pain patients referred to a Danish multidisciplinary pain center. Pain 1997;73:393–400.
[3] Glickman-Simon R. Persistent pain and palliative care. Medscape coverage of the American College of Physicians 2006 Annual Session [Web site]. 2006. Available at: http://www.medscape.com/viewarticle/535720. Accessed January 24, 2007.
[4] Siddall PJ, Cousins MJ. Persistent pain as a disease entity: implications for clinical management. Anesth Analg 2004;99:510–20.
[5] Department of Health and Human Services, National Institutes of Health. New directions in pain research: [Web site]. September 4, 1998. Available at: http://grants.nih.gov/grants/guide/pa-files/PA-98-102.html. Accessed February 21, 2007. It is the third leading cause of absence from work.
[6] Katz WA. Musculoskeletal pain and its socioeconomic implications. Clin Rheumatol 2002; 21:S2–4.
[7] Ortho-McNeil Pharmaceutical. 1999 National pain survey [Web site]. 2003. Available at: http://www.chiro.org/LINKS/FULL/1999NationalPainSurvey.html. Accessed February 21, 2007.
[8] Allen H, Hubbard D, Sullivan S. The burden of pain on employee health and productivity at a major provider of business services. J Occup Environ Med 2005;47:658–70.
[9] Stewart WF, Ricci JA, Chee E, et al. Lost productive time and cost due to common pain conditions in the US workforce. JAMA 2003;290:2443–54.
[10] Hu XH, Markson LE, Lipton RB, et al. Burden of migraine in the United States: disability and economic costs. Arch Intern Med 1999;159:813–8.
[11] Ricci JA, Stewart WF, Chee E, et al. Pain exacerbation as a major source of lost productive time in US workers with arthritis. Arthritis Rheum 2005;53:673–81.
[12] Rizzo JA, Abbott TA III, Berger ML. The labor productivity effects of chronic backache in the United States. Med Care 1998;36:1471–88.
[13] Barkin RL, Schwer WA, Barkin SJ. Recognition and management of depression in primary care: a focus on the elderly. A pharmacotherapeutic overview of the selection process among the traditional and new antidepressants. Am J Ther 2000;7:205–26.
[14] Merskey H. Logic, truth and language in concepts of pain. Qual Life Res 1994;3(Suppl 1): S69–76.
[15] IASP Pain Terminology. Available at: http://www.iasppain.org/AM/Template.cfm?Section=Pain_Definitions&Template=/CM/HTMLDisplay.cfm&ContentID=1728. Accessed March 15, 2008.

[16] Recommendations for the medical management of osteoarthritis of the hip and knee: 2000 update. American College of Rheumatology Subcommittee on Osteoarthritis guidelines. Arthritis Rheum 2000;43:1905–15.

[17] Katz WA, Rothenberg R. The importance of improving function in patients with pain. J Clin Rheumatol 2005;11:S8–10.

[18] American Geriatrics Society Panel on Chronic Pain in Older Persons. The management of chronic pain in older persons. J Am Geriatr Soc 1998;46:635–51.

[19] Burton DG, Allen MC, Bird JL, et al. Bridging the gap: ageing, pharmacokinetics and pharmacodynamics. J Pharm Pharmacol 2005;57:671–9.

[20] Elliott TE, Renier CM, Palcher JA. Chronic pain, depression, and quality of life: correlations and predictive value of the SF-36. Pain Med 2003;4:331–9.

[21] Laursen BS, Overvad K, Olesen AS, et al. Ongoing pain, sexual desire, and frequency of sexual intercourse in females with different chronic pain syndromes. Sex Disabil 2006;24: 27–37.

[22] McBeth J, Silman AJ, Macfarlane GJ. Association of widespread body pain with an increased risk of cancer and reduce cancer survival. Mortality: a prospective, population-based study. Arthritis Rheum 2003;48(6):1686–92.

[23] Sherwood A, Blumenthal JA, Trivedi R, et al. Relationship of depression to death or hospitalization in patients with heart failure. Arch Intern Med 2007;67:367–73.

[24] Katz WA. Use of nonopioid analgesics and adjunctive agents in the management of pain in rheumatic diseases. Curr Opin Rheumatol 2002;14:63–71.

[25] Fishman SM, Teichera D. Challenges and choices in drug therapy for chronic pain. Cleve Clin J Med 2003;70:119–38.

[26] Maizels M, McCarberg B. Antidepressants and antiepileptic drugs for chronic non-cancer pain. Am Fam Physician 2005;71:483–90.

[27] Barkin RL, Fawcett J. The management challenges of chronic pain: the role of antidepressants. Am J Ther 2000;7:31–47.

[28] Potter M, Schafer S, Gonzalez-Mendez E, et al. Opioids for chronic nonmalignant pain. Attitudes and practices of primary care physicians in the UCSF/Stanford Collaborative Research Network. University of California, San Francisco. J Fam Pract 2001;50:145–51.

[29] World Health Organization. Cancer pain relief, 2nd ed. With a guide to opioid availability, 1996 availability. 2nd edition. Geneva: United Nations, World Health Organization; 1996.

[30] Furlan AD, Sandoval JA, Mailis-Gagnon A, et al. Opioids for chronic noncancer pain: a metaanalysis of effectiveness and side effects. CMAJ 2006;174(11):1589–94.

[31] Turk DC, Brody MC, Okifuji EA. Physicians' attitudes and practices regarding the long-term prescribing of opioids for non-cancer pain. Pain 1994;59:201–8.

[32] Passik SD, Weinreb HJ. Managing chronic malignant pain: overcoming obstacles to the use of opioids. Adv Ther 2000;17:70–83.

[33] Glajchen M. Chronic pain: treatment barriers and stategies for clinical practice. J Am Board Fam Pract 2001;14:211–8.

[34] Portnoy RK, Foley KM. Chronic use of opioid analgesics in non-malignant pain: report of 38 cases. Pain 1986;25:171–86.

[35] Ekman EF, Korman LA. Acute pain following musculoskeletal injuries and orthopaedic surgery: mechanisms' and management. Instr Course Lect 2005;54:21–33.

[36] Simpson KH. Opioids for persistent non-cancer pain: recommendations for clinical practice. Br J Anaesth 2004;92(3):326–8.

[37] Turk DC, Okifuji A. What factors affect physicians' decisions to prescribe opioids for chronic noncancer pain. Clin J Pain 1997;13:330–6.

[38] Yaksh TL, Hua XY, Kalcheva I, et al. The spinal biology in humans and animals of pain states generated by persistent small afferent input. Proc Natl Acad Sci 1999;96:7680–6.

[39] Grahmann PH, Jackson KC, Lipman AG. Clinical beliefs about opioid use and barriers in chronic nonmalignant pain. J Pain Palliat Care Pharmacother 2004;18(2):7–28.

[40] DURAGESIC. Fentanyl transdermal system [package insert]. Titusville (NJ): Janssen Pharmaceutical Products, LP; 2005.
[41] ULTRAM. Tramadol hydrochloride tablets [package insert]. Raritan (NJ): Ortho-McNeil Pharmaceutical; 2004.
[42] Gutstein HB, Akil H. Opioid analgesics. In: Brunton L, Lazo JS, Parker KL, editors. Goodman & Gilman's the pharmacological basis of therapeutics. New York: McGraw-Hill; 2006. p. 547–90.
[43] Barkin RL, Lubenow TR, Bruehl S, et al. Management of chronic pain: part I. Dis Mon 1996;42:389–454.
[44] Cherny NI. Opioid analgesics: comparative features and prescribing guidelines. Drugs 1996;51:713–37.
[45] Avouac J, Gossec L, Dougados M. Efficacy and safety of opioids for osteoarthritis: a meta-analysis of randomized controlled trials. Osteoarthritis Cartilage 2007;15(8):957–65.
[46] Caudill-Slosberg MA, Schwartz LM, Woloshin S. Office visits and analgesic prescriptions for musculoskeletal pain in US: 1980 vs. 2000. Pain 2004;109(3):514–9.
[47] Goodwin JK, Kraemer JJ, Bajwa ZH. The use of opioids in the treatment of osteoarthritis: when, why, and how? Curr Pain Headache Rep 2005;9(6):360–8.
[48] Griessinger N, Sittl R, Jost R, et al. The role of opioid analgesics in rheumatoid disease in the elderly population. Drugs Aging 2003;20(8):571–83.
[49] Available at: http://www.news-medical.net/print_article.asp?id=30532. Accessed March 16, 2008.
[50] Solomon DH, Avorn J, Wang PS, et al. Prescription opioid among older adults with arthritis or low back pain. Arthritis Rheum 2006;55(1):35–41.
[51] Fanciullo GJ, Ball PA, Girault G, et al. An observational study on the prevalence and pattern of opioid use in 25,479 patients with spine and radicular pain. Spine 2002;27:201–5.
[52] Martell BA, O'Connor PG, Kerns RD, et al. Systematic review: opioid treatment for chronic back pain: prevalence, efficacy, and association with addiction. Ann Intern Med 2007;146(2):116–27.
[53] Available at: http://www.ama-cmeonline.com/pain_mgmt/. Accessed March 1, 2008.
[54] Burgess FW, Krantz MJ, Barkin RL. Methadone: unintended mortality due to overdose and arrhythmia. Pain Medicine News 2007 (May/June);1–6.
[55] Barkin RI, Barkin SJ, Barkin DS. Propoxyphene (dextropropoxyphene): a critical review of a weak opioid analgesic that should remain in antiquity. Am J Ther 2006;13:534–42.
[56] Wang D, Teichtahl H. Opioids sleep architecture and sleep-disordered breathing. Sleep Med Rev 2007;11(1):35–46.
[57] Zhang W, Moskowitz RW, Nuki G, et al. OARSI recommendations for the management of hip and knee osteoarthritis, Part II: OARSI evidence-based, expert consensus guidelines. Osteoarthr Cartil 2008;16:137–62.
[58] Zhang W, Doherty M, Arden N, et al. EULAR evidence based recommendations for the management of hip osteoarthritis: report of a task force of the EULAR Standing Committee for International Clinical Studies including Therapeutics (ESCISIT). Ann Rheum Dis 2005;64:669–81.
[59] Katz WA, Schnitzer TJ, Almekinders LC, et al. Emerging paradigms on the management of musculoskeletal pain: focus on osteoarthritis and low back pain. Clinical Courier 2006; 24(34):1–10.
[60] Straub RH, Wolff C, Fassold A, et al. Anti-inflammatory role of endorphins in osteoarthritis, rheumatoid arthritis and adjuvant-induced poly arthritis. Arthritis Rheum 2008;58(2): 456–66.
[61] Dominick KL, Bosworth HB, Dudley TK, et al. Patterns of opioid analgesic prescription among patients with osteoarthritis. J Pain Palliat Care Pharmacother 2004;18(1):31–46.
[62] Bjordal JM, Klovning A, Ljunggren AE, et al. Short-term efficacy of pharmacotherapeutic interventions in osteoarthritic knee pain: a meta-analysis of randomized placebo-controlled studies. Eur J Pain 2007;11(2):125–38.

[63] Peloso PM, Bellamy N, Bensen W, et al. Double blind randomized placebo control trial of controlled release codeine in the treatment of osteoarthritis of the hip or knee. J Rheumatol 2000;27(3):764–71.
[64] Markenson JA, Croft J, Zhang PG, et al. Treatment of persistent pain associated with osteoarthritis with controlled-release oxycodone tablets in a randomized controlled study. Clin J Pain 2005;21(6):524–35.
[65] Matsumoto AK, Babul N, Ahdieh H. Oxymorphone extended-release tablets relieve moderate to severe pain and improve physical function in osteoarthritis: results of a randomized, double-blind, placebo- active-controlled phase III trial. Pain Med 2005;6(5):357–66.
[66] Langford R, McKenna F, Ratcliffe S, et al. Transdermal fentanyl for improvement of pain and functioning in osteoarthritis: a randomized, placebo controlled trial. Arthritis Rheum 2006;54(6):1829–37.
[67] Cepeda MS, Camargo F, Zea C, et al. Tramadol for osteoarthritis: a systematic review and metaanalysis. J Rheumatol 2007;34(3):543–55.
[68] Adler L, McDonald C, O'Brien C, et al. A comparison of one-daily tramadol with normal release tramadol in the treatment of pain in osteoarthritis. J Rheumatol 2002;29(10):2196–9.
[69] Malone F, Coffiner M, Soonet B, et al. Efficacy and tolerability of sustained-release tramadol in the treatment of symptomatic osteoarthritis of the hip or knee: a multicenter, randomized, double-blind, placebo-controlled study. Clin Ther 2004;26(11):1174–82.
[70] Babul N, Noveck R, Chipman H, et al. Efficacy and safety of extended-release, once-daily tramadol in chronic pain: a randomized 12-week clinical trial in osteoarthritis. J Pain Symptom Manage 2004;28(1):59–71.
[71] Pavelka K, Le Loet X, Bjorneboe O, et al. Benefits of transdermal fentanyl inpatients with rheumatoid arthritis or osteoarthritis of the knee or hip: an open label study to assess pain control. Curr Med Res Opin 2004;20(12):1967–77.
[72] Herrero-Beaumont G, Bjorneboe O, Richarz U. Transdermal fentanyl for the treatment of pain caused by rheumatoid arthritis. Rheumatol Int 2004;24(6):325–32.
[73] Lee EY, Lee EB, Park BJ, et al. Tramadol 37.5-mg/acetaminophen 325-mg combination tablets added to regular therapy for rheumatoid arthritis pain: a 1-week study, randomized, double-blind, placebo-controlled trial. Clin Ther 2006;28(12):2052–60.
[74] Parkhill Al, Bidlack JM. Reduction of lipopolysaccharide-induced interleukin-6 production by kappa opioid U50,488 in a mouse monocyte-like cell line. Int Immunopharmacol 2006;6(6):1013–9.
[75] Walker JS. Anti-inflammatory effects of opioids. Adv Exp Med Biol 2003;521:148–50.
[76] Kalso E, Perrot S. On behalf of the Chronic Low Back Pain Panel. Recommendations on the use of strong opioids in low back pain before it becomes chronic. EULAR 2005. Vienna (Austria), June 8–11, 2005. [Abstract SAT0360]. Available at: http://www.medscape.com/viewarticle/538250_print. Accessed March 10, 2008.
[77] Deshpande A, Furlan A, Mailis-Gagnon A, et al. Opioids for chronic low-back pain. Cochrane Database Syst Rev 2007;(3):CD004959.10.1002/14651858.CD004959.pub3.
[78] Portenoy RK, Messina J, Xie F, et al. Fentanyl buccal (FBT) for relief of breakthrough pain in opioid-treated patients with chronic low back pain: a randomized placebo-controlled study. Curr Med Res Opin 2007;23(1):223–33.
[79] Wallace M, Skowronski R, Khanna S, et al. Efficacy and safety evaluation of once-daily OROS hydromorphone in patients with chronic low back pain: a pilot open-label study. Curr Med Res Opin 2007;23(5):981–9.
[80] Hale ME, Ahdieh H, Ma T, et al. Efficacy and safety of OPANA ER (oxymorphone extended release) for the relief of moderate to severe chronic low back pain in opioid-experienced patients: a 12-week, randomized, double-blind, placebo-controlled study. J Pain 2007;8(2):175–84.
[81] Raber M, Hofmann S, Junge K, et al. Analgesic efficacy and tolerability of tramadol 100 mg sustained-release capsules in patients with moderate to severe chronic low back pain. Clinical Drug Investigation 1999;17(6):415–23.

[82] Harris RE, Clauw DJ, Scott DJ, et al. Decreased central μ-opioid receptor availability in fibromyalgia. J Neurosci 2007;27:10000–6.
[83] Wolfe F, Anderson J, Harkness D, et al. A prospective, longitudinal, multicenter study of service utilization and costs in fibromyalgia. Arthritis Rheum 1997;40:1560–70.
[84] Kemple KL, Smith G, Wong-Ngan J. Opioid therapy in fibromyalgia—A four-year prospective evaluation of therapy selection, efficacy, and predictions of outcome. Arthritis Rheum 2003;48:S88.
[85] Chu LF, Clark DJ, Angst MS. Opioid tolerance and hyperalgesia in chronic pain patients after one month of oral morphine therapy: a preliminary prospective study. J Pain 2006;7:43–8.
[86] Russell IJ, Kamin M, Bennett RM, et al. Efficacy of tramadol in treatment of pain of fibromyalgia. J Clin Rheumatol 2000;6:250–7.
[87] Bennett RM, Kamin M, Karim R, et al. Tramadol and acetaminophen combination tablets in the treatment of fibromyalgia pain: a double-blind randomized, placebo-controlled study. Am J Med 2003;113:537–45.
[88] Barkin RI, Barkin D. Pharmacologic management of acute and chronic pain; focus on drug interactions and patients-specific pharmacotherapeutic selection. South Med J 2001;18: 790–804.
[89] Katz WA, Otis JAD, McCarberg B, et al. Pain management: balancing efficacy with safety and tolerability. Clinical Courier 2007;25(10):1–10.
[90] Drake MJ, Nixon PM, Crew JP. Drug-induced bladder and urinary disorders: incidence, prevention and management. Drug Saf 1998;19(1):45–55.
[91] Jovanovi-Cupi V, Martinovi Z, Nesi N. Seizures associated with intoxication and abuse of tramadol. Clin Toxicol (Phila) 2006;44(2):143–6.
[92] Byas-Smith MG, Chapman SL, Reed B, et al. The effect of opioids on driving and psychomotor performance in patients with chronic pain. Clin J Pain 2005;21(4):345–52.
[93] Gaertner J, Radbruch L, Giesecke T, et al. Assessing cognition and psychomotor function under long-term treatment with controlled release oxycodone in non-cancer pain patients. Acta Anaesthesiol Scand 2006;50(6):664–72.
[94] Abs R, Verhelst J, Van Buyten J, et al. Endocrine consequences of long-term intrathecal administration of opioids. J Clin Endorcrinol Metab 2000;85:2215–22.
[95] Deardorf W. Breaking the cycle of chronic pain and insomnia. [Web site]. August 23, 2005. Available at: http://www.spine-health.com/topics/conserv/nsomnia/insomnia1.html. Accessed February 10, 2008.
[96] Roehrs T, Roth T. Sleep and pain: interaction of two vital functions. Semin Neurol 2005; 25(1):106–16.
[97] Onen SH, Onen F, Courpron P, et al. How pain and analgesics disturb sleep. Clin J Pain 2005;21(5):422–31.
[98] Available at: http://www.painmed.org/pdf/definition.pdf. Accessed March 1, 2008.
[99] Available at: http://www.ampain.org/advocacy/opioids.htm. Accessed March 1, 2008.
[100] Available at: http://www.emedicine.com/med/topic1673.htm. Accessed March 1, 2008.
[101] Ballantyne JC, Mao J. Opioid therapy for chronic pain. N Engl J Med 2003;349:1943–53.
[102] Available at: http://www.ama-cmeonline.com/pain_mgmt/module04/index.htm. Accessed March 1, 2008.
[103] Bloodworth D. Opioids in the treatment of chronic pain: legal framework and therapeutic indications and limitations. Phys Med Rehabil Clin N Am 2006;17(2):355–79.
[104] Chan KT, Fishman SM. Legal aspects of chronic opioid therapy. Curr Pain Headache Rep 2006;10(6):426–30.
[105] Wilsey B, Fishman DM, Rose JS, et al. Pain management in the ED. Am J Emerg Med 2004;221(1):51–7.
[106] Rupp T, Dekaney KA. Inadequate analgesia in emergency medicine. Ann Emerg Med 2004;43(4):494–503.
[107] Hoffman DE, Tarzian AJ. Achieving the right balance in oversight of physician opioid prescribing for pain: The role of state medical boards. J Law Med Ethics 2003;31:21–40.

[108] Quigley C. Opioid switching to improve pain relief and drug tolerability. Cochrane Database Syst Rev 2004;(3):CD004847.
[109] Clinical practice guidelines for the management of opioid therapy for chronic pain. Appendix E. Mar.2003. Washington, DC. Available at: http://www.ihs.gov/NonMedicalPrograms/NC4/Documents/ChronicpainguidelinesVA2003.pdf.
[110] American Medical Association. Pain management: Part 3. Management of persistent nonmalignant pain. 2006.
[111] Katz WA, Barkin RL. Dilemmas in chronic/persitent pain management. Am J Ther, accepted for publication.

ELSEVIER
SAUNDERS

Rheum Dis Clin N Am
34 (2008) 415–432

RHEUMATIC
DISEASE CLINICS
OF NORTH AMERICA

Topical Agents in the Treatment of Rheumatic Pain

R. Andrew Moore, MA, DPhil, CChem, FRSC, DSc*,
Sheena Derry, MA,
Henry J. McQuay, MA, DM, FRCA, FRCP (Edin)

Nuffield Department of Anaesthetics, University of Oxford, John Radcliffe Hospital, The Churchill, Headington, Oxford OX3 9DU, UK

Topical analgesics are viewed differently in different parts of the world. Outside of North America and the United Kingdom, they have been available and used extensively for rheumatic pain for many years. Although available in the United Kingdom, prescribing guidance has for many years been that topical analgesics are ineffective, and that any effect is "just the rubbing." This was completely reversed by draft guidance from the National Institute for Health and Clinical Excellence in July 2007 [1], which recommended that:

1. Topical nonsteroidal anti-inflammatory drugs should be a core treatment for knee and hand osteoarthritis.
2. Topical capsaicin should be considered as an adjunct to core therapy for knee and hand osteoarthritis.
3. Rubefacients are not recommended.

These recommendations are clearly in line with the best evidence available from systematic reviews of the literature, and reflect recent guidance from European League Against Rheumatism (EULAR) for hand osteoarthritis [2], and Osteoarthritis Research Society International (OARSI) for hip and knee osteoarthritis [3]. In the United States the Food and Drug Administration has approved topical diclofenac in a prescription form for osteoarthritic pain.

RAM and HJM have received lecture and consultancy fees from pharmaceutical companies with interests in analgesic drugs, including topical analgesics. The authors have received research support from charities and government sources at various times, some of which has related to topical analgesics. No author has any direct stock holding in any pharmaceutical company.

* Corresponding author.
E-mail address: andrew.moore@pru.ox.ac.uk (R.A. Moore).

0889-857X/08/$ - see front matter
doi:10.1016/j.rdc.2008.03.006

Previous concerns about the lack of longer, larger, and better studies in arthritis have been largely overturned with the publication of larger and better trials. A number of small new pharmaceutical companies have been active in the area of topical analgesics, and a significant number of new trials have been conducted. Frustratingly, most of the results are not in the public domain.

This article examines the evidence that is currently publicly available, and examines topical rubefacients, capsaicin, and nonsteroidal anti-inflammatory drugs (NSAIDs). Most of the evidence is for NSAIDS. For rubefacients and capsaicin neither the amount or quality of evidence, nor the size of the effect, makes them of any major interest for rheumatic pain. Although this article concentrates on information predominantly from systematic reviews and meta-analyses, supplemented by randomized trials, it does not rate the strength of evidence. The reason is that many systematic reviews are misleading because they are of poor quality, and judging the strength of evidence by study architecture alone has every possibility of being wrong.

Definitions

Classifying topical analgesics is helpful, although a number of authorities lump topical agents together. The British National Formulary, for instance, lists and classifies rubefacients and topical NSAIDs together [4]. The *Pharmaceutical Journal* more helpfully distinguishes three main categories of topical analgesics [5]:

1. Rubefacients: traditional formulations based on salicylate and nicotinate esters, capsaicin and capsicum extracts, and derivatives.
2. NSAIDs: diclofenac, felbinac, ibuprofen, ketoprofen, piroxicam, naproxen, flurbiprofen, and other NSAIDs.
3. A miscellaneous group: including benzydamine, mucopolysaccharide polysulphate, salicylamide, and cooling sprays.

Some compounds, such as salicylates, are related pharmacologically to aspirin and NSAIDs, but in the form that they are used in topical products (often as amine derivatives) their principal action is to act as skin irritants (called "counterirritants" in many texts, to "counter" pain). These agents cause a reddening of the skin by causing the blood vessels of the skin to dilate, giving a soothing feeling of warmth. The term "counterirritant" refers to the idea that irritation of the sensory nerve endings alters or offsets pain in the underlying muscle or joints that are served by the same nerves. Topical capsaicin probably works by a different mechanism and because of this capsaicin and rubefacients are reviewed separately here. Topical NSAIDs act by penetrating deep into underlying structures to inhibit cyclooxygenase enzymes responsible for development of inflammatory processes.

The concentration of components of topical analgesics can vary considerably, and dose-response relationships are largely unknown. Concentration may define prescription or over-the-counter status.

Topical rubefacient (salicylate)

Rubefacients are believed to work by counterirritation, to relieve pain in muscles, joints, and tendons and in nonarticular musculoskeletal conditions, rather than as NSAIDs inhibiting cyclooxygenase responsible for prostaglandin biosynthesis and the development of inflammation.

The information on topical rubefacients (all as salicylate) comes from a 2004 systematic review [6]. No further trials for topical rubefacients were found on more recent searches to March 2008. Twelve randomized, double-blind trials with 862 patients reported outcomes of clinical success, representing approximately a 50% reduction in pain, using a hierarchy of outcomes. Outcomes used were those closest to 14 days (but at least 7 days) for chronic conditions.

Six placebo-controlled trials in arthritis, or rheumatic conditions, and including back pain had information on 429 comparisons from 403 patients (26 patients were in a crossover study). The mean percentage of patients with at least 50% pain relief was 54% with topical salicylate and 36% with placebo. Treatment with rubefacient was significantly better than placebo with a number needed to treat (NNT) [7] of 5.3 (95% confidence interval [CI], 3.6–10) for at least 50% pain relief at 14 days in chronic conditions compared with placebo. Better trials had less effect. For the three trials (253 patients) with adequate validity scores measured using a validated pain validity scale there was no difference between topical salicylate and placebo (Table 1).

The evidence for efficacy of topical salicylates in rheumatic pain is poor. Short but otherwise valid chronic pain studies showed no difference between topical salicylate and placebo, whereas acute pain studies that did show some efficacy in a small number of patients could easily be overturned if any negative studies emerged. There is no good evidence for using topical rubefacients in rheumatic pain.

Topical capsaicin

Capsaicin is the active compound present in chili peppers, responsible for making them hot when eaten. It binds to nociceptors in the skin, causing an initial excitation of the neurones and a period of enhanced sensitivity to noxious stimuli, usually perceived as itching, pricking, or burning sensations. This is followed by a refractory period with reduced sensitivity and, after repeated applications, persistent desensitization; the ability of capsaicin to desensitize nociceptors is exploited for therapeutic pain relief.

For postherpetic neuralgia and diabetic neuropathy, treatment is with 0.075% cream three to four times daily for 8 weeks (followed by review), and for osteoarthritis treatment is with 0.025% cream four times daily. The information on topical capsaicin comes from a 2004 systematic review [8]. No additional trials for topical capsaicin were found on more recent searches to March 2008.

Table 1
Summary of evidence for topical nonsteroidal anti-inflammatory drugs, capsaicin, and rubefacient from placebo-controlled trials of higher quality and validity, compared with placebo at 14 days treatment

	Number of		Percent with treatment success		
Topical treatment	Trials	Patients	Active	Placebo	NNT (95%CI)
Rubefacient					
NSAID	10	1197	40	17	4.4 (3.6–5.6)
Capsaicin	3	368	38	25	8.1 (4.6–34)
Rubefacient	3	253	51	41	No significant benefit

Duration: 14 days, except capsaicin, which was 4 weeks. Comparator: placebo preparations rubbed on in same way as active.

Abbreviations: CI, confidence interval; NNT, number needed to treat; NSAID, nonsteroidal anti-inflammatory drugs.

Six randomized double-blind trials (521 patients) in osteoarthritis or back or jaw pain contained relevant information about 3 or 4 weeks of treatment. In three trials (368 patients) with a placebo comparison the mean treatment response at 3 to 4 weeks was 38%, whereas the mean response to placebo was 25% (see Table 1). The NNT compared with placebo at 4 weeks was 8.1 (95% CI, 4.6–34).

In all trials combined (musculoskeletal and neuropathic pain), local adverse events occurred more frequently with capsaicin cream than with placebo, with a number needed to harm of 2.5 (95% CI, 2.1–15) compared with placebo. Over half (54%) of patients had a local adverse event with capsaicin creams, and 13% of patients withdrew because of adverse events. Coughing was reported in 29 (8%) of 372 patients treated with capsaicin 0.075%, but in none of the placebo-controlled trials using 0.025% capsaicin.

Topical capsaicin can be distinguished from placebo in both neuropathic pain and in musculoskeletal pain. The quality and validity of the trials were high, although those in musculoskeletal pain were short, at 4 weeks. Only a small proportion of patients were helped by capsaicin, and adverse event rates were high. Topical capsaicin is an unlikely first or even second choice treatment, but helps some people.

Topical nonsteroidal anti-inflammatory drugs

The usefulness of topical NSAIDs has been questioned, and results of systematic reviews can differ. One systematic review [9] updated a previous review [10] by accepting only higher-quality trials (randomized, double blind); omitting salicylates; and adding newer trials. It concluded that topical NSAIDs were effective in rheumatic pain using a 2-week end point. Another review of topical NSAIDs in musculoskeletal pain [11] published in 2004 concluded that there was no evidence of superior efficacy beyond 2 weeks of use. It is worth looking at how this latter conclusion was reached, because the idea that topical NSAIDs work only for 2 weeks has gained considerable currency.

1. The review [11] used a subset of trials, with diagnosis of osteoarthritis of the hand, knee, or hip.
2. Four studies included in the meta-analysis used topical salicylates, which are not classified as NSAIDs, and are ineffective.
3. Outcomes are converted to mean effect sizes for reporting. This gives an overall smoothed out average result but can allow different outcomes to be pooled. Pooling mean results from a skewed distribution are known to lead to mistakes [12].
4. One trial appeared as three trials in the calculations. It was actually three doses of eltenac (0.1%, 0.3%, and 1%) versus placebo in a single trial. Topical eltenac, even at the highest dose, did not show significant benefit over placebo in two trials that used it, and there is no evidence that it is effective by any route of administration. Eltenac was the only topical NSAID tested beyond 2 weeks in the review.
5. The only evidence beyond 2 weeks is from trials of eltenac or salicylate, none of which had any effect at 1 week, 2 weeks, 3 weeks, or 4 weeks. Trials where topical NSAIDs worked were no longer than 2 weeks.

In August 2004, just weeks after the meta-analysis claiming no effect beyond 2 weeks, a large (248 patient) randomized trial of topical diclofenac and placebo for 4 weeks in patients with osteoarthritis of the knee was published [13]. Statistical benefit over placebo was found for pain, physical function, stiffness, pain on walking, and global assessment. Other large and long duration studies showing long-term efficacy of topical NSAIDs in osteoarthritis, up to at least 12 weeks, have been published subsequently.

All the systematic reviews [9–11] have highlighted the deficiency in older trials of topical NSAIDs in rheumatic pain, namely that they are of limited duration compared with modern requirements. The main results of the latest and widest systematic review are examined first, followed by results of trials published since that review (from 2003 onward).

Topical nonsteroidal anti-inflammatory drugs compared with topical placebo

Eighteen placebo-controlled trials had information on 2032 patients with osteoarthritis, musculoskeletal pain, rheumatism, back pain, and some other conditions [9]. Fourteen trials with information from 1502 patients were analyzed for efficacy. Overall, 48% of patients receiving topical NSAID reported success (defined as at least 50% pain relief) compared with 26% with placebo. Topical NSAIDs as a class were significantly better than placebo, with an NNT of 4.6 (95% CI, 3.8–5.9). There were 10 studies (1197 patients) with higher quality and validity scores indicating minimal bias, and these had an NNT of 4.4 (see Table 1).

There was no statistically significant difference between topical NSAID and topical placebo for the number of patients experiencing local adverse events (6%); systemic adverse events (3%); or the number withdrawing because of an adverse event (1%). With topical NSAID or topical placebo, local adverse events were usually described as rash, itching, or stinging, and were predominantly mild.

Topical nonsteroidal anti-inflammatory drugs compared with oral nonsteroidal anti-inflammatory drugs

Three trials, with 764 patients, directly compared a topical NSAID with an oral NSAID (diclofenac, 100 mg daily, in one trial and ibuprofen, 1200 mg daily, in two trials). Overall rates of treatment success were similar for topical NSAID (37%) and oral NSAID (37%), with no statistically significant difference (relative benefit 1.1; 95% CI, 0.9–1.3).

Eight of the active controlled trials (1461 patients) provided some information on adverse events. In two active controlled trials comparing topical with oral NSAID, local adverse events occurred more frequently (8%) with topical than with oral NSAID (3%). Systemic adverse events and adverse event withdrawals did not differ between topical and oral NSAID.

Subsequent topical nonsteroidal anti-inflammatory drugs randomized trials in rheumatic pain

The systematic review showed that topical NSAIDs were clearly better than placebo in chronic musculoskeletal pain, but there was insufficient information on different topical NSAID preparations to tell whether any one topical NSAID was better than another. The limited studies comparing topical with oral NSAIDs detected no difference. Topical NSAIDs were not associated with any higher rate of adverse events, either local or systemic, compared with placebo, but had higher rates of local adverse events compared with oral NSAIDs. Trials included in the 2004 review [9] were of high quality and validity, minimizing the possibility of bias. The short duration of the studies, however, predominantly 2-week outcomes, is a weakness for rheumatic pain, where longer duration trials are now expected. Have subsequent studies in rheumatic pain provided additional illumination? The authors performed a literature search for randomized trials of topical diclofenac, ketoprofen, ibuprofen, indomethacin, and piroxicam in rheumatic painful conditions published since 2003 to update the reviews.

Table 2 gives details of six randomized trials [13–18] involving topical NSAID in rheumatic pain published since the last systematic review in 2004. All of the trials were of high quality, being properly randomized and double blind. They were large, so that five comparisons with placebo added information on 1286 patients, and one with 622 patients, compared topical with oral NSAID. Together these trials increased the total number of patients in placebo and active comparisons by 70% over the previous systematic review.

All the trials involved topical diclofenac, four with a dimethyl sulfoxide solution formulation (Pennsaid [13–16]); one a gel formulation [17]; and one a plaster [18]. These latter two had relatively short durations of 2 and 3 weeks, but three of the Pennsaid trials lasted 6 or 12 weeks. The four Pennsaid trials have been the subject of a separate meta-analysis [19].

All five trials comparing topical diclofenac with placebo concluded that topical diclofenac was significantly better than placebo on a range of outcome measures, including pain, stiffness, physical function, and patient global assessment. The trial that compared topical diclofenac with 150 mg daily of oral diclofenac found no difference in efficacy (Fig. 1). Trials that used the OMERACT-OARSI definition of responder also found topical diclofenac to be better than placebo, and no different from 150 mg daily oral diclofenac. A responder is defined as a patient with greater than or equal to 50% improvement in pain or function that was greater than or equal to 20 mm on a 100-mm VAS, or greater than or equal to 20% improvement in at least two of pain, function, or patient global assessment that was greater than or equal to 10 mm on a 100-mm visual analog scale [20].

Adverse events in the trials using a solution of diclofenac with dimethyl sulfoxide (Pennsaid) typically found that local adverse reactions of dry skin and rash occurred more frequently with topical diclofenac than with vehicle control in about a third of patients with Pennsaid. Much the same was found in the comparison of topical with oral diclofenac [15]; application site reactions occurred almost uniquely in patients using active topical diclofenac, with dry skin (27%), rash (12%), and pruritus (6%) the most common.

Gastrointestinal adverse events with topical diclofenac were rare and occurred no more frequently with topical diclofenac than with placebo. Gastrointestinal adverse events occurred significantly more often for dyspepsia, abdominal pain, and diarrhea with oral than topical diclofenac, and were more likely to be severe with oral than topical diclofenac [15]. Overall, the number needed to harm for severe dyspepsia, abdominal pain, or diarrhea for oral compared with topical diclofenac for 12 weeks was 11 (95% CI, 8–19). Laboratory changes were also more common for oral compared with topical diclofenac; elevations in liver enzymes and reduced hemoglobin gave number needed to harm values of 7 to 14. Clinically significant elevations of three times the upper limit of normal or more occurred more frequently with oral diclofenac (1%, 5%, and 4% for aspartate transaminase, alanine transaminase, and γ-glutamyltransferase) than topical diclofenac (0.4%, 1.1%, and 1.4%, respectively).

The evidence from the more recent trials, all of which were of good reporting quality, supports that from previous systematic reviews. Topical NSAIDs are consistently better than placebo, with no evidence that they are inferior to oral NSAIDs. The most and the best evidence is for topical diclofenac.

Table 2
Details of randomized, double-blind, trials of topical nonsteroidal anti-inflammatory drugs published since 2003 and 2004

Reference	Design, drugs, doses	Main results
Bookman et al [13]	248 men and women with radiologically confirmed OA knee, with baseline flare after therapy discontinuation Mean age 63 y Topical diclofenac solution four times daily (diclofenac plus DMSO carrier); vehicle control (DMSO carrier but no diclofenac); or placebo solution, no massage 4 wk Various outcomes, including WOMAC, and patient global assessment	At least 50% reduction in pain was not reported Significant improvement topical diclofenac compared with vehicle control and placebo in pain, physical functioning, patient global assessment, stiffness, pain on walking Significant increase in dry skin and rash with topical diclofenac; more discontinuations with placebo, mainly because of lack of effect
Roth and Shainhouse [14]	326 men and women with radiologically confirmed OA knee, with baseline flare after therapy discontinuation Age 41–85 y Topical diclofenac solution four times daily or placebo solution, no massage 12 wk Various outcomes, including WOMAC, and patient global assessment	At least 50% reduction in pain was not reported Significant improvement with topical diclofenac compared with placebo in pain, physical functioning, patient global assessment, stiffness, pain on walking Significant increase in dry skin and rash with topical diclofenac; more discontinuations with placebo, mainly because of lack of effect

Tugwell et al [15]	622 men and women with radiologically confirmed OA knee, with baseline flare after therapy discontinuation Age 40–85 y Topical diclofenac solution three times daily or oral diclofenac, 50 mg three times daily for 12 wk Various outcomes, including WOMAC, and patient global assessment	No major differences between topical or oral diclofenac for the major outcomes; similar proportion of clinical responders according to OMERACT-OARSI criteria, and more laboratory changes, especially in liver enzymes and hemoglobin, with oral diclofenac Significantly more gastrointestinal adverse events with oral than topical diclofenac Significantly more local adverse events (dry skin, rash) with topical than oral diclofenac
Baer et al [16]	216 men and women with radiologically confirmed OA knee, with baseline flare after therapy discontinuation Age 40–85 y Topical diclofenac solution four times daily or placebo solution, no massage 6 weeks Various outcomes, including WOMAC, and patient global assessment	At least 50% reduction in pain with 44% with diclofenac, 25% with placebo (ITT analysis) Significant improvement with topical diclofenac compared with placebo in pain, physical functioning, patient global assessment, stiffness, pain on walking Significant increase in dry skin with topical diclofenac; more discontinuations with placebo, mainly because of lack of effect
Niethard et al [17]	238 men and women with radiologically confirmed OA knee, with baseline flare after therapy discontinuation Age 45 or older Topical diclofenac gel or placebo gel for 3 weeks Various outcomes, including WOMAC, and patient global assessment	Significant improvement for topical diclofenac over placebo for pain, physical functioning, and stiffness, as well as proportion of OMERACT-OARSI responders, and patient global score
Bruhlmann et al [18]	258 patients with radiologically confirmed symptomatic knee OA from two randomized trials Topical diclofenac plaster or placebo plaster for 2 wk Outcomes were Lesquesne index and pain	Significant reductions in both outcomes for topical diclofenac compared with placebo; NNT for at least 50% pain relief calculated to be 3

Abbreviations: DMSO, dimethyl sulfoxide; ITT, intention to treat; OA, osteoarthritis; WOMAC, Western Ontario and McMaster Osteoarthritis Questionnaire.

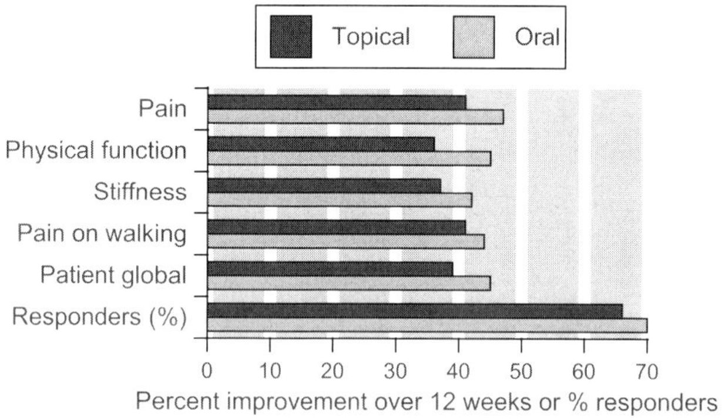

Fig. 1. Main efficacy outcomes with topical and oral diclofenac over 12 weeks. (*Data from* Tugwell PS, Wells GA, Shainhouse JZ. Equivalence study of a topical diclofenac solution (Pennsaid) compared with oral diclofenac in symptomatic treatment of osteoarthritis of the knee: a randomized controlled trial. J Rheumatol 2004;31:2002–12.)

Safety of topical nonsteroidal anti-inflammatory drugs

Gastrointestinal and renal safety

Randomized trials can give useful information about common adverse events, which are usually mild and reversible. Risk of rare, serious, and often irreversible adverse events is often better estimated in observational studies. For topical NSAIDs, two major case-control studies inform on rare but serious gastrointestinal harm and renal failure [21,22]. Both were conducted in about 400,000 people living in Tayside, Scotland, where there is excellent record linkage.

Cases were patients with diagnostic code for upper gastrointestinal bleeding and perforation, or acute renal failure. Controls were from the community or hospital. Community controls were matched for age and gender and were selected randomly for each case (up to six controls for each case). Up to two hospital controls were also selected, matched for age and gender, and generated randomly for each case. They had been admitted to hospital for any reason other than gastrointestinal bleeding and perforation. Previous exposure to any oral and topical NSAIDs, gastrointestinal healing drugs, or aspirin was examined for association with admission for gastrointestinal bleeding. Topical NSAID in these studies had a wide definition that also included rubefacients (salicylates).

For gastrointestinal bleeding [21] there were 1101 cases and 6593 controls. After adjustment for use of other drugs using conditional logistic regression, the conclusion was that topical NSAIDs were never significantly associated with higher bleeding rates irrespective of controls used, or duration of exposure. Oral NSAIDs were significantly associated with higher bleeding rates irrespective of controls used or duration of exposure, and ulcer-healing drugs were predominantly significantly associated with higher bleeding rates.

For acute renal failure [22] there were 207 cases and 1238 controls. After adjustment for use of other drugs using conditional logistic regression, the conclusion was that topical NSAIDs probably carry no risk of acute renal failure, whereas oral NSAIDs were associated with an approximate doubling of the risk of hospitalization for acute renal failure; aspirin may carry a similar increased risk.

Photosensitivity

All NSAIDs can potentially induce phototoxic reactions. The main NSAID with known phototoxic adverse reactions is ketoprofen, which can undergo UV-catalyzed chemical changes that render toxic reactions more likely. On irradiation photosensitizers can be transformed into haptens with a benzophenone moiety, leading to an immune response after binding to a tissue antigen. These sensitivity reactions usually regress after discontinuation of the drug, but can occasionally be prolonged [23].

A review [24] collected about 100 case reports of photocontact dermatitis after application of topical ketoprofen, and epidemiologic data from Italy, France, and Sweden. The best estimate of rate is 1 to 2 per 10,000 patients treated.

Supporting evidence for efficacy of topical nonsteroidal anti-inflammatory drugs

Topical NSAIDs, either prescribed or bought without prescription, are often used for soft tissue injuries, or strains or sprains. A systematic review [25] sought evidence for their effectiveness in these conditions.

Placebo-controlled trials

Twenty-six trials with information from 2853 patients were analyzed for efficacy at 7 days. In 19 of the 26 trials topical NSAID was significantly better than placebo. Topical NSAIDs as a class were significantly better than placebo, with an NNT of 3.8 (95% CI, 3.4–4.4). In 22 of 26 studies with higher quality and validity scores that minimized bias, the NNT was also 3.8.

Efficacy estimates were also made for five individual drugs studied in at least three trials. All were significantly better than placebo, but in the case of indomethacin only just so. Ketoprofen had the lowest (best) NNT of 2.6 (95% CI, 2.2–3.3). The result for ketoprofen was significantly better than for ibuprofen, felbinac, piroxicam, and indomethacin (Fig. 2); there was no information on diclofenac.

Topical compared with oral nonsteroidal anti-inflammatory drugs

Three trials, with 433 patients, compared a topical NSAID with an oral NSAID (indomethacin, 75 mg daily, in one trial and ibuprofen, 1200 mg daily, in two trials). Overall rates of treatment success at 7 days were similar

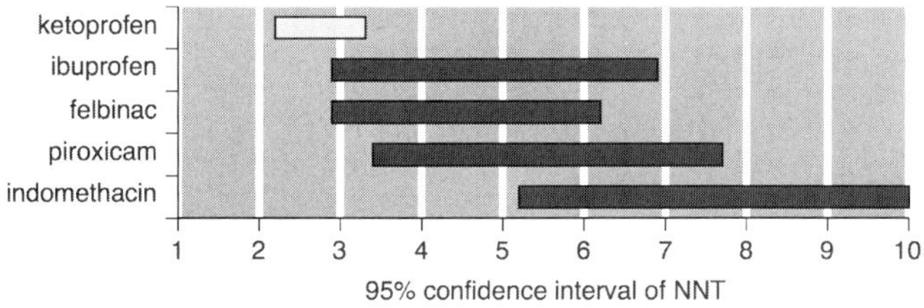

Fig. 2. Efficacy of individual topical NSAIDs measured at 7 days for strains and sprains (95% CI of number needed to treat compared with placebo). NNT, number needed to treat. (*Data from* Mason L, Moore RA, Edwards JE, et al. Topical NSAIDs for acute pain: a meta-analysis. BMC Fam Pract 2004;5:10.)

for topical NSAID (57%) and oral NSAID (62%), with no statistically significant difference (relative benefit 0.9; 95% CI, 0.8–1.1).

Adverse events

There was no statistically significant difference between the numbers of patients experiencing one or more local adverse events (4%), one or more systemic adverse events (2.5%), or the numbers of patients withdrawing because of an adverse event (0.8%), with topical NSAIDs than with placebo. Systemic adverse events and adverse event withdrawals did not differ between topical and oral NSAID.

Trials included in this review were of high quality and validity, minimizing the possibility of bias. The outcomes chosen were at 1 week, which is appropriate for soft tissue injuries, and for strains and sprains. This systematic review confirms the results of a previous review. Topical NSAIDs are effective for pain relief in such conditions as strains and sprains.

Is there any science behind topical nonsteroidal anti-inflammatory drugs?

For topical NSAIDs there is information on background biology. That information allows one to investigate the evidence about skin penetration, plasma, and tissue levels of NSAIDs after topical application (Fig. 3).

Penetrating the skin

For topical NSAIDs to be effective, they have to at least penetrate the skin. Only when the drug has entered the lower layers of the skin can it be absorbed by blood and transported to the site of action, or penetrate deeper into areas where inflammation occurs. Diffusion through skin can be measured using in vivo microdialysis techniques [26], and depends on several factors, including the skin or membrane itself, the drug, and any other materials that are used either to increase or decrease diffusion. The literature

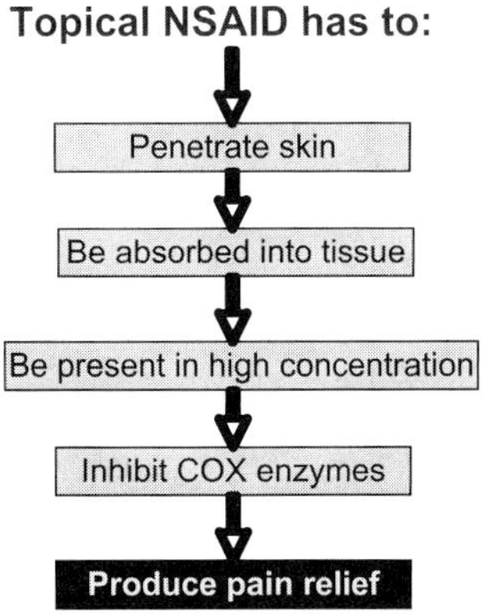

Fig. 3. Actions needed for topical NSAIDs to work.

on NSAID diffusion through the skin (not quoted) indicates the following to be important:

1. Importance of the drug: Theoretic and experimental results suggest that a balance between lipid and aqueous solubility is needed to optimize penetration. Use of prodrug esters has been suggested as a way of enhancing permeability [27].
2. Importance of formulation: Several studies indicated that formulation can make a huge difference to drug permeation. Creams are generally less effective than gels or sprays, but newer formulations, such as microemulsions, have greater potential. Considerable efforts are being expended on enhancing skin permeation by using better formulations.
3. Although transdermal penetration of topical NSAID can be good, it can also be highly variable [28]. This is probably a result, in part, of variable skin blood flow; increased blood flow removes topically applied drug and reduces the chance of high local concentrations in underlying tissues. Increased blood flow can be caused by rubbing, occlusion, and use of menthol. Reduced blood flow [29] and high tissue binding enhance local penetration from topical application [30–32].
4. The main determinant of flux across the skin is probably small molecular size [33].

For a topical NSAID to be effective, it has not only to reach inflamed tissue, but also to be there in sufficient concentration to produce a relevant anti-inflammatory activity. The ratio of penetration to concentration in tissue has been called an index of topical anti-inflammatory activity [34]. Theoretic considerations indicate that four drugs are particularly good candidates: (1) diclofenac, (2) ketorolac, (3) ketoprofen, and (4) indomethacin; piroxicam and tenoxicam are not, and ibuprofen was not tested. It is interesting to compare this theoretic approach with results from use of topical NSAIDs for strains and sprains, where indirect comparison suggests that ketoprofen and ibuprofen had the best activity, whereas piroxicam and indomethacin had the worst.

Plasma and tissue concentrations

Topical NSAID administration results in peak plasma concentrations that are much lower than after oral administration of standard NSAID doses [35]. Plasma concentrations after topical administration have been generally found to be less than 5% of those in plasma. Drug concentrations in adipose tissue and skeletal muscle after topical administration are the same or higher than those after oral administration, at least with topical diclofenac [36].

The largest and most detailed study involved single and multiple applications of topical ketoprofen plaster in patients having knee operations [37]. Mean plasma ketoprofen concentrations were no higher than about 20 ng/mL. These levels were achieved within 6 hours of the first application, but fell away rapidly after the last application was removed following 5 days of multiple applications. After oral ketoprofen, peak plasma concentrations were at least two orders of magnitude higher, at 2600 ng/mL 2 hours after a single 50-mg dose, and were at least twice as high as the maximum value after topical application at 14 hours after an oral dose.

Synovial fluid concentrations of NSAIDs after topical application were generally lower than those found in plasma. The largest study [37] of ketoprofen found that the ratio of synovial fluid to plasma concentration was of the order of 0.6 to 0.8 at most times after the first or last dose. Synovial fluid concentrations are likely to reflect blood concentrations because this is a highly vascular compartment. When topical diclofenac was applied to one knee in a randomized double-blind trial [38], the concentration of diclofenac in synovial fluid in the untreated knee was almost the same as that in the treated knee.

Concentrations of NSAID in tissue after topical administration tended to be higher. For instance, after 3 days of application of topical ketoprofen, concentrations in the knee capsule were 2.4 μg/g, and after 3 days of topical ibuprofen were 7 to 9 μg/g in capsule and tendon. After a single dose, other studies found concentrations about a thousandfold higher than plasma concentrations in subcutaneous tissue, muscle, and tendon sheath. In the largest single study [37], very high concentrations of ketoprofen were found in meniscus and cartilage after topical administration, about four to seven times greater than were found after oral administration (Fig. 4), despite plasma concentrations around 100 times higher with oral than topical use. By comparison, concentrations of ketoprofen in meniscus and cartilage after oral administration were well below those of synovial fluid and synovial tissue.

Discussion

The evidence is quite strong that topical NSAIDs are effective for a considerable proportion of patients with rheumatic pain. As Table 1

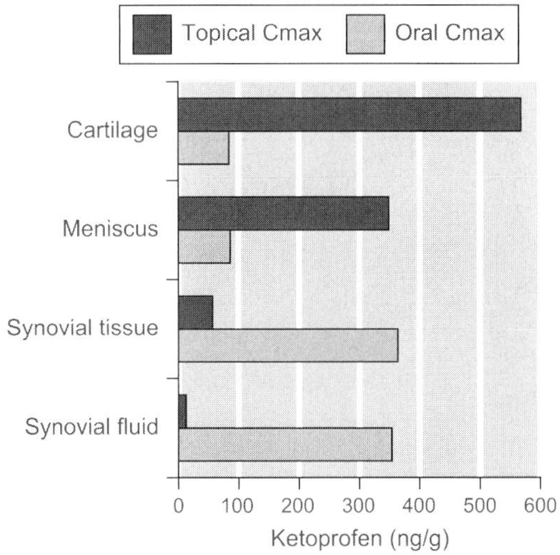

Fig. 4. Concentration of ketoprofen in knee tissues following topical and oral administration. Cmax, maximum concentration.

demonstrates, information from placebo comparisons in high-quality and validity trials with low risk of bias provided a high degree of comfort for the efficacy of topical NSAIDs, and this has been supported by a considerable additional body of data, especially from longer trials. Topical capsaicin is much less effective, and is supported by only a small amount of evidence of limited quality. Topical rubefacients have no supporting evidence of efficacy.

Topical NSAIDs are without the gastrointestinal adverse events of oral NSAIDS, and should be better tolerated. Topical NSAIDs are safer when compared with oral NSAIDs with less risk of gastrointestinal bleeding or renal failure. Differences in tolerability and safety probably reflect considerably lower plasma concentrations with topical NSAIDs.

Oral NSAIDs are known to cause gastrointestinal bleeding [39], renal failure [40,41], and congestive cardiac failure [42,43]. These have major humanitarian and cost implications, especially in ageing populations. Projections show the number of citizens aged 65 years and older in the United States will almost double from 37 million in 2006 to 63 million by 2025, and there will be a third of a million over the age of 100 years by 2020 [44]. The need for safe and effective analgesics will not go away. For many people, topical NSAIDs are likely to be a safe starting point.

This may be what patients want. A study 100 consecutive patients living in the community with osteoarthritis of the knee collected preference data on treatment choices and usefulness was assessed using conjoint analysis [45]. Patients were given information about treatment efficacy, common adverse events, route and frequency of administration, onset of action, and risk of ulcer for five treatments: (1) nonselective NSAIDs, (2) coxibs,

(3) opioids, (4) glucosamine (all oral), and (5) capsaicin cream. They were experienced patients.

None preferred a traditional nonselective NSAID, in any scenario. This is likely to reflect an aversion to their common adverse events, especially in a group that was predominantly female, averaging 70 years of age. Topical NSAIDs were not tested, but topical capsaicin was a choice for about a quarter.

It is probable that a strong health economic case could be made for using topical NSAIDs in rheumatic pain, especially compared with oral NSAIDs and coxibs. That argument has not yet been made.

What's missing?

There are several gaps in knowledge that need to be filled.

1. A greater degree of clarity over classifying topical analgesics. Clinical trials that mix up topical NSAIDs and rubefacients as if they were they same [46], with a similar mechanism of action, do not increase knowledge, and merely confuse matters.
2. Publication of what seems to be a large number of well-conducted and longer-duration trials that have been completed, but are not yet in the public domain.
3. More safety studies, or publication of long-term safety studies performed for Food and Drug Administration approval, as was done for diclofenc gel [47].
4. Better help to know which patient to treat with which therapy. Logic dictates that persons with single joint problems are better served by topical rather than oral NSAIDs, but more robust evidence is welcomed.

References

[1] Osteoarthritis: the care and management of osteoarthritis in adults. London: Royal College of Physicians; 2008.

[2] Zhang W, Doherty M, Leeb BF, et al. EULAR evidence based recommendations for the diagnosis of hand osteoarthritis: report of a task force of the EULAR Standing Committee for International Clinical Studies Including Therapeutics (ESCISIT). Ann Rheum Dis 2007;66: 377–88.

[3] Zhang W, Moskowitz RW, Nuki G, et al. OARSI recommendations for the management of hip and knee osteoarthritis. Part II: OARSI evidence-based, expert consensus guidelines. Osteoarthritis Cartilage 2008;16:137–62.

[4] British National Formulary. March 2006. p. 531.

[5] Li Wan Po A. Topical analgesics. PJ practice checklist. The Pharmaceutical Journal 2006.

[6] Mason L, Moore RA, Edwards JE, et al. Systematic review of efficacy of topical rubefacients containing salicylates for the treatment of acute and chronic pain. BMJ 2004;328:995–8.

[7] McQuay HJ, Moore RA. Using numerical results from systematic reviews in clinical practice. Ann Intern Med 1997;126:712–20.

[8] Mason L, Moore RA, Derry S, et al. Systematic review of topical capsaicin for the treatment of chronic pain. BMJ 2004;328:991–4.

[9] Mason L, Moore RA, Edwards JE, et al. Topical NSAIDs for chronic musculoskeletal pain: systematic review and meta-analysis. BMC Musculoskelet Disord 2004;5:28.
[10] Moore RA, Tramèr MR, Carroll D, et al. Quantitative systematic review of topically applied non-steroidal anti-inflammatory drugs. BMJ 1998;316:333–8.
[11] Lin J, Zhang W, Jones A, et al. Efficacy of topical non-steroidal anti-inflammatory drugs in the treatment of osteoarthritis: meta-analysis of randomised controlled trials. BMJ 2004; 329:324–7.
[12] McQuay H, Carroll D, Moore A. Variation in the placebo effect in randomised controlled trials of analgesics: all is as blind as it seems. Pain 1996;64:331–5.
[13] Bookman AA, Williams KS, Shainhouse JZ. Effect of a topical diclofenac solution for relieving symptoms of primary osteoarthritis of the knee: a randomized controlled trial. CMAJ 2004;171:333–8.
[14] Roth SH, Shainhouse JZ. Efficacy and safety of a topical diclofenac solution (Pennsaid) in the treatment of primary osteoarthritis of the knee: a randomized, double-blind, vehicle-controlled clinical trial. Arch Intern Med 2004;164:2017–23.
[15] Tugwell PS, Wells GA, Shainhouse JZ. Equivalence study of a topical diclofenac solution (Pennsaid) compared with oral diclofenac in symptomatic treatment of osteoarthritis of the knee: a randomized controlled trial. J Rheumatol 2004;31:2002–12.
[16] Baer PA, Thomas LM, Shainhouse Z. Treatment of osteoarthritis of the knee with a topical diclofenac solution: a randomised controlled, 6-week trial [ISRCTN53366886]. BMC Musculoskelet Disord 2005;6:44.
[17] Niethard FU, Gold MS, Solomon GS, et al. Efficacy of topical diclofenac diethylamine gel in osteoarthritis of the knee. J Rheumatol 2005;32:2384–92.
[18] Brühlmann P, de Vathaire F, Dreiser RL, et al. Short-term treatment with topical diclofenac epolamine plaster in patients with symptomatic knee osteoarthritis: pooled analysis of two randomised clinical studies. Curr Med Res Opin 2006;22:2429–38.
[19] Towheed TE. Pennsaid therapy for osteoarthritis of the knee: a systematic review and metaanalysis of randomized controlled trials. J Rheumatol 2006;33:567–73.
[20] Pham T, van der Heijde D, Lassere M, et al. Outcome variables for osteoarthritis clinical trials: The OMERACT-OARSI set of responder criteria. J Rheumatol 2003; 30:1648–54.
[21] Evans JM, McMahon AD, McGilchrist MM, et al. Topical non-steroidal anti-inflammatory drugs and admission to hospital for upper gastrointestinal bleeding and perforation: a record linkage case-control study. BMJ 1995;311:22–6.
[22] Evans JM, McGregor E, McMahon AD, et al. Non-steroidal anti-inflammatory drugs and hospitalization for acute renal failure. QJM 1995;88:551–7.
[23] Albès B, Marguery MC, Schwarze HP, et al. Prolonged photosensitivity following contact photoallergy to ketoprofen. Dermatology 2000;201:171–4.
[24] Bagheri H, Lhiaubet V, Montastruc JL, et al. Photosensitivity to ketoprofen: mechanisms and pharmacoepidemiological data. Drug Saf 2000;22:339–49.
[25] Mason L, Moore RA, Edwards JE, et al. Topical NSAIDs for acute pain: a meta-analysis. BMC Fam Pract 2004;5:10.
[26] Kreilgaard M. Assessment of cutaneous drug delivery using microdialysis. Adv Drug Deliv Rev. 2002;54(Suppl 1):S99–121.
[27] Sloan KB, Wasdo S. Designing for topical delivery: prodrugs can make the difference. Med Res Rev 2003;23:763–93.
[28] Dehghanyar P, Mayer BX, Namiranian K, et al. Topical skin penetration of diclofenac after single- and multiple-dose application. Int J Clin Pharmacol Ther 2004;42:353–9.
[29] Higaki K, Nakayama K, Suyama T, et al. Enhancement of topical delivery of drugs via direct penetration by reducing blood flow rate in skin. Int J Pharm 2005;288:227–33.
[30] Roberts MS, Cross SE. A physiological pharmacokinetic model for solute disposition in tissues below a topical application site. Pharm Res 1999;16:1392–8.

[31] Roberts MS, Cross SE. Percutaneous absorption of topically applied NSAIDs and other compounds: role of solute properties, skin physiology and delivery systems. Inflammopharmacology 1999;7:339–50.
[32] Cross SE, Roberts MS. Use of in vitro human skin membranes to model and predict the effect of changing blood flow on the flux and retention of topically applied solutes. J Pharm Sci 2007; [Epub ahead of print].
[33] Magnusson BM, Anissimov YG, Cross SE, et al. Molecular size as the main determinant of solute maximum flux across the skin. J Invest Dermatol 2004;122:993–9.
[34] Cordero JA, Camacho M, Obach R, et al. In vitro based index of topical anti-inflammatory activity to compare a series of NSAIDs. Eur J Pharm Biopharm 2001;51:135–42.
[35] Heyneman CA, Lawless-Liday C, Wall GC. Oral versus topical NSAIDs in rheumatic diseases: a comparison. Drugs 2000;60:555–74.
[36] Brunner M, Dehghanyar P, Seigfried B, et al. Favourable dermal penetration of diclofenac after administration to the skin using a novel spray gel formulation. Br J Clin Pharmacol 2005;60:573–7.
[37] Rolf C, Engström B, Beauchard C, et al. Intra-articular absorption and distribution of ketoprofen after topical plaster application and oral intake in 100 patients undergoing knee arthroscopy. Rheumatology (Oxford) 1999;38:564–7.
[38] Radermacher J, Jentsch D, Scholl MA, et al. Diclofenac concentrations in synovial fluid and plasma after cutaneous application in inflammatory and degenerative joint disease. Br J Clin Pharmacol 1991;31:537–41.
[39] Hernández-Diaz S, García Rodriguez LA. Association between nonsteroidal anti-inflammatory drugs and upper gastrointestinal tract bleeding and perforation: an overview of epidemiological studies published in the 1990s. Arch Intern Med 2000;160:2093–9.
[40] Griffin MR, Yared A, Ray WA. Nonsteroidal antiinflamatory drugs and acute renal failure in elderly persons. Am J Epidemiol 2000;151:488–96.
[41] Henry D, Page J, Whyte I, et al. Consumption of non-steroidal anti-inflammatory drugs and the development of functional renal impairment in elderly subjects: results of a case-control study. Br J Clin Pharmacol 1997;44:85–90.
[42] Page J, Henry D. Consumption of NSAIDs and the development of congestive heart failure in elderly patients: an underrecognized public health problem. Arch Intern Med 2000;160: 777–84.
[43] Heerdink ER, Leufkens HG, Herings RM, et al. NSAIDs associated with increased risk of congestive heart failure in elderly patients taking diuretics. Arch Intern Med 1998;158: 1108–12.
[44] United States Census Bureau. Available at: http://www.census.gov/. Accessed February 29, 2008.
[45] Fraenkel L, Bogardus ST Jr, Concato J, et al. Treatment options in knee osteoarthritis: the patient's perspective. Arch Intern Med 2004;164:1299–304.
[46] Underwood M, Ashby D, Cross P, et al. Advice to use topical or oral ibuprofen for chronic knee pain in older people: randomised controlled trial and patient preference study. BMJ 2008;336:138–42.
[47] Eurek Alert! Available at: http://www.eurekalert.org/pub_releases/2007-10/fi-vgr102107.php. Accessed February 29, 2008.

ELSEVIER
SAUNDERS

Rheum Dis Clin N Am
34 (2008) 433–453

RHEUMATIC
DISEASE CLINICS
OF NORTH AMERICA

Antidepressant Use in Painful Rheumatic Conditions

Serge Perrot, MD, PhD[a,*], Rose-Marie Javier, MD[b], Marc Marty, MD[c], Claire Le Jeunne, MD[a], Françoise Laroche, MD[d]

[a]*Service de Médecine Interne et Thérapeutique, Consultation de la Douleur, Hôtel Dieu, Université Paris Descartes, 1 Place du Parvis Notre Dame, 75004 Paris, France*
[b]*Service de Rhumatologie, Hôpital Hautepierre, Avenue Moliere, 67200 Strasbourg, France*
[c]*Service de Rhumatoloie, Hôpital Henri Mondor, c-51 Avenue du Marechal de Passigny, 94010 Créteil Cedex, France*
[d]*Centre d'Evaluation et de Traitement de la Douleur, Hôpital St. Antoine, d-184 Rue du Fauborg St. Antoine, 75581 Paris Cedex 12, France*

Pain is the main symptom of most rheumatologic conditions. In some cases, standard analgesics (acetaminophen, nonsteroidal anti-inflammatory drugs, and opioids), are ineffective and other drugs, such as antidepressants, are required. Antidepressants are increasingly prescribed for conditions such as fibromyalgia, rheumatoid arthritis, spondylarthropathies, low back pain, and osteoarthritis. However, the results obtained with antidepressants are highly variable [1–4] and the use of antidepressants for analgesia remains controversial. This article reviews the evidence supporting the use of antidepressants in painful rheumatologic conditions, with a view to helping rheumatologists understand the background of antidepressant use in their daily practice [5–7]. This work was also performed to develop clinical guidelines on the use of antidepressants in rheumatologic conditions (Antidepressants in Rheumatology recommendations [8]), based on literature analysis in five European languages (French, English, Spanish, Italian, and German) from 1966 to June 2007. Each article was classified using Jadad's method, awarding a score from 0 to 5 [9], and graded in terms of its evidence category, as described by Shekelle and colleagues [10]. Selecting articles with Jadad's score of 2 or more, the authors kept 78 clinical studies and 12 meta-analyses and literature reviews for analysis.

* Corresponding author.
E-mail address: serge.perrot@htd.aphp.fr (S. Perrot).

doi:10.1016/j.rdc.2008.03.004 ***rheumatic.theclinics.com***

Analysis of the identified articles

Evaluation criteria were grouped into seven categories: study design, number of patients, average dose of antidepressants administered, study duration, outcome measurement, and calculation of analgesic effect size (ES). Pain was considered the main outcome variable in these studies. Analgesic ES was determined by calculating the standardized difference between two means (antidepressant analgesic effect versus placebo analgesic effect). ES is the difference between these two means divided by the pooled estimate standard deviation. This article uses the mean change between baseline and the end of the study for quantitative pain data, if such data are available. In cases in which the change between baseline and the end of the study was not described in the original article, ES was calculated based on the value obtained at the end of the trial, despite the limitations associated with this information. Pain assessed by visual analog scale was retained as the main parameter if available. If visual analog scale pain was not available, the pain dimension of the fibromyalgia impact questionnaire or pain assessment of the McGill pain questionnaire was used. If no sufficient data on pain parameters were available for the calculation of ES, the conclusions of the investigators are reported. ES is reported in the tables with 95% confidence limits. Most of the studies included a small number of subjects, so a correction procedure, using Hedge's adjusted G effect measure, was applied to calculate effect size. The authors considered the ES to be large if it exceeded 1, moderate if it was between 0.5 and 0.9, and small if it was between 0.30 and 0.50.

Classification of antidepressants

Antidepressants are usually classified according to their mechanism of action (eg, effect on monoamines) and their chemical structure (eg, tricyclic) (Table 1) [11]. Most animal studies involving acute nociceptive tests or persistent pain models (neuropathic or nociceptive) have concluded that antidepressants have an antinociceptive effect or an antihyperalgesic effect. The effects of antidepressants appear to depend on their activity on monoamines.

Mechanisms of action underlying the analgesic effects of antidepressants

Antidepressants are generally considered to have a central effect, reflecting their ability to cross the blood-brain barrier [11]. This has been demonstrated in animal and human studies and may involve both spinal and supraspinal mechanisms [12,13]. Animal studies have confirmed the involvement of monoaminergic pathways and have demonstrated that intact serotonin and noradrenalin systems and bulbospinal pathways are required for

Table 1
Classification of antidepressant drugs tested in painful conditions

Mode of action	Name/structure	
Imipraminic	Tricyclic	Amitriptyline, clomipramine, desipramine, dothiepin, doxepine
Imipraminic	Tetracyclic	Maprotiline
Selective serotonin reuptake inhibitors	SSRIs	Fluoxetine, citalopram, paroxetine, sertraline
Serotonin and noradrenalin reuptake inhibitors	SNRIs	Venlafaxine, milnacipran, duloxetine
Noradrenergic and specific Serotonergic antidepressants	NaSSAs	Mirtazapine
Selective norepinephrine reuptake inhibitor	SNERI	Bupropion, reboxetine
Monoamine oxidase inhibitors	MAOI	Moclamide
Others		Mianserin, nefazodone, tianeptin

tricyclic antidepressants (TCAs) (the most frequently studied antidepressants) to exert their antinociceptive effects [11,14]. In studies of human subjects with neuropathic pain, TCAs seem to be more effective than serotonin and noradrenalin reuptake inhibitors (SNRIs), which are, in turn, more effective than selective serotonin reuptake inhibitors (SSRIs) [15]. The "number of patients needed to treat" (NNT) to obtain at least one neuropathic patient with a 50% improvement is two to three for TCAs, about four for venlafaxine (an SNRI), and seven for SSRIs.

However, other mechanisms have also been suggested for TCAs. These mechanisms include a possible effect on opioid receptors, as suggested by several preclinical and clinical studies in which naloxone was shown to inhibit the analgesic effect of TCAs [16]. They may also exert an effect by interacting with excitatory amino acids, as they may act as antagonists of N-methyl-D-aspartic acid (NMDA). It has also been suggested that TCAs may act by blockading sodium channels or inhibiting neuronal adenosine uptake, as adenosine can generate both spinal and supraspinal analgesia. Other mechanisms may also be involved and further investigation is required to resolve this issue.

Some studies have considered a possible peripheral site of action for antidepressants (reviewed in Ref. [12]). The first studies have found no evidence of such a site of action, but more recent studies based on models of inflammatory, neuropathic, or visceral pain have suggested that some TCAs and fluoxetine may have a peripheral antinociceptive effect [17]. The mechanisms put forward to account for such a peripheral effect differ from those for centrally mediated action. The inhibition of monoamine reuptake, which induces a pain-facilitating effect in the periphery, cannot be involved. None of the other known pharmacologic actions of antidepressants, particularly those of TCAs (antagonism of alpha-1 adrenergic action; antagonism of H_1 histaminergic and muscarinic receptors; opioidergic activation; NMDA receptor antagonism; adenosine reuptake; ion channel blockade) are likely to account completely for the peripheral effects of these drugs. Further studies with specific tools are required to determine more precisely the action of these drugs in the periphery. Thus, the precise mechanism by which antidepressants relieve chronic pain is unclear. Active research is required in this area to identify differences between drugs in terms of their mode of action, as a function of the chronic pain condition considered [13].

Clinical pharmacology of antidepressants for the treatment of painful conditions

Evaluation of the dose-response effect in chronic pain

There is no clear evidence for a dose-dependent response to antidepressant treatment in terms of pain relief. However, the authors identified no studies dealing specifically with rheumatic pain. Conflicting data have been obtained concerning the possible relationship between concentration and analgesic effect, but current therapeutic plasma concentration ranges seem to give an acceptable response for TCAs. Several studies in which TCAs were administered for various types of neuropathic pain reported a relationship between serum drug concentration and analgesic effect [18]. A curvilinear concentration-response relationship has been reported for some TCAs (see references in [19]). Low doses of TCAs are frequently used for pain management [20], probably because of the distressing side effects potentially associated with the use of higher doses, which might interfere with pain reduction or compliance (see references in [1,21]). A study on imipramine treatment in neuropathic pain demonstrated that the plasma drug concentration at which an individual maximal analgesic effect was obtained in responders (global pain relief $> 25\%$) ranged from 50 nmol/L to 1,400 nmol/L, remaining below 400 nmol/L in most cases [22]. Conflicting data have been obtained for the newer antidepressants, with some studies suggesting that plasma concentration and effect are correlated (eg, for paroxetine in neuropathic pain) and others reporting no such correlation (eg, for fluoxetine and citalopram for neuropathic pain) (see references in [23]).

Onset of action in chronic pain

The analgesic response seems to begin before the antidepressant response. An analgesic response is usually observed within 1 week of starting treatment, whereas the antidepressant response usually occurs after 2 weeks (see [1]). A recent randomized, controlled trial of duloxetine in subjects with diabetic neuropathic pain showed a difference between the treated and placebo groups, beginning at week one [24]. However, some studies have demonstrated a considerable time lag before effective neuropathic pain management (eg, Ref. [25]) because of the length of the titration period.

Evaluation of different routes and patterns of administration

The advantages of the various routes of administration are unclear in human beings. Because of a marked first-pass effect, oral bioavailability ranges from 20% to 80% (see [19]). Genetic polymorphism may also play a role in the pronounced pharmacokinetic variability observed with these drugs [26]. Parenteral administration overcomes the problem of first-pass metabolism and results in high plasma concentrations. However, apart from a possible indication in patients unable to swallow, the parenteral route seems to have no other real advantage, despite reports that this route may accelerate the onset of the therapeutic effect [27]. In experimental conditions in animals, the intravenous route gave better results (91% analgesic effects) than the intraperitoneal, subcutaneous, and oral routes (67%, 54%, and 50% analgesia, respectively) (see [11]).

In experimental models of pain and in conditions involving persistent pain (eg, polyarthritis, nerve injury), repeated administrations of antidepressants were more effective than a single acute administration (see references in [11]). There is now considerable evidence that antidepressants do not increase serotonin (5-HT) release at the beginning of treatment because of an activation of somatic 5-HT_{1A} autoreceptors, potentially accounting for their delayed action. Chronic treatment with antidepressants leads to the desensitization of these presynaptic receptors. It may therefore be possible to accelerate the onset of action by combining a specific 5-HT_{1A} antagonist and an antidepressant. This approach has been shown to be more effective in animals with sustained, neurogenic pain [28,29]. In some studies in human beings, the thymoleptic activity of antidepressant has been shown to be enhanced by the concomitant administration of a specific 5-HT_{1A} antagonist [30,31].

Evidence for the clinical efficacy of antidepressants in various painful conditions

Several meta-analyses and reviews of studies dealing with various chronic nonmalignant painful conditions [1,6,32–37] have reported an analgesic effect of antidepressants. Onghena and van Houdenhove [1] found in their meta-analysis a mean ES of 0.64 for patients with chronic pain treated with antidepressants. Tricyclic drugs appeared to be more efficient than heterocyclic drugs (ES equals 0.69 ± 0.1 versus $0.36 + 0.17$). By contrast, serotonergic drugs were not found to be significantly more effective than noradrenergic drugs (ES equals 0.32 ± 0.21 versus 0.4 ± 0.16). Drugs inhibiting both monoamines less selectively (mixed action) were significantly more effective than drugs inhibiting a single monoamine selectively (ES equals 0.73 ± 0.12). These investigators also dealt with rheumatic pain separately, and showed that the ES for rheumatic pain was smaller (0.37 ± 0.19) than that for neuropathic pain. No difference was observed between sedative and nonsedative drugs. Similar results were obtained in other studies.

A critical review of the use of antidepressants in the management of pain, including that experienced by patients with rheumatic conditions [38], found that there was little reason to replace TCAs by SSRIs in pain management. Too few comparative trials have been performed for definitive conclusions to be drawn, but there is a clear trend against the use of SSRIs. McQuay and colleagues [34] compared the effects of various antidepressants on neuropathic pain and found that TCAs were more effective than SSRIs. Similarly, Sindrup and colleagues [33] concluded that TCAs, when administered at optimal doses, were the most effective antidepressants for the treatment of neuropathic pain. The number of patients that must be treated to obtain one patient with a significant response to the active drug (ie, pain reduced by 50%) was two to three. This NNT value was the lowest obtained for any of the various drugs (SSRIs, gabapentin, carbamazepine, capsaicin) tested for this indication [35]. These results were confirmed by two recent meta-analyses [15,39].

Only paroxetine and citalopram were found to have a positive effect on neuropathic pain in some studies included in a review comparing SSRIs with TCAs [23]. Mixed-action antidepressants, such as venlafaxine, milnacipran, and duloxetine, have considerable potential for pain management, because they have both serotonergic and adrenergic effects and are better tolerated than TCAs (lower levels of undesirable blocking of cholinergic, adrenergic, and histaminergic receptors). Venlafaxine has been shown to control neuropathic pain effectively after surgical treatment for breast cancer [40] and in painful neuropathies [41,42] and fibromyalgia [43]. In painful neuropathies [44], the NNT obtained with venlafaxine was greater than that for imipramine (indicating lower efficacy). One recent comparative review also showed a lower percentage of responders to venlafaxine than to imipramine [44]. Duloxetine has been shown to be effective in patients with diabetic neuropathic pain [45,46].

Evidence of analgesic effects of antidepressants in specific musculoskeletal conditions

Antidepressants for treating fibromyalgia syndrome

The authors identified 52 studies on the use of antidepressants in fibromyalgia, including 28 controlled trials, most of which involved TCAs, and five meta-analyses and reviews (Table 2) [54,72–75]. A major placebo effect was identified in early studies of the effects of TCAs on pain in fibromyalgia, and no long-lasting effect of antidepressants has been demonstrated for this condition [72–74]. This effect is similar to that reported for most of the drugs tested for fibromyalgia treatment [72] and may reflect a particular aspect of fibromyalgia syndrome.

Tricyclic antidepressants

Despite their widespread use, TCAs have only a moderate analgesic effect and only a minority of patients display sustained, marked improvement [47–53,55,56,59–61,66,76–78]. When possible to calculate, the authors found an analgesic ES of TCAs in fibromyalgia of 0.23 (confidence interval or CI: −0.35; 0.81) [47] to 1.34 (CI: −0.70; 1.98) [60], with a mean analgesic ES of around 0.50, similar to the results obtained in previous studies of the effects of TCAs in chronic pain conditions [1]. Amitriptyline is the most widely used drug for which an effect on pain, fatigue, sleep, and general condition has been demonstrated [47,49,56,60]. Amitriptyline and cyclobenzaprine begin to act after 1 week, and have a greater effect on sleep disorders and fatigue than on pain [56,66,77], even at low doses [56,60]. Most studies reported the use of TCAs at lower doses than those used to treat depression, as TCAs have been reported to have an effect on fibromyalgia at low doses independently of mood disorders [61]. The adverse effects of TCAs are also a limiting factor for increasing doses in fibromyalgia syndrome.

Selective serotonin reuptake inhibitors

Several studies have assessed the effects of SSRIs, which may be better tolerated than TCAs. Citalopram has a small analgesic ES, from 0.18 (−0.43; 0.78) [58] to 0.45 (−0.23; 1.12). Paroxetine [71,79], even at high doses (up to 62.5 mg per day), has only a weak significant effect on pain and function in fibromyalgia, with an ES of 0.19 (−0.7; 0.56). Fluoxetine has a stronger analgesic ES than citalopram and paroxetine. This ES is dose-related, ranging from 0.45 (−0.38; 1.29) for a dose of 20 mg [57] to 1.08 (0.41; 1.74) at higher doses [59], greater than those used to treat patients with depression. Attempts have been made to combine TCAs and SSRIs [55,59], and this combination has been reported to have a greater analgesic ES. Such combinations seem to be synergic, possibly because of greater drug bioavailability. In conclusion, SSRIs are better tolerated but less effective than TCAs for the treatment of fibromyalgia, making it necessary to increase the dose to obtain significant pain relief and improvement.

Serotonin and noradrenalin reuptake inhibitors

Several studies on fibromyalgia have focused on newer antidepressants, the SNRIs: venlafaxine [43,80], duloxetine [68,69], or milnacipran [70]. With the exception of those dealing with venlafaxine, the methodology and quality of these studies was mostly good, with studies performed over long periods (at least 3 months). Duloxetine (60 mg–120 mg daily, analgesic ES of 0.53 [0.27; 0.79]) and milnacipran (100 mg–200 mg daily, analgesic ES of 0.54 [0.09; 1.03]) have been found to be similarly effective against pain in fibromyalgia. These treatments were significantly more effective than

Table 2
Randomized controlled studies of antidepressants in fibromyalgia syndrome

Author	Treatment	Study design	N of patients	Duration	Analgesic effect size or authors' conclusion	Quality score (Jadad)
Carette [47]	Amitriptyline 50 mg versus placebo	DB, PLA	48	9 weeks	ES: 0.23 [−0.35; 0.81]	3
Bibolotti [48]	Clomipramine 75 mg versus maprotiline 75 mg versus placebo	DB, XO	37	3 weeks	ES not calculable; significant analgesic effect	3
Goldenberg [49]	Amitriptyline 25 mg and naproxen 1,000 mg versus placebo	DB, PLA	62	6 weeks	ES not calculable; no significant effect	3
Bennett [50]	Cyclobenzaprine 10 mg–40 mg versus placebo	DB, PLA	63	12 weeks	ES not calculable; significant analgesic effect	4
Caruso [51]	Dothiepin 75 mg versus placebo	DB, PLA	60	8 weeks	ES not calculable; dothiepin superior to placebo	4
Scudds [52]	Amitriptyline 10 mg–50 mg versus placebo	DB, XO, PLA	36	4 weeks	ES not calculable; amitriptyline superior to placebo	3
Quimby [53]	Cyclobenzaprine up to 40 mg versus placebo	DB	45	3 weeks	ES not calculable; no significant analgesic effect	2
Jaeschke [54]	Amitryptiline 5 mg–50 mg versus placebo	DB, XO, PLA	22	2 weeks	ES not calculable	
Cantini [55]	Fluoxetine 20 mg and cyclobenzaprine 10 mg versus cyclobenzaprine 10 mg	DB	21	12 weeks	Combination better than cyclobenzaprine alone	3
Carette [56]	Amitriptyline 10 mg–50 mg versus cyclobenzaprine 10 mg–30 mg versus placebo	DB, PLA	204	6 months	Amitriptyline ES: 0.30 [−0.10; 0.69]; cyclobenzaprine ES: 0.38 [−0.03; 0.78]	4
Wolfe [57]	Fluoxetine 20 mg versus placebo	DB, PLA	42	6 weeks	ES: 0.45 [−0.38; 1.29]	5
Norregaard [58]	Citalopram 20 mg versus placebo	DB, PLA	42	8 weeks	ES: 0.18 [−0.43; 0.78]	4
Goldenberg [59]	Amitriptyline 25 mg fluoxetine 20 mg versus combination versus placebo	DB, PLA, XO	80	4–6 weeks	Amitriptyline ES: 0.71[0.07; 1.35]; fluoxetine ES: 1.08[0.41; 1.74]; fluoxetine + amiptriptyline ES: 1.63[0.89; 2.39]	3
Ginsberg [60]	Amitriptyline 25 mg (sustained release) versus placebo	DB, PLA	46	8 weeks	ES: 1 34 [−0.70; 1.98].	4

Hannonen [61]	Moclobemide 450 mg–600 mg versus amitriptyline versus placebo	DB, PLA	90	12 weeks	Moclobemide: ES: 0.26 [−0.25; 0.76]; amitriptyline ES: 0.25 [−0.25; 0.75]	5
Olin [62]	Ritanserin versus placebo	DB, PLA	51	16 weeks	ES not calculable; No significant effect.	3
Anderberg [63–65]	Citalopram 20 mg–40 mg versus placebo	DB, PLA	35	4 months	ES 0.45 [−0.23; 1.12]	5
Heymann [66]	Amitriptyline 25 mg versus nortriptyline versus placebo	DB, PLA	118	8 weeks	Amitriptyline ES: 0.54 [0.06; 1.02]; nortriptyline ES: 0.13 [−0.35; 0.60]	3
Arnold [67]	Fluoxetine up to 60 mg versus placebo	DB, PLA	51	12 weeks	ES: 0.90 [0.33;−1.48]	4
Arnold [68]	Duloxetine 120 mg bid versus placebo	DB, PLA	205	12 weeks	ES: 0.22[−0.06; 0.49]	5
Arnold [69]	Duloxetine 60 mg, versus duloxetine 120 mg versus placebo	DB, PLA	348	12 weeks	Duloxetine 60 mg ES: 0.53 [0.27; 0.79]; duloxetine 120 mg ES: 0.54 [0.28; 0.80]	5
Gendreau [70]	Milnacipran 200 mg versus milnacipran 100 mg × 2 versus placebo	DB, PLA	125	12 weeks	Minalcipran 200 mg ES: 0.35 [−0.12; 1.03]; ninalcipran 400 mg ES: 0.56 [0.09; 1.03]	5
Patkar [71]	Paroxetine 12.5 mg–62.5 mg versus placebo	DB, PLA	116	12 weeks	ES: 0.19 [−0.17; 0.56]	5

Abbreviations: bid, twice a day; DB, double-blind; pla, placebo; XO, crossover.

placebo, not only against pain but also for the fibromyalgia impact questionnaire, Tender Points assessments, Clinical Global Impression of Change (assessed both by the patient and the physician), sleep, and fatigue. These effects are independent of depressive symptoms, demonstrating that the analgesic effect is not related to any antidepressive effect of these treatments.

The effects on fibromyalgia of several other antidepressants, including moclobemide, a monoamine oxidase inhibitor [61], and ritanserin [62], have been studied. Moclobemide had no significant effect, and the methodologic quality of the study on ritanserin was too low for any conclusions to be drawn about possible significant effects.

Antidepressants in low back pain

Eleven [81–91] randomized, controlled trials on the use of antidepressants to treat low back pain have been published, and seven reviews have specifically examined the analgesic and functional effects of antidepressants in low back pain (Table 3) [92–98]. TCAs are the antidepressants most frequently tested in low back pain, with only two studies dealing with an SSRI, paroxetine [88,89], one with a noradrenalin reuptake inhibitor (NRI), bupropion [91], and none with SNRIs. Most of these studies were of poor methodologic quality, even lower than for fibromyalgia. Analysis of these studies suggests that antidepressants are no more effective than placebo for the relief of low back pain. Only 3 of the 11 studies demonstrated a significant analgesic effect. Nortriptyline [87], at a dose of 50 mg to 150 mg per day, has a small analgesic ES of 0.45 (0.00; 0.90), amitryptiline, 150 mg [86] has a moderate analgesic ES of 0.63 (−0.01; 1.27), like maprotiline, with an ES of 0.64 (0.06; 1.20). Antidepressants also tend to improve function and everyday activities, although this trend was not found to be statistically significant [81,85]. One study indicated that imipramine was more effective than placebo, but only in terms of the "numbers of days the patient had to lie down" and "number of days with at least some restriction of normal activity" [82]. Another study [83] showed that amitriptyline was better than placebo, comparing the use of rescue analgesics in the two treatment groups.

In conclusion, tricyclic and tetracyclic antidepressants appear to provide moderate relief of symptoms in patients with chronic low back pain, regardless of the patient's depression status. SSRIs seem to be less effective than TCAs [84,88], but the doses tested have been equivalent to those used to treat depression, rather than higher, as tested for fibromyalgia. The effects of antidepressants on health-related quality of life, mood, and functional status in patients with low back pain are unclear [92,97].

Osteoarthritis and inflammatory rheumatic diseases

The authors identified 15 randomized, controlled trials on osteoarthritis (OA), rheumatoid arthritis (RA), and ankylosing spondylitis (AS) (Table 4).

Table 3
Randomized, controlled studies of antidepressants in low back pain

Author	Treatment	Study design	N of patients	Duration (weeks)	Analgesic effect size or authors' conclusion	Quality score (Jadad)
Jenkins [81]	Imipramine 75 mg versus placebo	RCT, DB, PLA	44	4	ES not calculable; no significant effect	2
Alcoff [82]	Imipramine 150 mg versus placebo	RCT, DB, pla	40	8	ES not calculable; no significant effect	2
Pheasant [83]	Amitriptyline 50 mg versus placebo	RCT, DB, PLA, XO	16	16	ES not calculable; amitriptyline superior to placebo	2
Goodkin [84]	Trazodone 50 mg–600 mg versus placebo	DB, PLA	42	6	ES: 0.19 [−0.43; 0.81]	5
Treves [85]	Clomipramine 70 mg–75 mg versus placebo	RCT, DB, PLA	68	48	ES not calculable; clomipramine superior to placebo	2
Stein [86]	Amitriptyline 150 mg versus acetaminophen 2 g	RCT, DB	39	5	ES: 0.63 [−0.01; 1.27]	3
Atkinson [87]	Nortriptyline 50 mg–150 mg versus placebo	RCT, DB, PLA	78	8	ES: 0.45 [0.00; 0.90]	5
Atkinson [88]	Maprotiline 150 mg versus paroxetine 30 mg versus placebo	RCT, DB, PLA	173	8	Maprotiline: ES: 0.64 [0.06; 1.20]; paroxetine: ES: 0.14 [−0.40; 0.69]	5
Dickens [89]	Paroxetine 20 mg versus placebo	RCT,DB, PLA, XO	92	8	ES not calculable; no significant effect	2
Schreiber [90]	Amitriptyline 50 mg–75 mg; fluoxetine 20 mg	RCT, SB, no PLA	40	6	ES not calculable; no significant difference	2
Katz [91]	Bupropion 150 mg–300 mg versus placebo	RCT, DB, PLA, XO	44	6	ES not calculable; no significant effect	3

Abbreviation: RCT, randomized, controlled trial.

Table 4
Randomized, controlled studies of antidepressants in osteoarthritis and inflammatory rheumatic diseases

Author	Treatment	Study design	Number of patients	Duration (weeks)	Analgesic effect size or authors' conclusions	Quality score (Jadad)
McDonald [99]	Imipramine 75 mg versus placebo	DB, PLA, XO	24 OA, RA, AS	6	ES not calculable	2
Thorpe [100]	Dibenzepin 240 mg versus placebo	DB, PLA	OA = 31 RA = 13	13	ES not calculable; dibenzepin superior to placebo	4
Gingras [101]	Imipramine 50 mg–75 mg versus placebo	DB, PLA, XO	65 OA, RA, AS	8	ES not calculable; imipramine superior to placebo.	3
McNeil [102]	Imipramine 75 mg versus placebo	DB, PLA	20 RA	6	ES not calculable; Imipramine superior to placebo	2
Ganvir [103]	Clomipramine 25 mg versus placebo	DB, PLA	74 OA	8	ES: 0 [−0.81; 0.81]	2
Grace [104]	Amitriptyline 25 mg–75 mg versus placebo	DB, PLA	36 RA	12	ES not calculable; no significant effect	2
McFarlane [105]	Trimipramine 25 mg–75 mg versus placebo	DB, PLA	36 RA	12	ES: 1.22 [0.40; 2.04]	4
Wheatley [106]	Mianserine versus nomifensine versus placebo	DB, PLA	111 OA, RA, AS	8	ES not calculable; no significant effect	2
Franck [107]	Amitriptyline 1 mg/kg–3 mg/kg versus desipramine versus trazodone versus placebo	DB, PLA, XO	99 RA	32	ES not calculable; amitriptyline superior to placebo.	2

Sarzi-Puttini [108]	Dothiepin 75 mg + ibuprofen 1,800 mg versus placebo + ibuprofen 1,800 mg	DB PLA	60 RA	6	ES not calculable	0
Usha Rani [109]	Fluoxetine 20 mg versus amitriptyline 25 mg versus placebo	DB, PLA	59 LBP, OA, RA, FM	4	Fluoxetine: ES: 1.04 [0.37; 1.71]; amitriptyline ES: 0.35 [−0.30; 0.99]	2
Koh [110]	Amitriptyline 10 mg–30 mg versus placebo	DB, PLA	88 AS	2	ES: 0 [−0.35; 0.48]	3
Ash [111]	Dothiepin 75 mg–150 mg versus placebo	DB PLA	48 RA and depression	10	ES: 0.72 [0.14; 1.34]	4
Bird [112]	Amitriptyline 75 mg–150 mg versus paroxetine 20 mg–40 mg	DB PLA	191 RA	8	ES not calculable; No significant effect	4

Abbreviations: FM, fibromyalgia; LBP, low back pain.

Fourteen of these studies were placebo-controlled and one compared amitriptyline with paroxetine. Only eight of these 15 trials were considered to meet minimum standards for methodologic quality to demonstrate efficacy [99,103–105,107,108,110–112], and ES was calculated in only five studies because of a lack of available data. A significant analgesic ES was found in three studies, with trimipramine [104], amitriptyline [101], and dothiepin [108].

In most of these trials, subjects with different joint diseases were pooled (OA, RA, and AS). In some studies, subjects with depressive disorders associated with joint diseases were included [107,108]. However, in the study performed by Lin [113], in a large and diverse population of older adults with arthritis (mostly OA) and comorbid depression, the benefits of improvements in depression care extended beyond the reduction of depressive symptoms, with decreases in pain and improvements in functional status and quality of life also observed.

In conclusion, TCAs may have analgesic effects in patients with RA, with or without depressive symptoms. Low doses of amitriptyline (10 mg–30 mg daily) may be sufficient for an analgesic effect [102,114] in RA. Amitriptyline may be effective for the reduction of symptoms in AS after 1 week of treatment. This analgesic effect has not been confirmed with other antidepressants [106], but no study on SNRIs has ever been published for these conditions. No specific studies have been performed on OA either, with OA cases being pooled with RA and AS; it is therefore difficult to determine whether antidepressants are beneficial for pain related to osteoarthritis [51,100,101,103,109].

Side effects of antidepressants and their management

The side effects of antidepressants are related to their pharmacologic properties [115–118]. The blockade of muscarinic cholinergic receptors may lead to dysuria, constipation, mouth dryness, drowsiness, eye accommodation disorders, tachycardia, memory disorders, and confusion. The blockade of $\alpha 1$-noradrenergic receptors may induce orthostatic hypotension, tachycardia, and dizziness. The blockade of histaminic H_1 receptors may result in sedation, somnolence, and weight gain. Trembling, tachycardia, and impotence have also been attributed to noradrenalin reuptake inhibition. Serotonin reuptake inhibition may cause nausea, somnolence, drowsiness, and fatigue, and may induce a serotonergic syndrome. New antidepressants, such as venlafaxine, minalcipran, and duloxetine may also induce specific side effects (eg, hypertension for venlafaxine) but have no anticholinergic effects and do not blockade alpha and histaminic H_1 receptors.

Imipraminic drugs

Imipraminic drugs, including TCAs in particular, my cause side effects in 30% to 100% of patients treated for painful conditions [11,34]. Side effects are more frequent in fibromyalgia, occurring in 70% to 95% of cases [47,75]. The side effects parallel the analgesic effects and, in most cases, are dose-dependent [114,119]. Rapid washout may lead to severe symptoms, such as nausea, vomiting, and trembling [120,121]. Before starting TCA treatment, the physician should check for orthostatic hypotension and perform an ECG. No recommendations have yet been published with a view to preventing the side effects of TCAs. The effects of combined treatment with tramadol should also be monitored [122,123].

Selective serotonin reuptake inhibitors

SSRIs have been shown to be generally well tolerated. The most frequent side effects are digestive disorders (nausea, vomiting, diarrhea, and other disorders) particularly at the start of treatment. In exceptional cases, these compounds may also induce a serotonergic syndrome. This may account for the lower frequency of patients stopping treatment with SSRIs than with TCAs [109,112,120] in pain studies. Some studies of SSRIs in patients with fibromyalgia have shown these drugs to be as well tolerated as placebo [55,57,58], increasing the likelihood of their being prescribed. Furthermore, no tests are required before starting SSRI treatment.

Summary

Antidepressants have been shown to have analgesic effects in rheumatologic conditions and should be tested in patients with chronic pain, especially when classic analgesic treatments have failed [21,95,124]. This article shows that antidepressants are effective in specific pain syndromes, such as fibromyalgia. The results obtained for RA, AS, OA, and low back pain are less convincing, existing studies being of poor methodologic quality, and further studies are needed. TCAs appear to be more effective, although less well tolerated, than SSRIs. SSRIs have weak analgesic effects, and it may be necessary to use these drugs at higher doses to obtain more marked analgesic effects. The newer antidepressants, SNRIs (venlafaxine, milnacipran, duloxetine), and SNERIs (selective norepinephrine or noradrenalin reuptake inhibitors; reboxetine) appear to be promising treatments for fibromyalgia and their use for other chronic pain indications is in development. Further pharmacologic studies on pain, and studies of the pathophysiology of pain in musculoskeletal conditions, are required. Efforts should be made to identify the most appropriate antidepressant for use in each painful chronic rheumatologic condition.

References

[1] Onghena P, van Houdenhove B. Antidepressant-induced analgesia in chronic non-malignant pain: a meta-analysis of 39 placebo-controlled studies. Pain 1992;49:205–19.

[2] Lynch EM. Antidepressants as analgesics: a review of randomised controlled trials. J Psychiatry Neurosci 2001;26:30–6.
[3] Zitman FG, Linssen A, Edelbroek PM, et al. Clinical effectiveness of antidepressants and antipsychotics in chronic benign pain. Clin Neuropharmacol 1992;15(S1):377A–8.
[4] Barkin RL, Fawcett J. The management challenges of chronic pain: the role of antidepressants. Am J Ther 2000;7:31–47.
[5] Egbunike IG, Chaffe BJ. Antidepressants in the management of chronic syndromes. Pharmacotherapy 1990;10:262–70.
[6] Phillip M, Fickinger M. Psychotropic drugs in the management of chronic pain syndromes. Pharmacopsychiatry 1993;26:221–34.
[7] Sindrup SH. Antidepressants as analgesics. In: Yaksh TL, Lynch C 3rd, Zapol WM, et al, editors. Anesthesia; biologic foundations. Philadelphia: Lippincott-Raven; 1997.
[8] Perrot S, Maheu E, Javier RM, et al. Guidelines for the use of antidepressants in painful rheumatic conditions. Eur J Pain 2006;10:185–92.
[9] Jadad AR, Moore RA, Carroll D, et al. Assessing the quality of reports of randomized clinical trials: is blinding necessary? Control Clin Trials 1996;17:1–12.
[10] Shekelle PG, Woolf SH, Eccles M, et al. Clinical guidelines: developing guidelines. BMJ 1999;318:593–6.
[11] Eschalier A, Ardid D, Dubray C. Tricyclic and other antidepressants as analgesics. In: Sawynok J, Cowan A, editor. Novel Aspects of pain management: opioids and beyond. 1999; 15:303–319.
[12] Sawynok J, Esser MJ, Reid AR. Antidepresssants as analgesics: an overview of central and peripheral mechanisms of action. J Psychiatry Neurosci 2001;26:21–9.
[13] Blier P, Abbott FV. Putative mechanisms of action of antidepressant drugs in affective and anxiety disorders and pain. J Psychiatry Neurosci 2001;26:37–43.
[14] Bryson HM, Wilde MI. Amitriptyline. A review of its pharmacological properties and therapeutic use in chronic pain states. Drugs Aging 1996;8:459–76.
[15] Finnerup NB, Otto M, McQuay HJ, et al. Algorithm for neuropathic pain treatment: an evidence based propos. Pain 2005;118:289–305.
[16] Mico JA, Ardid D, Berrococo E, et al. Antidepressants and pain. Trends Pharmacol Sci 2006;27:348–54.
[17] Hood SD, Argyropoulos SV, Nutt DJ. Arthritis and serotoninergic antidepressants. J Clin Psychopharmacol 2001;24:458–61.
[18] Sindrup SH, Grodum E, Gram LF, et al. Concentration response relationship of paroxetine treatment in diabetic neuropathy: a patient-blinded dose escalation study. Ther Durg Monit 1991;13:408–14.
[19] Furlanut M, Benetello P, Spina E. Pharmacokinetic optimisation of tricyclic antidepressant therapy. Clin Pharmacokinet 1993;24:301–18.
[20] McQuay HJ, Carroll D, Glynn CJ. Low-dose amitriptyline in the treatment of chronic pain. Anaesthesia 1992;47:646–52.
[21] Sullivan MD, Robinson JP. Antidepressant and anticonvulsant medication for chronic pain. Phys Med Rehabil Clin N Am 2006;17:381–400.
[22] Rasmussen PV, Jensen TS, Sindrup SH, et al. TDM-based imipramine treatment in neuropathic pain. Ther Drug Monit 2004;26:352–60.
[23] Ansari A. The efficacy of newer antidepressants in the treatment of chronic pain: a review of current literature. Harv Rev Psychiatry 2000;7:257–77.
[24] Wernicke JF, Pritchett YL, D'Souza DN, et al. A randomized controlled trial of duloxetine in diabetic peripheral neuropathic pain. Neurology 2006;67(8):1411–20.
[25] Max MB, Zeigler D, Shoaf SE, et al. Effects of single oral dose of desipramine on postoperative morphine analgesia. J Pain Symptom Manage 1992;7:454–62.
[26] Rollins DE, Alvin G, Bertilsson L, et al. Interindividual differences in amitriptyline demethylation. Clin Pharmacol Ther 1980;1:121–9.

[27] Pollock BG, Perel JM, Shostac M, et al. Understanding the response lag to tricycles: application of pulse loading regimens with intravenous clomipramine. Psychopharmacol Bull 1986;22:214–9.
[28] Ardid D, Alloui A, Brousse G, et al. Potentiation of the antinociceptive effect of clomipramine by a 5-ht_{1A} antagonist in neuropathic pain in rats. Br J Pharmacol 2001;132:1118–26.
[29] Marchand F, Pelissier T, Eschalier A, et al. Blockade of supraspinal 5-HT1a receptors potentiates the inhibitory effect of venlafaxine on wind-up activity in mononeuropathic rats. Brain Res 2004;1008:288–92.
[30] Artigas F, Perez V, Alvarez E. Pindolol induces a rapid improvement of depressed patients treated with serotonin reuptake inhibitors. Arch Gen Psychiatry 1994;51:248–51.
[31] Blier P, Bergeron R. Effectiveness of pindolol with selected antidepressant drugs in the treatment of major depression. J Clin Psychopharmacol 1995;15:217–22.
[32] Magni G. The use of antidepressants in the treatment of chronic pain. A review of the current evidence. Drugs 1991;42:730–48.
[33] Sindrup SH, Brosen K, Gram LF. Antidepressant in pain treatment: antidepressant or analgesic effect? Clin Neuropharmacol 1992;15:636A–7A.
[34] McQuay HJ, Tramèr M, Nye BA, et al. A systematic review of antidepressants in neuropathic pain. Pain 1996;68:217–27.
[35] Sindrup Soren H, Jensen Troels S. Efficacy of pharmacological treatments of neuropathic pain: an update and effect related to mechanism of drug action. Pain 1999;83:389–400.
[36] Richardson PH, de Wiliams A. Meta-analysis of antidepressant-induced analgesia in chronic pain: comment. Pain 1993;52:247–9.
[37] Fishbain DA, Cutler RB, Rosomoff HL, et al. Do antidepressants have an analgesic effect in psychogenic pain and somatoform pain disorder: a meta-analysis. Psychosom Med 1998; 60:503–9.
[38] Smith AJ. The analgesic effects of selective serotonin reuptake inhibitors. J Psychopharmacol 1998;12:407–13.
[39] Attal N, Cruccu G, Hanpaa M, et al. EFNS guidelines on pharmacological treatment of neuropathic pain. Eur J Neurol 2006;13:1153–60.
[40] Tasmuth T, Hartel B, Kalso E. Venlafaxine in neuropathic pain following treatment of breast cancer. Eur J Pain 2002;6:17–24.
[41] Sindrup SH, Bach FW, Madsen C, et al. Venlafaxine versus imipramine in painful polyneuropathy: a randomized, controlled trial. Neurology 2003;60:1284–9.
[42] Rowbotham MC, Goli V, Kuntz NR, et al. Velafaxine extended release in the treatment of painful diabetic neuropathy: a double-blind, placebo-controlled study. Pain 2004;110: 697–706.
[43] Sayar K, Aksu G, Ak I, et al. Venlafaxine treatment of fibromyalgia. Ann Pharmacother 2003;37:1561–5.
[44] Sindrup SH, Otto M, Finnerup NB, et al. Antidepressants in the treatment of neuropathic pain. Basic Clin Pharmacol Toxicol 2005;96:399–409.
[45] Goldstein DJ, Lu Y, Detke MJ, et al. Duloxetine vs placebo in patients with painful diabetic neuropathy. Pain 2005;116:109–18.
[46] Raskin J, Wang F, Pritchett YL, et al. Duloxetine for patients with diabetic peripheral neuropathic pain: a 6-month open-label safety study. Pain Med 2006;7:373–85.
[47] Carette S, McCain GA, Bell DA, et al. Evaluation of amitriptyline in primary fibrositis. A double-blinded, placebo-controlled study. Arthritis Rheum 1986;29:655–9.
[48] Bibolotti E, Borghi C, Pasculli E, et al. The management of fibrositis. A double-blind comparison of maprotiline (Ludiomil) clorimipramine and placebo. Clin Trials J 1986;23: 269–80.
[49] Goldenberg DL, Felson DT, Dinerman H. A randomised, controlled trial of amitriptyline and naproxene in the treatment of patients with fibromyalgia. Arthritis Rheum 1986;29: 1371–7.

[50] Bennett RM, Gatter RA, Campbell SM, et al. A comparison of cyclobenzaprine and placebo in the management of fibrositis. A double-blind controlled study. Arthritis Rheum 1988;31(12):1535–42.
[51] Caruso I, Sarzi Puttini PC, Boccassini L, et al. Double-blind study of dothiepin versus placebo in the treatment of primary fibromyalgia syndrome. J Int Med Res 1987;15: 154–9.
[52] Scudds RA, McCain GA, Rollman GB, et al. Improvements in pain responsiveness in patients with fibrositis after successful treatment with amitriptyline. J Rheumatol Suppl 1989; 19:98–103.
[53] Quimby LG, Gratwick GM, Whitney CD. Block SR A randomized trial of cyclobenzaprine for the treatment of fibromyalgia. J Rheumatol Suppl 1989;19:140–3.
[54] Jaeschke R, Adachi J, Guyatt G, et al. Clinical usefulness of amitriptyline in fibromyalgia: the results of 23 N-of-1 randomized controlled trials. J Rheumatol 1991;18:447–51.
[55] Cantini F, Bellandi F, Niccoli L, et al. Fluoxetina associata a ciclobenzaprina nel trattamento della fibromialgia. Minerva Med 1994;85:97–100.
[56] Carette S, Bell MJ, John Reynolds W, et al. Comparison of amitriptyline, cyclobenzaprine, and placebo in the treatment of fibromyalgia. Arthritis Rheum 1994;37:32–40.
[57] Wolfe F, Cathey MA, Hawley DJ. A double-blind placebo controlled trial of fluoxetine in fibromyalgia. Scand J Rheumatol 1994;23:255–9.
[58] Norregard J, Volkmann H, Danneskiold-Samsoe B. A randomized controlled study of citalopram in the treatment of fibromyalgia. Pain 1995;61:445–9.
[59] Goldenberg D, Mayskiy M, Mossey C, et al. A randomized, double-blind crossover trial of fluoxetine and amitriptyline in the treatment of fibromyalgia. Arthritis Rheum 1996;39: 1852–9.
[60] Ginsberg F, Mancaux A, Joos E, et al. A randomized placebo-controlled trial of sustained-release amitriptyline in primary fibromyalgia. J Musculoskeletal Pain 1996;4:37–47.
[61] Hannonen P, Malminiemi K, Yli-Kerttula U, et al. A randomized, double-blind, placebo-controlled study of moclobemide and amitriptyline in the treatment of fibromyalgia in females without psychiatric disorder. Br J Rheumatol 1998;37:1279–86.
[62] Olin R, Klein R, Berg PA. A randomised double-blind 16-week study of ritanserin in fibromyalgia syndrome: clinical outcome and analysis of autoantibodies to serotonin, gangliosides and phospholipids. Clin Rheumatol 1998;17:89–94.
[63] Anderberg UA, Marteinsdottir I, von Knorring L. Citalopram in patients with fibromyalgia—a randomised, double-blind, placebo-controlled study. Eur J Pain 2000;4:27–35.
[64] Geller SA. Treatment of fibrositis with fluoxetine hydrochloride (Prozac®). Am J Med 1989;87:594–5.
[65] Cortet B, Houvenagel E, Forzy G, et al. Evaluation de l'efficacité d'un traitement sérotoninergique (chlorhydrate de fluoxetine). Etude ouverte au cours de la fibromyalgie. Rev Rhum Mal Osteoartic 1992;59:497–500.
[66] Heymann RE, Helfenstein M, Feldman D. A double-blind, randomised, controlled study of amitriptyline, nortriptyline and placebo in patients with fibromyalgia. An analysis of outcome measures. Clin Exp Rheumatol 2001;19:697–702.
[67] Arnold LM, Hess EV, Hudson JI, et al. A randomized, placebo-controlled, double-blind, flexible-dose study of fluoxetine in the treatment of women with fibromyalgia. Am J Med 2002;112:191–7.
[68] Arnold LM, Lu Y, Crofford LJ, et al. A double-blind, multicenter trial comparing duloxetine with placebo in the treatment of fibromyalgia patients with or without major depressive disorder. Arthritis Rheum 2004;50:2974–84.
[69] Arnold LM, Rosen A, Pritchett YL, et al. A randomised, double-blind, placebo-controlled trial of duloxetine in the treatment of women with fibromyalgia with or without major depressive disorder. Pain 2005;119:5–15.
[70] Gendreau RM, Thorn MD, Gendreau JF, et al. Efficacy of milnacipran in patients with fibromyalgia. J Rheumatol 2005;32:1975–85.

[71] Patkar AA, Masand PS, Krulewicz S, et al. A randomized, controlled, trial of controlled-release paroxetine in fibromyalgia. Am J Med 2007;120:448–54.
[72] White KP, Harth M. An analytical review of 24 controlled clinical trials of fibromyalgia syndrome (FMS). Pain 1996;64:211–9.
[73] O'Malley PG, Balden E, Tornkins G, et al. Treatment of fibromyalgia with antidepressants. A meta-analysis. J Gen Intern Med 2000;15:659–66.
[74] Arnold LM, Keck PE, Welge JA. Antidepressant treatment of fibromyalgia. A meta-analysis and review. Psychosomatics 2000;41:104–13.
[75] Moret C, Briley M. Antidepressants in the treatment of fibromyalgia. Neuropsychiatr Dis Treat 2006;2:537–48.
[76] Hamaty D, Valentine JL, Howard R, et al. The plasma endorphin, prostaglandin and catecholamine profile of patients with fibrositis treated with cyclobenzaprine and placebo: a 5-month study. J Rheumatol Suppl 1989;19:164–8.
[77] Reynolds WJ, Moldofsky H, Saskin P, et al. The effects of cyclobenzaprine on sleep physiology and symptoms in patients with fibromyalgia. J Rheumatol 1991;18:452–4.
[78] Fossaluzza V, De Vita S. Combined therapy with cyclobenzaprine and ibuprofen in primary fibromyalgia syndrome. Int J Clin Pharmacol Res 1992;XII:99–102.
[79] Ataoglu S, Ataoglu A, Erdoan F, et al. Comparison of paroxetine, amitriptyline in the treatment of fibromyalgia. Turkish Journal of Medical Sciences 1997;27:535–9.
[80] Dwight MM, Arnold LD, O'Brien H, et al. An open trial of venlafaxine treatment of fibromyalgia. Psychosomatics 1998;39:14–7.
[81] Jenkins DG, Ebbutt AF, Evans CD. Tofranil in the treatment of low back pain. J Int Med Res 1976;4:28–40.
[82] Alcoff J, Jones E, Rust P, et al. Controlled trial of imipramine for chronic low back pain. J Fam Pract 1982;14:841–6.
[83] Pheasant H, Bursk A, Godfarb J, et al. Amitriptyline and chronic low back pain. Spine 1983;8:552 7.
[84] Goodkin K, Gullion DM, Agras WS. A randomized, double-blind, placebo controlled trial of trazodone hydrochloride in chronic low back pain syndrome. J Clin Psychopharmacol 1990;10:269–78.
[85] Trèves R, Montane de la Roque P, Dumond JJ, et al. Etude prospective de l'action antalgique de la clomipramine versus placebo dans les lombosciatalgies rebelles (68 cas). Rev Rhum 1991;58:549–52.
[86] Stein D, Peri T, Edelstein E, et al. The efficacy of amitriptyline and acetaminophen in the management of acute low back pain. Psychosomatics 1996;36:63–70.
[87] Atkinson JH, Slater MA, Williams RA, et al. A placebo-controlled randomised clinical trial of nortriptyline for chronic low back pain. Pain 1998;76:287–96.
[88] Atkinson JH, Slater MA, Wahlgreen DR, et al. Effects of noradrenergic and serotoninergic antidepressants on chronic low back pain. Pain 1999;83:137–45.
[89] Dickens C, Jayson M, Sutton C, et al. The relationship between pain and depression in a trial using paroxetine in sufferers of chronic low back pain. Psychosomatics 2000;41: 490–9.
[90] Schreiber S, Vinokur S, Shavelzon V, et al. A randomized trial of fluoxetine versus amitriptyline in musculoskeletal pain. Isr J Psychiatry Relat Sci 2001;38:88–94.
[91] Katz J, Pennella-Vaughan J, Hetzel RD, et al. A randomised placebo-controlled trial of bupropion sustained release in chronic low back pain. J Pain 2005;6:656–61.
[92] Ward NG. Tricyclic antidepressants for chronic low back pain. Spine 1986;11:661–5.
[93] Turner JA, Denny MC. Do antidepressant agents relieve chronic low back pain? J Fam Pract 1993;37:545–53.
[94] van Tulder MW, Koes BW, Bouter LM. Conservative treatment of acute and chronic nonspecific low back pain. Spine 1997;22:2128–56.
[95] Fishbain D. Evidence-based data on pain relief with antidepressants. Ann Med 2000;32: 305–16.

[96] Salerno SM, Browning R, Jackson JL. The effect of antidepressant treatment on chronic back pain. Arch Intern Med 2002;162:19–24.
[97] Staiger TO, Gaster B, Sullivan MD, et al. Systematic review of antidepressants in the treatment of chronic low back pain. Spine 2003;28:2540–5.
[98] Schnitzer TJ, Ferraro A, Hunsche E, et al. A comprehensive review of clinical trials on the efficacy and safety of drugs for the treatment of low back pain. J Pain Symptom Manage 2004;28:72–95.
[99] McDonald Scott WA. The relief of pain with an antidepressant in arthritis. Practitioner 1969;202:802–7.
[100] Thorpe P, Marchant-Williams R. The role of an antidepressant, dibenzepin (Noveril), in the relief of pain in chronic arthritic states. Med J Aust 1974;1:264–6.
[101] Gringras M. A clinical trial of tofranil in rheumatic pain in general practice. J Int Med Res 1976;4(Suppl 2):41–9.
[102] MacNeill AL, Dick WC. Imipramine and rheumatoid factor. J Int Med Res 1976; 4(Suppl 2):23–7.
[103] Ganvir P, Beaumont G, Seldrup J. A comparative trial of clomipramine and placebo as adjunctive therapy in arthralgia. J Int Med Res 1980;8(Suppl):60–6.
[104] Grace EM, Bellamy N, Kassam Y, et al. Controlled, double-blind, randomized trial of amitriptyline in relieving articular pain and tenderness in patients with rheumatoid arthritis. Curr Med Res Opin 1985;9:426–9.
[105] Macfarlane JG, Jalali S, Grace EM. Trimipramine in rheumatoid arthritis: a randomized double-blind trial in relieving pain and joint tenderness. Curr Med Res Opin 1986;10(2): 89–93.
[106] Wheatley D. Antidepressants in elderly arthritics. Practitioner 1986;230:477–81.
[107] Frank RG, Kashani JH, Parker JC, et al. Antidepressant analgesia in rheumatoid arthritis. J Rheumatol 1988;15:1632–8.
[108] Sarzi Puttini P, Cazzola M, Boccassini L, et al. A comparison of dothiepin versus placebo in the treatment of pain in rheumatoid arthritis and the association of pain with depression. J Int Med Res 1988;16:331–7.
[109] Usha Rani P, Naidu MU, Prasad VB, et al. An evaluation of antidepressants in rheumatic pain conditions. Anesth Analg 1996;83:371–5.
[110] Koh WH, Pande I, Samuels A, et al. Low-dose amitriptyline in ankylosing spondylitis: a short-term, double-blind, placebo-controlled study. J Rheumatol 1997;4:2158–61.
[111] Ash G, Dickens CM, Creed FH, et al. The effects of dothiepin on subjects with rheumatoid arthritis and depression. Rheumatology (Oxford) 1999;38:959–67.
[112] Bird H, Broggini M. Paroxetine versus amitriptyline for treatment of depression associated with rheumatoid arthritis: a randomized, double blind, parallel group study. J Rheumatol 2000;27:2791–7.
[113] Lin EH, Katon W, Von Korff M, et al. Effect of improving depression care on pain and functional outcomes among older adults with arthritis: a randomized controlled trial. JAMA 2003;290:2428–9.
[114] McQuay HJ, Carroll D, Glynn CJ. Dose-response for analgesic effect of amitriptyline in chronic pain. Anaesthesia 1993;48:281–5.
[115] Baldessarini RJ. Drugs and the treatment of psychiatric disorders. In: Goodman Gilman A, Rall TTW, Nies AS, et al, editors. The Pharmacological basis of therapeutics, vol. 8. New York: Pergamon Press; 1990. p. 383–435.
[116] Loo J, Poirier MF, Brochier T, et al. Editions techniques, Encycl. Med Chir. (Paris-France). Psychiatrie 1995;37-860-B-72:14.
[117] Glassman AH, Bigger JT. Cardiovascular effects of therapeutic doses of tricyclic antidepressants. Arch Gen Psychiatry 1981;36:815–9.
[118] Thayssen P, Bjerre M, Kragh-Sørensen P, et al. Cardiovascular effects of imipramine and nortriptyline in elderly patients. Psychopharmacology 1981;74:360–4.

[119] Watson C, Peter N. Antidepressant drugs as adjuvant analgesics. J Pain Symptom Manage 1994;9:392–405.
[120] Sindrup SH, Gram LF, Brøsen K, et al. The selective serotonin reuptake inhibitor paroxetine is effective in the treatment of diabetic neuropathy symptoms. Pain 1990;42:135–44.
[121] Rosenbaum JF, Fava M, Hoog SL. Selective serotonin reuptake inhibitors discontinuation syndrome. A randomized clinical trial. Biol Psychiatry 1998;44:77–87.
[122] Reus VI, Rawitscher L. Possible interaction of tramadol and antidepressants. Am J Psychiatry 2000;157:839.
[123] Gardner JS, Blough D, Drinkard CR, et al. Tramadol and seizures: a surveillance study in a managed care population. Pharmacotherapy 2000;20:1423–31.
[124] Curatolo M, Bogduk N. Pharmacologic pain treatment of musculoskeletal disorders: current perspectives and future prospects. Clin J Pain 2001;17:25–32.

ELSEVIER
SAUNDERS

Rheum Dis Clin N Am
34 (2008) 455–467

RHEUMATIC
DISEASE CLINICS
OF NORTH AMERICA

Complementary Treatments in Rheumatic Diseases

Edzard Ernst, MD, PhD, FRCP, FRCPEd

Complementary Medicine, Peninsula Medical School, Universities of Exeter and Plymouth, 25 Victoria Park Road, Exeter EX2 4NT, UK

Many rheumatic patients use complementary treatments, making it an important topic [1]. The subject of complementary treatments is also perplexing and controversial. The confusion starts with the definition of complementary treatments. They are commonly defined negatively as, for example, not plausible, not scientific, or not accepted, which is hardly satisfactory. Our positive definition, on the other hand, is hardly explicit: "Complementary medicine is diagnosis, treatment and/or prevention that complements mainstream medicine by contributing to a common whole, by satisfying a demand not met by orthodoxy or by diversifying the conceptual frameworks of medicine" [2]. So perhaps it is best to simply list some of the most important modalities and their descriptions (Table 1) and explain that most have several "characteristics" in common:

- They accommodate a whole person approach.
- They permit a high degree of individualization.
- They have image of being natural and safe.
- They have a long history of use.

Closer scrutiny discloses these "characteristics" as postulates or perhaps even advertising slogans, which may or may not be true. What, for instance, is natural about sticking needles into patients' skin (as in acupuncture)? And hemlock is clearly natural, but is it safe?

Our perplexity continues when we ask why so many people try complementary therapies. Arguably, conventional medicine is today better than ever, so why turn one's back on it? One answer to this complex question is that most users of complementary medicine use it not instead of but as an adjunct to mainstream health care. Furthermore, most users of complementary medicine have more than one reason for doing so (Box 1).

E-mail address: edzard.ernst@pms.ac.uk

doi:10.1016/j.rdc.2008.03.007 ***rheumatic.theclinics.com***

Table 1
Some of the most popular complementary therapies

Name	Description
Acupuncture	Insertion of a needle into the skin and underlying tissues in special sites, known as points, for therapeutic or preventive purposes
Aromatherapy	The controlled use of plant essences for therapeutic purposes
Bach flower remedies	A therapeutic system that uses specially prepared plant infusions to balance physical and emotional disturbances
Biofeedback	The use of apparatus to monitor, amplify, and feed back information on physiologic responses so that a patient can learn to regulate these responses; it is a form of psychophysiological self-regulation
Chelation therapy	A method for removing toxins, minerals, and metabolic wastes from the bloodstream and vessel walls using intravenous ethylene diamine tetra-acetic acid infusions
Chiropractic	A system of health care based on the belief that the nervous system is the most important determinant of health and that most diseases are caused by spinal subluxations that respond to spinal manipulation
Craniosacral therapy	A proprietary form of therapeutic manipulation that is tissue-, fluid-, membrane-, and energy-orientated and more subtle than any other type of cranial work
Herbalism	The medical use of preparations that contain exclusively plant material
Homoeopathy	A therapeutic method using preparations of substances whose effects when administered to healthy subjects correspond to the manifestations of the disorder (symptoms, clinical signs, and pathologic states) in the unwell patient
Hypnotherapy	The induction of a trancelike state to facilitate the relaxation of the conscious mind and make use of enhanced suggestibility to treat psychologic and medical conditions and effect behavioral changes
Massage	A method of manipulating the soft tissue of whole body areas using pressure and traction
Naturopathy	An eclectic system of health care that integrates elements of complementary and conventional medicine to support and enhance self-healing processes
Osteopathy	Form of manual therapy involving massage, mobilization, and spinal manipulation
Reflexology	A therapeutic method that uses manual pressure applied to specific areas, or zones, of the feet (and sometimes the hands or ears) believed to correspond to areas of the body; the method is meant to relieve stress and prevent and treat physical disorders
Relaxation therapy	Techniques for eliciting the "relaxation response" of the autonomic nervous system
Spiritual healing	The direct interaction between one individual (the healer) and a second (sick) individual with the intention of bringing about an improvement or cure of the illness
Yoga	A practice of gentle stretching, exercises for breath control, and meditation as a mind–body intervention

Box 1. Positive and negative motivations for trying complementary therapies

Positive motivations

Hope that complementary therapies will improve well-being and provide other positive outcomes
Belief that complementary therapies are congruent with personal philosophies
- Offers spiritual dimension
- Is consistent with emphasis on holism
- Accommodates active role of patient
- Supports explanation that is intuitively acceptable
- Is natural

Desire for personal control over treatment
Satisfaction with relationship with therapist
- Creates sense of being on equal terms
- Provides time for discussion
- Allows for emotional factors

Is accessible

Negative motivations

Dissatisfaction with certain aspects of conventional medicine
- Found conventional medicine ineffective
- Worried about adverse effects of conventional medicine
- Experienced poor communication with health care practitioner
- Unable to schedule sufficient time with health care practitioner

Total rejection of conventional medicine
- Has antiscience or antiestablishment attitude

Desperation

In this article, I address the question: Which complementary therapies are effective for reducing pain in which rheumatic conditions? As this is a vast field, I confine myself to treatments that are, according to the totality of the available trial data, likely to be effective. Also, I focus on just six conditions relevant to rheumatologists: back pain, fibromyalgia, myofascial pain, neck pain, osteoarthritis, and rheumatoid arthritis. I base my deliberations on a recent book written by myself and colleagues. The book evaluated the entire field of complementary medicine in a transparent and evidence-based fashion [3].

Back pain

Acupuncture/acupressure

Two current meta-analyses have generated cautiously positive results [4,5]. An analysis by the author and colleagues included 33 randomized controlled trials (RCTs), of which 22 could be submitted to a meta-analysis. Some of these RCTs were of high methodological quality. The results indicated that, for chronic low back pain, acupuncture is effective. A recent, three-armed RCT ($n = 298$) compared acupuncture with "minimal acupuncture" or a waiting list control group [6]. Its results showed no difference between acupuncture and placebo but both generated more pain relief than no treatment at all. Another RCT suggested that the beneficial effects of acupuncture last for 2 years, but this finding clearly requires independent confirmation [7]. An RCT ($n = 129$) of acupressure versus physical therapy showed greater pain reduction with acupressure when applied regularly for 1 month [8].

Herbal medicine

A range of herbal remedies has shown promising results in alleviating back pain [9]. The remedy that has been most thoroughly investigated is devil's claw (*Harpagophytum procumbens*). A systematic review included four RCTs, some with good methodological quality, and concluded that devil's claw is effective [10].

Massage

A Cochrane review of massage therapy included eight RCTs [11]. Their quality was satisfactory on average. The results were somewhat contradictory but, overall, the investigators arrived at a cautiously positive conclusion [11], suggesting that regular massage therapy does alleviate back pain.

Spinal manipulation

Spinal manipulation is almost considered an established treatment for back pain. Its effectiveness is therefore rarely questioned. However, a Cochrane review of all types of manipulation failed to show that these approaches are superior to other treatment options [12]. It included 39 RCTs, some of which were of acceptable quality. Spinal manipulation was better that sham, ineffective, or harmful interventions, but not better than conventional approaches. More recent RCTs demonstrated positive effects of spinal manipulation on back pain [13] and suggested that chiropractic care is associated with higher costs [14]. A large ($n = 681$) RCT with long-term follow-up tested the effects of chiropractic with or without physical therapy [15]. The differences in outcomes between medical and chiropractic care were "not clinically meaningful." An RCT with 252 patients suffering from osteoarthritic back pain suggested that chiropractic care with heat is more effective in reducing pain than heat alone [16]. An RCT ($n = 102$) of chiropractic spinal manipulation for acute sciatica suggested that manipulation, in comparison with sham manipulation, generates greater pain relief [17].

Fibromyalgia

Acupuncture

The systematic review by the author and colleagues included five RCTs of acupuncture. Most were of low methodological quality. Our conclusion was therefore cautious [18]:

> The notion that acupuncture is an effective systematic treatment for fibromyalgia is not supported by the results from rigorous clinical trials. On the basis of this evidence, acupuncture cannot be recommended for fibromyalgia.

Biofeedback

Several RCTs have suggested that fibromyalgia patients can benefit from various mind–body therapies. Yet appropriate attention controls have rarely been used, and the data are therefore not as conclusive as one would hope. In one study, 12 patients received 15 sessions of either biofeedback or sham biofeedback over 5 weeks [19]. Persistent improvements in pain intensity and morning stiffness were found. In another RCT (n = 119), biofeedback with relaxation was compared with exercise, a combination of biofeedback and exercise, and attention control [20]. Biofeedback was superior to the control group only in terms of tender points and enhanced self-efficacy of function.

Exercise

Exercise therapy might be considered entirely mainstream by most rheumatologists. (For this reason I have omitted it in the section on back pain.) However, as a treatment for fibromyalgia, it seems less commonly used and it thus is included here. A Cochrane review [21] of 17 RCTs produced good evidence for aerobic exercise to increase physical capacity and alleviate pain. This was recently confirmed in a further systematic review evaluating the health benefits of exercise for any indication [22]. A subsequent RCT with 79 female fibromyalgia patients showed that a home-based exercise program is an effective, low-cost approach for reducing pain and improving function [23]. A further RCT suggests that group exercise can be usefully combined with pain and stress management and education [24].

Myofascial pain

Acupuncture

A Cochrane review aimed to determine the effectiveness of dry needling for myofascial pain syndrome in the lower back [5]. It concluded that dry needling appears to be a useful adjunct to other therapies. For treating myofascial trigger-point pain, a systematic review concluded that a positive effect is likely [25]. Superficial needling followed by stretching was found to be more effective than stretching alone or no treatment at all [26].

For temporomandibular joint dysfunction, a systematic review included six RCTs, which overall suggested that acupuncture might be an effective option [27]. Subsequent studies reported mixed results in pain reduction compared with placebo/sham acupuncture [28–37]. Overall, the evidence for acupuncture as a treatment of myofascial pain is therefore encouraging, but not fully convincing.

Biofeedback

A systematic review of various types of biofeedback for temporomandibular disorders identified six RCTs [38]: two for surface electromyographic training of the masticatory muscles, two for surface electromyographic training combined with adjunctive cognitive–behavioral therapy techniques, and two for biofeedback-assisted relaxation training. The totality of this evidence suggested that these types of biofeedback training are probably effective.

Neck pain

Acupuncture

A systematic review of 14 RCTs of acupuncture as a treatment of neck pain of various causes failed to provide evidence that acupuncture is effective beyond a placebo effect [39]. Subsequent RCTs generated both positive [34,36,40–45] and negative results [46]. Other RCTs yielded ambiguous findings. Acupuncture turned out to be less effective than spinal manipulation but superior to medication [47], or acupuncture, compared with placebo, produced a statistically significant, but not clinically significant, effect [48]. A further RCT suggested that acupuncture/acupressure is better than sham treatment for a mixed group of patients suffering from chronic neck or shoulder pain [49]. A recent systematic review that included some of these new trials found "modest" evidence in support of a specific effect of acupuncture [50], a conclusion that may be, according to the totality of the best available evidence, slightly optimistic.

Spinal manipulation

A Cochrane review included 33 RCTs of spinal manipulation and mobilization for neck pain and found no strong evidence for the effectiveness of spinal manipulation for neck pain [51], a finding that was confirmed also by other nonchiropractic reviewers [52]. However, systematic reviews investigated by chiropractors [53,54] arrive at more optimistic conclusions. A recent large RCT ($n = 350$) suggested that adding spinal manipulation to an exercise regimen was not followed by clinical improvements after the end of the 6-week intervention nor at a 6-month follow-up [55]. Other RCTs suggested that spinal manipulation may have immediate and long-term analgesic effects in patients with neck pain [56,57] and that osteopathic spinal manipulation generates results similar to those of a single dose of intramuscular ketorolac for acute neck pain [58]. Considering this level of uncertainty and the well-documented risks of upper spinal manipulation [59], there seems to be good reasons to be cautious.

Osteoarthritis

Acupuncture

Acupuncture is widely used for treating the pain of osteoarthritis. The systematic review by the author and colleagues identified evidence of effectiveness of acupuncture for peripheral joint osteoarthritis [60]. Ten trials tested manual acupuncture and 8 trials tested electroacupuncture. The sham-controlled RCTs suggested that manual acupuncture has specific effects in reducing pain. Other systematic reviews support these findings [61–64]. More recently, however, several negative studies have emerged and, in 2008, the United Kingdom National Institute of Clinical Excellence (NICE) recommended not to use acupuncture for treating osteoarthritis because the totality of the evidence is not convincing [65].

Herbal medicine

A number of studies have assessed the effectiveness of Phytodolor (a proprietary preparation that contains *Populus tremula, Fraxinus excelsior*, and *Solidago virgaurea*) in painful arthritic conditions. A systematic review identified six RCTs [66], most of which were of good quality. These trials suggested reduced pain, increased mobility, and reduced consumption of nonsteroidal anti-inflammatory drugs (NSAIDs).

A systematic review assessed all RCTs of capsaicin cream (0.025%–0.075%) [66]. It identified three RCTs ($n = 135$) that suggested beneficial effects on pain and articular tenderness. A meta-analysis indicated that it was better than placebo for treating osteoarthritis.

Supplements

Chondroitin sulfate [67] and glucosamine [68] appear to be effective and have fewer adverse effects than NSAIDs. A meta-analysis [69] evaluated the data for both supplements and concluded that, although the effect sizes are likely to be exaggerated by publication bias and quality issues, some degree of effectiveness appears probable for both preparations. A further comprehensive meta-analysis suggested structural effectiveness for glucosamine and symptomatic effectiveness for glucosamine and chondroitin in knee osteoarthritis [70], which also seems to be effective in long-term treatment [71–73]. Several negative trials have, however, emerged recently [74–76]. The recent NICE guidelines therefore do not recommend these supplements for osteoarthritis. Whether these supplements prevent further cartilage loss in patients is currently not clear [77,78].

The effectiveness of *S*-adenosylmethionine has been assessed in a meta-analysis of 11 RCTs [79]. There were beneficial effects on joint function when compared with placebo and the supplement appears to be as effective as NSAIDs in improving functional limitations.

Rheumatoid arthritis

Diet

Trials from Scandinavia showed encouraging effects for fasting followed by a vegetarian diet. A systematic review included four such studies [80]. A meta-analysis of these data suggested long-term improvements in pain and related outcomes. Both fasting and strict vegetarian diets are associated with the risk of malnutrition. Thus adequate medical supervision is necessary.

Herbal medicine

Several herbal mixtures have been tested in clinical trials with positive results for rheumatoid arthritis patients. Of these preparations, only Phytodolor (see above) has been submitted to independently replicated clinical trials [81]. The totality of this evidence shows a positive effect on pain from rheumatoid arthritis.

Supplements

The results of a meta-analysis of RCTs of fish oil for rheumatoid arthritis suggested a reduction in tender joints and in morning stiffness [82], a finding that was confirmed by subsequent double-blind RCTs [83,84]. Another RCT reported no clinical benefit over placebo for a supplement containing omega-3 fatty acids [85]. Overall, the size of the effect is modest. Interestingly, α-linolenic acid (eg, from flaxseed oil), which is the precursor of omega-3 polyunsaturated fatty acids, does not seem to have the same clinical effects [86].

Tai chi

A Cochrane review assessed the evidence for or against tai chi as a treatment of rheumatoid arthritis [87]. It included 10 RCTs with a total of 1035 patients. In terms of swollen/tender joints, tai chi seems to have no detrimental effects on the disease activity of rheumatoid arthritis, whereas it appears to have a clinically important benefit in terms of range of motion of the affected joints. This overall result was supported by another systematic review that assessed the effects of tai chi on various chronic conditions [88].

Summary

Many rheumatic patients try some form of complementary treatment. Even though the area is clearly underresearched, encouraging evidence is now emerging for some of these modalities. Rheumatologists should be aware of these data to advise their patients responsibly.

References

[1] Eisenberg D, David RB, Ettner SL, et al. Trends in alternative medicine use in the United States; 1990–1997. JAMA 1998;280:1569–75.
[2] Ernst E, Resch KL, Mills S, et al. Complementary medicine—a definition. Br J Gen Pract 1995;45:506.
[3] Ernst E, Pittler MH, Wider B, et al. Complementary therapies for pain management. An evidence-based approach. London: Elsevier; 2007.
[4] Manheimer E, White A, Berman B, et al. Meta-analysis: acupuncture for low back pain. Ann Intern Med 2005;142:651–63.
[5] Furlan AD, van Tulder M, Cherkin D, et al. Acupuncture and dry-needling for low back pain: an updated systematic review within the framework of the Cochrane collaboration. Spine 2005;30:944–63.
[6] Brinkhaus B, Witt CM, Jena S, et al. Acupuncture in patients with chronic low back pain: a randomized controlled trial. Arch Intern Med 2006;166:450–7.
[7] Thomas KJ, MacPherson H, Ratcliffe J, et al. Longer term clinical and economic benefits with chronic low back pain. Health Technol Assess 2005;9:1–109.
[8] Hsieh LL, Kuo CH, Lee LH, et al. Treatment of low back pain by acupressure and physical therapy: randomised controlled trial. BMJ 2005;332:696–700.
[9] Ernst E, Chrubasik S. Phyto-anti-inflammatories: a systematic review of randomized, placebo-controlled, double-blind trials. Rheum Dis Clin North Am 2000;26:13–27.
[10] Gagnier JJ, Chrubasik S, Manheimer E. Harpagophytum procumbens for osteoarthritis and low back pain: a systematic review. BMC Complement Altern Med 2004;4:13.
[11] Furlan AD, Brosseau L, Imamura M, et al. Massage for low-back pain: a systematic review within the framework of the Cochrane Collaboration Back Review Group. Spine 2002;27:1896–910.
[12] Assendelft WJJ, Morton SC, Yu Emily I, et al. Spinal manipulative therapy for low-back pain. Cochrane Database Syst Rev 2004;(1):CD000447.
[13] Geisser ME, Wiggert EA, Haig AJ, et al. A randomized, controlled trial of manual therapy and specific adjuvant exercise for chronic low back pain. Clin J Pain 2005;21:463–70.
[14] Kominski GF, Heslin KC, Morgenstern H, et al. Economic evaluation of four treatments for low back pain: results from a randomized controlled trial. Med Care 2005;43:428–35.
[15] Hurwitz EL, Morgenstern H, Kominski GF, et al. A randomized trial of chiropractic and medical care for patients with low back pain: eighteen-month follow-up outcomes from the UCLA low back pain study. Spine 2006;31:611–21.
[16] Beyerman KL, Palmerino MB, Zohn LE, et al. Efficacy of treating low back pain and dysfunction secondary to osteoarthritis: chiropractic care compared with moist heat alone. J Manipulative Physiol Ther 2006;29:107–14.
[17] Santilli V, Beghi E, Finucci S. Chiropractic manipulation in the treatment of acute back pain and sciatica with disc protrusion: a randomized double-blind clinical trial of active and simulated spinal manipulations. Spine J 2006;6:131–7.

[18] Mayhew E, Ernst E. Acupuncture for fibromyalgia—a systematic review of randomized clinical trials. Rheumatology 2006 Dec 19. Rheumatology (Oxford) 2008;46:801–4 [epub ahead of print].
[19] Ferraccioli G, Gherilli L, Scita F, et al. EMG-biofeedback training in fibromyalgia syndrome. J Rheumatol 1987;14:820–5.
[20] Buckelew SP, Conway R, Parker J, et al. Biofeedback/relaxation training and exercise interventions for fibromyalgia. Arthritis Care Res 1998;11:196–209.
[21] Busch A, Schachter CL, Peloso PM, et al. Exercise for treating fibromyalgia syndrome. Cochrane Database Syst Rev 2002;(2):CD003786.
[22] Karmisholt K, Gotzsche PC. Physical activity for secondary prevention of disease. Systematic reviews of randomised clinical trials. Dan Med Bull 2005;52:90–4.
[23] Da Costa D, Abrahamowicz M, Lowensteyn I, et al. A randomized clinical trial of an individualized home-based exercise treatment programme for women with fibromyalgia. Rheumatology (Oxford) 2005;44:1422–7.
[24] Lemstra M, Olszynski WP. The effectiveness of multidisciplinary rehabilitation in the treatment of fibromyalgia: a randomized controlled trial. Clin J Pain 2005;21:166–74.
[25] Cummings TM, White AR. Needling therapies in the management of myofascial trigger point pain: a systematic review. Arch Phys Med Rehabil 2001;82:986–92.
[26] Edwards J, Knowles N. Superficial dry needling and active stretching in the treatment of myofascial pain—a randomised controlled trial. Acupunct Med 2003;21:80–6.
[27] Ernst E, White A. Acupuncture as a treatment for temporomandibular joint dysfunction. Arch Otolaryngol Head Neck Surg 1999;125:269–72.
[28] Schmid-Schwap M, Simma-Kletschka I, Stockner A, et al. Oral acupuncture in the therapy of craniomandibular dysfunction syndrome—a randomised controlled trial. Wien Klin Wochenschr 2006;118:36–42.
[29] Goddard G, Karibe H, McNeill C, et al. Acupuncture and sham acupuncture reduce muscle pain in myofascial pain patients. J Orofac Pain 2002;16:71–6.
[30] Zhou FH, Zhao HY. [Acupuncture and ultrasound therapy for temporomandibular disorders]. Di Yi Jun Yi Da Xue Xue Bao 2004;24:720–1 [in Chinese].
[31] Kamanli A, Kaya A, Ardicoglu O, et al. Comparison of lidocaine injection, botulinum toxin injection, and dry needling to trigger points in myofascial pain syndrome. Rheumatol Int 2005;25:604–11.
[32] Ilbuldu E, Cakmak A, Disci R, et al. Comparison of laser, dry needling, and placebo laser treatments in myofacial pain syndrome. Photomed Laser Surg 2004;22:306–11.
[33] Chu J. Does EMG (dry needling) reduce myofascial pain symptoms due to cervical nerve root irritation? Electromyogr Clin Neurophysiol 1997;37:259–72.
[34] Irnich D, Behrens N, Gleditsch JM, et al. Immediate effects of dry needling and acupuncture at distant points in chronic neck pain: results of a randomized, double-blind, sham-controlled crossover trial. Pain 2002;99:83–9.
[35] Birch S, Jamison RN. Controlled trial of Japanese acupuncture for chronic myofascial neck pain—assessment of specific and nonspecific effects of treatment. Clin J Pain 1998;14:248–55.
[36] Irnich D, Behrens N, Molzen H, et al. Randomised trial of acupuncture compared with conventional massage and 'sham' laser acupuncture for treatment of chronic neck pain. BMJ 2001;322:1574–8.
[37] Ceccheerelli F, Bordin M, Gagliardi G, et al. Comparison between superficial and deep acupuncture in the treatment of the shoulder's myofascial pain: a randomized and controlled study. Acupunct Electrother Res 2001;26:229–38.
[38] Crider A, Glaros AG, Gevirtz RN. Efficacy of biofeedback-based treatments for temporomandibular disorders. Appl Psychophysiol Biofeedback 2005;30:333–45.
[39] White AR, Ernst E. A systematic review of randomized controlled trials of acupuncture for neck pain. Rheumatology (Oxford) 1999;38:143–7.
[40] Sator-Katzenschlager SM, Szeles JC, Scharbert G, et al. Electrical stimulation of auricular acupuncture points is more effective than conventional manual auricular acupuncture in chronic cervical pain: a pilto study. Anesth Analg 2003;97:1469–73.

[41] Konig A, Radke S, Molzen H, et al. [Randomised trial of acupuncture compared with conventional massage and 'sham' laser acupuncture for treatment of chronic neck pain—range of motion analysis]. Z Orthop Ihre Grenzgeb 2003;141:395–400 [in German].
[42] Seidel U, Uhlemann C. Behandlung der zervikalen Tendomyose. Deutsche Zeitschrift fur Akupunktur 2002;45:258–69.
[43] Nabeta T, Kawakita K. Relief of chronic neck and shoulder pain by manual acupuncture to tender points—a sham-controlled randomized trial. Complement Ther Med 2002;10: 217–22.
[44] He D, Veierstad KB, Hostmark AT, et al. Effect of acupuncture treatment on chronic neck and shoulder pain in sedentary female workers: a 6-month and 3-year follow-up study. Pain 2004;109:299–307.
[45] Heikkila H, Johansson M, Wenngren BI. Effects of acupuncture, cervical manipulation and NSAID therapy on dizziness and impaired head repositioning of suspected cervical origin: a pilot study. Man Ther 2000;5:151–7.
[46] Zu XM, Polus BA. A controlled trial on acupuncture for chronic neck pain. Am J Chin Med 2002;30:13–28.
[47] Giles LG, Muller R. Chronic spinal pain: a randomised clinical trial comparing medication, acupuncture, and spinal manipulation. Spine 2003;28:1490–502.
[48] White P, Lewith G, Prescott P, et al. Acupuncture versus placebo for the treatment of chronic mechanical neck pain. Ann Intern Med 2004;141:911–9.
[49] He D, Hostmark AT, Veierstad KB, et al. Effect of intensive acupuncture on pain-related social and psychological variables for women with chronic neck and shoulder pain—an RCT with six month and three year follow up. Acupunct Med 2005;23:52–61.
[50] Irnich D. Acupuncture for neck pain—review of recent randomised controlled trials. Deutsche Zeitschrift fur Akupunktur 2005;48:40–3.
[51] Gross AR, Hoving JL, Haines TA, et al. A Cochrane review of manipulation and mobilization for mechanical neck disorders. Spine 2004;29:1541–8.
[52] Sarigiovannis P, Hollins B. Effectiveness of manual therapy in the treatment of non-specific neck pain: a review. Phys Ther Rev 2005;10:35–50.
[53] Bronfort G, Haas M, Evans RL, et al. Efficacy of spinal manipulation and mobilization for low back pain and neck pain: a systematic review and best evidence synthesis. Spine J 2004;4: 335–56.
[54] Haneline MT. Chiropractic manipulation and acute neck pain: a review of the evidence. J Manipulative Physiol Ther 2005;28:520–5.
[55] Dziedzic K, Hill J, Lewis M, et al. Effectiveness of manual therapy or pulsed shortwave diathermy in addition to advice and exercise for neck disorders: a pragmatic randomized controlled trial in physical therapy clinics. Arthritis Rheum 2005;53:214–22.
[56] Cleland JA, Childs MJ, McRae M, et al. Immediate effects of thoracic manipulation in patients with neck pain: a randomized clinical trial. Man Ther 2005;10:127–35.
[57] Palmgren PJ, Sadnstrom PJ, Lundqvist FJ, et al. Improvement after chiropractic care in cervicocephalic kinesthetic sensibility and subjective pain intensity in patients with nontraumatic chronic neck pain. J Manipulative Physiol Ther 2006;29:100–6.
[58] McReynolds TM, Sheridan BJ. Intramuscular ketorolac versus osteopathic manipulative treatment in the management of acute neck pain in the emergency department: a randomised clinical trial. J Am Osteopath Assoc 2005;105:57–68.
[59] Ernst E. Adverse effects of spinal manipulation: a systematic review. J R Soc Med 2007;100: 330–8.
[60] Kwon YD, Pittler MH, Ernst E. Acupuncture for peripheral joint osteoarthritis: a systematic review and meta-analysis. Rheumatology (Oxford) 2006;45:1331–7.
[61] Ezzo J, Hadhazy V, Birch S, et al. Acupuncture for osteoarthritis of the knee. Arthritis Rheum 2001;44:819–25.
[62] Soeken KL. Selected CAM therapies for arthritis-related pain: the evidence from systematic reviews. Clin J Pain 2004;20:13–8.

[63] Ernst E. Musculoskeletal conditions and complementary/alternative medicine. Best Pract Res Clin Rheumatol 2004;18:539–56.
[64] Weiner D, Ernst E. Complementary and alternative approaches to the treatment of persistent musculoskeletal pain. Clin J Pain 2004;20:244–55.
[65] National Collaborating Centre for Chronic Conditions. Osteoarthritis: national clinical guideline for care and management in adults. London: Royal College of Physicians; 2008.
[66] Long L. Herbal medicines for the treatment of osteoarthritis a systematic review. Rheumatology (Oxford) 2001;40:779–93.
[67] Leeb BF, Schweitzer H, Montag K, et al. A metaanalysis of chondroitin sulfate in the treatment of osteoarthritis. J Rheumatol 2000;27:205–11.
[68] Towheed TE, Anastassiades TP, Shea B, et al. Glucosamine therapy for treating osteoarthritis. Cochrane Database Syst Rev 2000;(2):CD002946.
[69] McAlindon TE, La Valley MP, Gulin JP, et al. Glucosamine and chondroitin for treatment of osteoarthritis. A systematic quality assessment and meta-analysis. JAMA 2000;283: 1469–75.
[70] Richy F, Bruyere O, Ethgen O, et al. Structural and symptomatic efficacy of glucosamine and chondroitin in knee osteoarthritis. Arch Intern Med 2003;163:1514–22.
[71] Poolsup N, Suthisisang C, Channark P, et al. Glucosamine long-term treatment and the progression of knee osteoarthritis: systematic review of randomised controlled trials. Ann Pharmacother 2005;39:1080–7.
[72] Uebelhart D, Malaise M, Marcolongo R, et al. Intermittent treatment of knee osteoarthritis with oral chondroitin sulfate: a one-year, randomized, double-blind, multicenter study versus placebo. Osteoarthritis Cartilage 2004;12:269–76.
[73] Cohen M, Wolfe R, Mai T, et al. A randomized double blind, placebo controlled trial of a topical cream containing glucosamine sulfate, chondroitin sulfate, and camphor for osteoarthritis of the knee. J Rheumatol 2003;30:523–8 [Erratum in: J Rheumatol 2003;30:2512].
[74] Cibere J, Kopec JA, Thorne A, et al. Randomized, double-blind, placebo-controlled glucosamine discontinuation trial in knee osteoarthritis. Arthritis Rheum 2004;51:738–45.
[75] McAlindon T, Formica M, LaValley M, et al. Effectiveness of glucosamine for symptoms of knee osteoartritis: results from an Internet-based randomized double-blind controlled trial. Am J Med 2004;117:643–9.
[76] Clegg DO, Reda DJ, Harris CL, et al. Glucosamine, chondroitin sulfate, and the two in combination for painful knee osteoarthritis. N Engl J Med 2006;354:795–808.
[77] Cibere J, Thorne A, Kopec JA, et al. Glucosamine sulfate and cartilage type II collagen degradation in patients with knee osteoarthritis: randomized discontinuation trial results employing biomarkers. J Rheumatol 2005;32:896–902.
[78] Michel BA, Stucki G, Frey D, et al. Chondroitins 4 and 6 sulfate in osteoarthritis of the knee: a randomized, controlled trial. Arthritis Rheum 2005;52:779–86.
[79] Soeken KL, Lee WL, Bausell RB, et al. Safety and efficacy of S-adenosylmethionine (SAMe) for osteoarthritis. J Fam Pract 2002;51:425–30.
[80] Müller H, de Toledo FW, Resch KL. Fasting followed by vegetarian diet in patients with rheumatoid arthritis: a systematic review. Scand J Rheumatol 2001;30:1–10.
[81] Ernst E. The efficacy of Phytodolor® for the treatment of musculoskeletal pain—a systematic review of randomized clinical trials. Natural Medicine Journal 1999;2:14–7.
[82] Fortin PR, Lew RA, Liang MH, et al. Validation of a meta-analysis: the effects of fish oil in rheumatoid arthritis. J Clin Epidemiol 1995;48:1379–90.
[83] Volker D, Fitzgerald P, Major G, et al. Efficacy of fish oil concentrate in the treatment of rheumatoid arthritis. J Rheumatol 2000;27:2343–6.
[84] Berbert AA, Kondo CR, Almendra CL, et al. Supplementation of fish oil and olive oil in patients with rheumatoid arthritis. Nutrition 2005;21:131–6.
[85] Remans PH, Sont JK, Wagenaar LW, et al. Nutrient supplementation with polyunsaturated fatty acids and micronutrients in rheumatoid arthritis: clinical and biochemical effects. Eur J Clin Nutr 2004;58:839–45.

[86] Nordstrom DCE, Honkanen VEA, Nasu Y, et al. Alpha-linolenic acid in the treatment of rheumatoid arthritis: a double-blind, placebo-controlled and randomized study: flaxseed vs safflower seed. Rheumatol Int 1995;14:231–4.
[87] Han A, Robinson V, Judd M, et al. Tai chi for treating rheumatoid arthritis. Cochrane Database Syst Rev 2004;(3):CD004849.
[88] Wang C, Collet JP, Lau J. The effect of tai chi on health outcomes in patients with chronic conditions: a systematic review. Arch Intern Med 2004;164:493–501.

ELSEVIER
SAUNDERS

Rheum Dis Clin N Am
34 (2008) 469–479

RHEUMATIC
DISEASE CLINICS
OF NORTH AMERICA

Dietary Omega-3 Fats for Treatment of Inflammatory Joint Disease: Efficacy and Utility

Susanna M. Proudman, MBBS, FRACP,
Leslie G. Cleland, MBBS, MD, FRACP,
Michael J. James, PhD*

Rheumatology Unit, Royal Adelaide Hospital, North Terrace, Adelaide, SA 5000, Australia

Effects of fish oil in rheumatoid arthritis and other inflammatory disorders

There have been 14 double-blind, randomized, controlled trials that examined the effects of fish oil on clinical outcomes in established rheumatoid arthritis (RA) (reviewed in Ref. [1]). Tender joint count was the most common outcome measure to have a statistically significant improvement with fish oil, compared with other outcomes. Ten of these trials were included in a meta-analysis and mega-analysis of outcomes after 12 weeks of fish oil supplementation. These analyses concluded that fish oil provides an improvement in tender joint count and duration of morning stiffness [2]. Focusing on pain relief, another meta-analysis examined 17 randomized, controlled trials that included assessment of the analgesic effects of omega-3 (ω-3) fatty acid supplementation in patients with RA or joint pain secondary to inflammatory bowel disease or dysmenorrhea. This indicated that fish oil decreased joint pain intensity, duration of morning stiffness, number of tender and swollen joints, and use of nonsteroidal anti-inflammatory drugs (NSAIDs) [3].

An important finding from these studies is that fish oil can have an NSAID-sparing effect. In three of the RA studies in which this was examined, fish oil decreased NSAID use [4–6]. In another two studies, there was a predetermined cessation of NSAIDs after a fixed interval; even with the provocation of an inflammatory disease such as RA, the results indicated an NSAID-sparing effect of fish oil ingestion [7,8]. The meta-analysis

* Corresponding author.
E-mail address: michael.james@health.sa.gov.au (M.J. James).

doi:10.1016/j.rdc.2008.03.003

that focused on pain outcomes concluded there was decreased NSAID use with fish oil [3].

Collectively, these studies provide evidence of symptomatic benefits of dietary fish oil in established RA, and that:

- The effects are generally delayed by 2 to 3 months after commencement of fish oil, similar to the lag seen with commencement of disease modifying anti-rheumatic drugs (DMARDs),
- There is a dose response for time of onset of symptomatic benefits [7],
- Symptomatic benefits were seen with doses between 2.6 g and 7.1 g per day of ω-3 fats, with no effect seen at 1 g per day [1], and
- Fish oil supplements are NSAID-sparing [3–8].

Fish oil supplements have also shown benefits in decreased relapse in Crohn's disease [9], reduced progression to renal failure in IgA nephropathy [10], and reduced disease activity scores in systemic lupus erythematosus [11]. A retrospective analysis of use of fish oil for discogenic neck or back pain showed that 60% ceased NSAID use [12].

The beneficial effects of fish oils in inflammatory disorders are attributed to their omega-3 fatty acid content. Understanding the chemistry of these fatty acids is critical to understanding the practical points regarding their clinical use.

Chemistry of omega-3 fatty acids

There can be the mistaken assumption, often created by marketers, that ω-3 fats in vegetable oils are the same as those in fish oils. The designation ω-3 applies to a class of fatty acids that have a double bond between carbon atoms 3 and 4, counted from the omega end of the carbon chain (Fig. 1). These fatty acids are essential for many functions, particularly in excitable tissues such as brain, retina, and myocardium, and because neither human beings nor fish can insert an ω-3 double bond, they are dietary essential fatty acids. Fish low in the food chain obtain ω-3 fatty acids from marine algae and human beings obtain them from fish and certain plant oils. However, the fish-derived ω-3 fatty acids, eicosapentaenoic acid (EPA) and docosahexaenoic acid (DHA), have longer carbon chains and are more unsaturated than the plant-derived ω-3 fatty acids, α-linolenic acid (ALA) and stearidonic acid (SDA) (Table 1). It is most likely that tissue content of EPA and DHA is responsible for the beneficial effects of dietary fish oil.

Biochemical actions of omega-3 fatty acids relevant to inflammatory disorders

The lipid inflammatory mediators, prostaglandin E_2 (PGE_2) and leukotriene B_4 (LTB_4) are products of the ω-6 20-carbon fatty acid, arachidonic acid

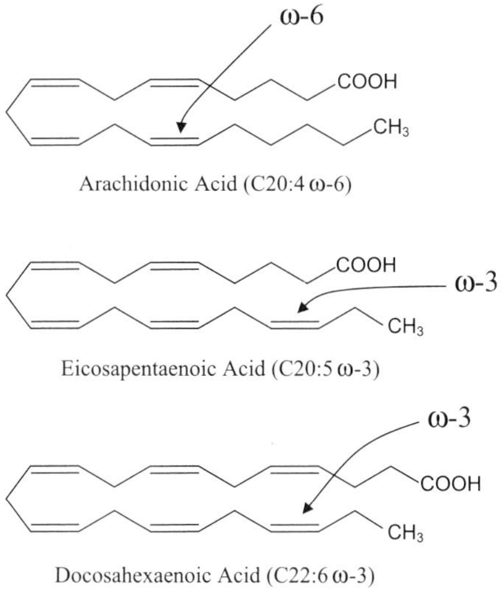

Fig. 1. Fatty acid structures. *Abbreviations:* CH_3, methyl group; COOH, carboxylic acid group.

(AA; 20:4ω-6), metabolized via the cyclooxygenase (COX) and 5-lipoxygenase (5-LOX) pathways, respectively. Hyperalgesia in response to peripheral inflammation appears to be caused by the actions of central nervous system (CNS) PGE_2 newly synthesized by both induced and constitutive CNS COX-2 in concert with induced PGE synthase [13–15]. However, PGE_2 produced at a peripheral site of inflammation is most likely COX-1 and COX-2 derived and is involved in oedemogenesis [16]. LTB_4 is a neutrophil chemoattractant and activator [17].

EPA and DHA are homologs of the PGE_2 and LTB_4 precursor, AA, and so they can be effective competitive inhibitors of AA metabolism (see Fig. 1). EPA and DHA have Ki values for COX of approximately 2 μM, which is similar to that of ibuprofen [18]. Indeed, dietary fish oil has been shown to inhibit PGE_2 and LTB_4 synthesis in healthy human beings [19,20] and patients with rheumatoid arthritis [21–23].

As well as inhibiting AA-derived proinflammatory eicosanoids, ω-3 long-chain fatty acids are substrates for anti-inflammatory eicosanoid formation.

Table 1
Sources and basic chemistry of omega-3 fatty acids

Name	Source	Carbons[a]	Double bonds	Abbreviation/ designation
α-linolenic acid	Canola, flaxseed oils	18	3	ALA; 18:3
Stearidonic acid	Echium, borage oils	18	4	SDA; 18:4
Eicosapentaenoic acid	Fish oils	20	5	EPA; 20:5
Docosahexaenoic acid	Fish oils	22	6	DHA; 22:6

[a] 18-carbon fatty acids are from vegetable oils; 20- and 22-carbon fatty acids are from fish oil.

DHA can be converted via 15-LOX or aspirin-treated COX-2 to 17(S)- and 17(R)-hydroxy derivatives, respectively, which are converted by 5-LOX to resolvin D1 (RvD1) and aspirin-triggered RvD1, respectively. Likewise, EPA can be converted via aspirin-treated COX-2 to RvE1. These resolvins have anti-inflammatory effects in murine peritonitis by down-regulating leucocyte recruitment and stimulating macrophage removal of apoptotic cells [24,25].

Omega-3 fatty acids can inhibit production of peptide, as well as lipid inflammatory mediators. Accordingly, dietary fish oil has been shown to inhibit tumor necrosis factor alpha (TNFα) and interleukin-1β synthesis in healthy human beings [19,20,26,27] and patients with rheumatoid arthritis [7,23]. Although the mechanisms are not known, the inhibitory effect of fish oil on TNFα in healthy males was dependent on the basal TNFα production and on a polymorphism in the TNF gene [28]. Thus, there are many potential biochemical fates of EPA and DHA that could have anti-inflammatory outcomes (Fig. 2). Collectively, these provide biologic plausibility for the clinical outcomes observed with fish oil use in RA.

Dietary omega-6 fatty acids: excess and interactions

The use of polypharmacy in modern medical practice has brought an appreciation of the care that is needed in handling drug interactions. These can decrease or increase actions of the drug under consideration. Likewise, this is a consideration in the therapeutic use of fish oil and it is one that requires an appreciation of other unsaturated fats in the diet.

In chemical terms, ω-3 fatty acids are polyunsaturated. However, the common or marketing use of the word "polyunsaturated" for fats in

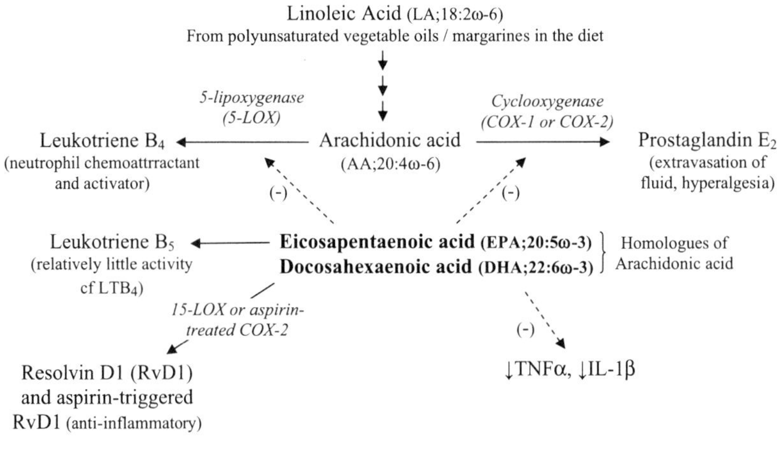

Fig. 2. Possible metabolic pathways for anti-inflammatory effects of the long-chain ω-3 fatty acids, eicosapentaenoic acid, and docosahexaenoic acid.

commercial cooking oils, margarines, and foods is restricted to ω-6 fatty acids, principally linoleic acid (LA). This is in soybean, peanut, cottonseed, corn, and sunflower oils and their margarine products (Fig. 3). The chemical similarity of ω-3 and ω-6 polyunsaturated fatty acids leads to competitive inhibition of metabolism of ω-3 by ω-6 fatty acids and vice versa. This is important when considering vegetable oil sources of ω-3 fatty acids to elevate tissue EPA and DHA.

Tissue levels of EPA and DHA are elevated mainly by dietary EPA and DHA (ie, fish oil), but they can be elevated also by dietary ALA and SDA (ie, plant oils). SDA is currently a sufficiently minor component of available plant oils that it can be ignored. ALA, once ingested, can be metabolized by unsaturation and elongation to EPA and, in theory, DHA. However, in practice, dietary ALA has led to elevation only of tissue EPA and not DHA [29,30]. In addition, for elevation of tissue EPA, dietary ALA was 14-fold less effective than dietary EPA [30]. However, there is considerable inter-individual variation, possibly with a genetic basis, in the ability to convert ALA and SDA to EPA (M. James, unpublished results, 2008). This suggests that there will be variation in the requirements for dietary EPA (and DHA) to elevate tissue EPA (and DHA).

A negative determinant of tissue EPA plus DHA levels is the intake of LA, the ω-6 fatty acid that is present in foods marketed as polyunsaturated. Because LA is the ω-6 homolog of ALA, it can decrease metabolism of the vegetable oil-derived ALA to EPA [31]. Dietary LA also decreases the level of tissue EPA plus DHA that has arisen from dietary EPA plus DHA [32]. In Western diets, LA is present at approximately 10-fold and 100-fold

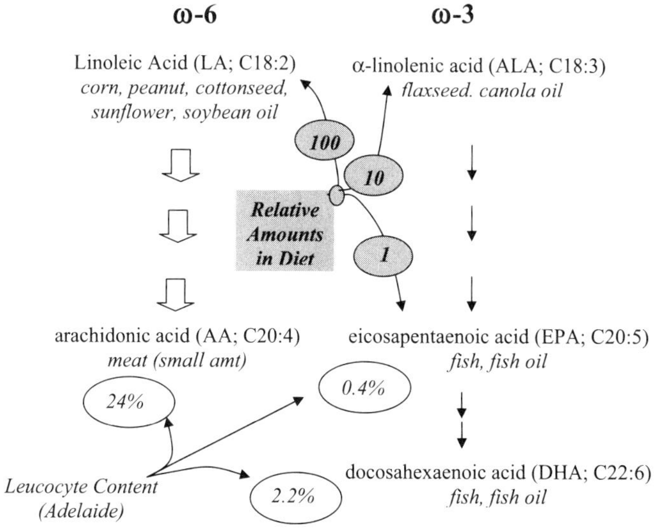

Fig. 3. Fatty acid sources, dietary, and tissue amounts in subjects not taking fish oil.

greater amounts than ALA and EPA plus DHA, respectively (see Fig. 3) [33]. Thus, the relatively high LA intake presents an important practical issue for dietary strategies aimed at elevating tissue EPA plus DHA.

Fish oil use in a rheumatology clinic

Doses of 3 g to 5 g per day EPA plus DHA are required for an anti-inflammatory effect. Such doses can be achieved realistically only with fish oil, even though fish and ω-3 containing vegetable oils can provide a valuable contribution. Typically, 10 mL to 15 mL per day of fish oil is needed for an anti-inflammatory dose of ω-3 fats, and this can be achieved most cheaply and efficiently with bottled fish oil.

A practical method for ingestion of 10 mL to 15 mL per day of fish oil has been developed [34]. The fish oil dose is floated onto an equivalent amount of fruit juice in a small glass, ingested in a single swallow, avoiding contact with the lips, and followed immediately by a small amount of juice. This avoids tasting the fish oil. The long-term (more than 3 years) use of this method by RA patients has been documented and shown to elevate tissue EPA and DHA levels by approximately sixfold and twofold, respectively and to decrease AA levels by 30% to 40% [35,36]. Over 3 years, fish oil use in a clinic setting was continued by 75% of RA patients [37].

Experience shows that patient instruction booklets for use of fish oil at anti-inflammatory doses provide a valuable complement to physician advice and instructions. The key points to be conveyed are:

- Vegetable oils containing the ω-3 fatty acid, ALA, can elevate tissue EPA, but
- Fish oil is much more effective than ω-3 containing vegetable oils, and fish oil elevates both tissue EPA and DHA, and
- Vegetable oils containing the ω-6 fatty acid, LA, decrease tissue EPA arising from dietary EPA or dietary ALA.

Thus, tissue levels of the anti-inflammatory ω-3 fatty acids, EPA plus DHA will be most efficiently increased by a combination of all of the following: fish oil supplements, fish meals, omega-3 containing vegetable oils (such as canola and flaxseed oil), and avoidance of omega-6 containing vegetable oils (such as peanut, cottonseed, sunflower, and soybean oil) by substituting monounsaturated vegetable oils, such as olive and canola oils.

Beyond symptomatic benefits of fish oil: considerations of cardiovascular benefits in rheumatoid arthritis

RA confers an approximate threefold increased risk of myocardial infarction and an approximate twofold increased risk of sudden cardiac death [38]. The increased cardiovascular risk is not explained by traditional risk factors and appears to be related to the extent of disease activity as measured by systemic inflammatory markers or extra-articular disease [39].

Cardiovascular risk may be further increased in RA patients because of the frequent use of NSAIDs for symptomatic relief. Using a United Kingdom general practice database for a case-controlled analysis, NSAID-use was associated with increased risk of myocardial infarction [40]. Using the Nurses' Health Study group for a cohort analysis, daily NSAID use was associated with an increased risk of a major cardiovascular event [41]. Because of their activity as anti-inflammatory agents, all NSAIDs can be considered to be COX-2 inhibitors and thus, inhibitors of the endothelial antithrombotic eicosanoid, prostacyclin, which is COX-2 derived [42].

Controlled intervention studies with the COX-1-sparing NSAIDs, such as celecoxib, rofecoxib, parecoxib, and valdecoxib, have demonstrated increased cardiovascular risk in subjects with or without RA [43–45]. Because the prothrombotic platelet eicosanoid, thromboxane A_2, is COX-1 derived, the increased cardiovascular risk with selective COX-2 inhibitors (ie, COX-1-sparing NSAIDs) was expected. However, all NSAIDs are COX inhibitors and have the potential to unfavorably perturb the prostacyclin/thromboxane balance. Some older NSAIDs, such as diclofenac and meloxicam, are intrinsically COX-2 selective [46]. Other older NSAIDs, even if intrinsically nonselective for the COX-isotypes, could have a selective prostacyclin inhibitory effect at periods within the dosing cycle, because of a combination of pharmacokinetics and variable pharmacodynamics [47]. With regard to the latter point, the relationship between COX-2 inhibition and inhibition of prostacyclin synthesis is more proportional than that between COX-1 inhibition and inhibition of platelet aggregation, where 95% inhibition of thromboxane synthesis is needed before platelet aggregation is substantially affected [47]. Thus, equivalent inhibition (eg, 50% inhibition) of both COX-2 and COX-1 could differentially inhibit antithrombotic COX functions, compared with prothrombotic COX functions.

In addition to the effects of NSAIDs on the pro- versus antithrombotic eicosanoid balance, all NSAIDs, no matter what their COX selectivity, can potentially alter renal function and elevate blood pressure [47].

In Australia at least, the government drug advisory bodies recommend NSAID use in as low a dose for as short a time as possible. In this context, the NSAID-sparing effect of fish oil becomes significant for the limitation of use of drugs that confer cardiovascular risk in a patient population already at increased cardiovascular risk. However, the significance of fish oil use in this cardiovascular risk context goes beyond its NSAID-sparing effect because the fish oil ω-3 fatty acids have cardio-protective effects.

Interest in the cardiovascular effects accelerated in response to an ecological study that found a very low incidence of acute myocardial infarction among Greenland Inuit consuming their traditional diet of marine mammals and fish, which provided a high intake of EPA and DHA [48,49]. Since that report, a large number of cohort studies (Zutphen, Chicago Western

Electric, United States Physicians Health, Nurses Health, Multiple Risk Factor Intervention Trial studies) [50–54] and dietary intervention studies (Diet and Reinfarction Trial, GISSI) [55,56] have demonstrated that fish and ω-3 fatty acids confer considerable health benefits in heart disease. In addition, case-controlled studies have found a 90% reduction in risk of primary cardiac arrest [57] or sudden cardiac death [58] in subjects within the highest versus the lowest quartile of erythrocyte ω-3 fatty acids. Given these outcomes, it is not surprising that the American Heart Association has recommended a daily intake of about 1 g of long chain ω-3 fatty acids in patients with documented cardiovascular disease [59].

Although their cardioprotective mechanisms are different, statins and dietary ω-3 fats have an equivalent effect size on cardiac mortality [60]. Whereas statins lower low density lipoprotein-cholesterol, ω-3 fatty acids are antithrombotic, have antiarrhythmic effects, can increase arterial compliance, and can lower plasma triglycerides and blood pressure [59]. These beneficial effects, examined in general populations and those with cardiovascular disease, are likely to be conferred in an RA population as well, on a full range of disease suppressive drugs. In a cohort of RA patients whose DMARD regimen was determined by an algorithm designed to be responsive to disease activity and intolerance, and which aimed to achieve maximal disease suppression, those who took regular anti-inflammatory doses of fish oil had lower platelet thromboxane production at 3 years of fish oil use. In addition, there was a decrease in triglycerides and a favorable increase in high-density lipoprotein-cholesterol in the fish oil group, whereas there was no change from baseline in those who chose not to take fish oil. The fish oil group also had higher remission rates [36]. It is notable that patients did not gain weight while taking anti-inflammatory doses of fish oil.

Summary and perspectives

Fish oil is not widely used in RA therapy, despite the following, all of which has been presented above:

- There is high level evidence (meta-analysis of randomized, controlled trials) for symptomatic benefits
- There is biologic plausibility for its clinical effects (inhibition of inflammatory mediator production, production of anti-inflammatory mediators)
- There is reduction in use of NSAIDs, which confer cardiovascular risk as well as the well-known risk of gastrointestinal adverse events
- There is a cardioprotective effect in a patient population that has an inherent increased cardiovascular risk that is probably augmented by NSAID use.

Given this catalog of activities, any of which would have been sufficient to launch commercially sponsored clinical trials of a patented drug, the lack of uptake of fish oil use in rheumatology clinics represents a failure of evidence-based practice. One of the probable reasons for the failure of uptake is that fish and fish oil are not patented; therefore, they lack the marketing finances that accompany the patented drugs used in rheumatology practice. The marketing budgets of the commercial sponsors allows the detailed presentation of the putative benefits of the patented drugs to practitioners in a manner that detracts attention from the academic evidence base. A dispassionate examination would indicate that the evidence for benefits of the commercially promoted agents, compared with those of ω-3 fatty acids, is not stronger or more numerous, it is simply louder.

References

[1] Cleland LG, James MJ, Proudman SM. The role of fish oils in the treatment of rheumatoid arthritis. Drugs 2003;63:845–53.
[2] Fortin PR, Lew RA, Liang MH, et al. Validation of a meta-analysis: the effects of fish oil in rheumatoid arthritis. J Clin Epidemiol 1995;48:1379–90.
[3] Goldberg RJ, Katz J. A meta-analysis of the analgesic effects of omega-3 polyunsaturated fatty acid supplementation for inflammatory joint pain. Pain 2007;129:210–23.
[4] Skoldstam L, Borjesson O, Kjallman A, et al. Effect of six months of fish oil supplementation in stable rheumatoid arthritis. A double blind, controlled study. Scand J Rheumatol 1992;21:178–85.
[5] Lau CS, Morley KD, Belch JJ. Effects of fish oil supplementation on non-steroidal anti-inflammatory drug requirement in patients with mild rheumatoid arthritis—a double blind placebo controlled study. Br J Rheumatol 1993;32:982–9.
[6] Geusens P, Wouters C, Nijs J, et al. Long-term effect of omega-3 fatty acid supplementation in active rheumatoid arthritis. Arthritis Rheum 1994;37:824–9.
[7] Kremer JM, Lawrence DA, Petrillo GF, et al. Effects of high-dose fish oil on rheumatoid arthritis after stopping nonsteroidal antiinflammatory drugs. Arthritis Rheum 1995;38:1107–14.
[8] Kjeldsen-Kragh J, Lund JA, Riise T, et al. Dietary omega-3 fatty acid supplementation and naproxen treatment in patients with rheumatoid arthritis. J Rheumatol 1992;19:1531–6.
[9] Belluzzi A, Brignola C, Campieri M, et al. Effect of an enteric-coated fish-oil preparation on relapses in Crohn's disease. N Engl J Med 1996;334:1557–60.
[10] Donadio JV. The emerging role of omega-3 polyunsaturated fatty acids in the management of patients with IgA nephropathy. J Ren Nutr 2001;11:122–8.
[11] Duffy EM, Meenagh GK, McMillan SA, et al. The clinical effect of dietary supplementation with omega-3 fish oils and/or copper in systemic lupus erythematosus. J Rheumatol 2004;31:1551–6.
[12] Maroon JC, Bost JW. [omega]-3 Fatty acids (fish oil) as an anti-inflammatory: an alternative to nonsteroidal anti-inflammatory drugs for discogenic pain. Surg Neurol 2006;65:326–31.
[13] Hori T, Oka T, Hosoi M, et al. Pain modulatory actions of cytokines and prostaglandin E2 in the brain. Ann NY Acad Sci 1998;840:269–81.
[14] Engblom D, Ek M, Saha S, et al. Prostaglandins as inflammatory messengers across the blood-brain barrier. J Mol Med 2002;80:5–15.
[15] Guay J, Bateman K, Gordon R, et al. Carrageenan-induced paw edema in rat elicits a predominant prostaglandin E2 (PGE2) response in the central nervous system associated with the induction of microsomal PGE2 synthase-1. J Biol Chem 2004;279:24866–72.
[16] Smith CJ, Zhang Y, Koboldt CM, et al. Pharmacological analysis of cyclooxygenase-1 in inflammation. Proc Natl Acad Sci U S A 1998;95:13313–8.

[17] Samuelsson B. Leukotrienes: mediators of immediate hypersensitivity reactions and inflammation. Science 1983;220:568–75.
[18] Lands WEM. Biosynthesis of prostaglandins. Annu Rev Nutr 1991;11:41–60.
[19] Mantzioris E, Cleland LG, Gibson RA, et al. Biochemical effects of a diet containing foods enriched with n-3 fatty acids. Am J Clin Nutr 2000;72:42–8.
[20] Caughey GE, Mantzioris E, Gibson RA, et al. The effect on human tumor necrosis factor α and interleukin-1β production of diets enriched in n-3 fatty acids from vegetable oil or fish oil. Am J Clin Nutr 1996;63:116–22.
[21] Cleland LG, French JK, Betts WH, et al. Clinical and biochemical effects of dietary fish oil supplements in rheumatoid arthritis. J Rheumatol 1988;15:1471–5.
[22] Sperling RI, Weinblatt M, Robin JL, et al. Effects of dietary supplementation with marine fish oil on leukocyte lipid mediator generation and function in rheumatoid arthritis. Arthritis Rheum 1987;30:988–97.
[23] Kremer JM, Lawrence DA, Jubiz W, et al. Dietary fish oil and olive oil supplementation in patients with rheumatoid arthritis. Arthritis Rheum 1990;33:810–20.
[24] Sun Y-P, Oh SF, Uddin J, et al. Resolvin D1 and its aspirin-triggered 17R epimer: stereochemical assignments, anti-inflamamatory properties, and enzymic inactivation. J Biol Chem 2007;282:9323–34.
[25] Serhan CN, Hong S, Gronert K, et al. Resolvins: a family of bioactive products of omega-3 fatty acid transformation circuits initiated by aspirin treatment that counter proinflammation signals. J Exp Med 2002;196:1025–37.
[26] Endres S, Ghorbani R, Kelley VE, et al. The effect of dietary supplementation with n-3 polyunsaturated fatty acids on the synthesis of interleukin-1 and tumor necrosis factor by mononuclear cells. N Engl J Med 1989;320:265–71.
[27] Meydani SN, Endres S, Woods MM, et al. Oral (n-3) fatty acid supplementation suppresses cytokine production and lymphocyte proliferation: comparison between young and older women. J Nutr 1991;121:547–55.
[28] Grimble RF, Howell WM, O'Reilly G, et al. The ability of fish oil to suppress tumor necrosis factor alpha production by peripheral blood mononuclear cells in healthy men is associated with polymorphisms in genes that influence tumor necrosis factor alpha production. Am J Clin Nutr 2002;76:454–9.
[29] Mantzioris E, James MJ, Gibson RA, et al. Dietary substitution with an α-linolenic acid-rich vegetable oil increases eicosapentaenoic acid concentrations in tissues. Am J Clin Nutr 1994; 59:1304–9.
[30] James MJ, Ursin VM, Cleland LG. Metabolism of stearidonic acid in human subjects: comparison with the metabolism of other n-3 fatty acids. Am J Clin Nutr 2003;77:1140–5.
[31] Emken EA, Adlof RO, Gulley RM. Dietary linoleic acid influences desaturation and acylation of deuterium-labeled linoleic and linolenic acids in young adult males. Biochim Biophys Acta 1994;1213:277–88.
[32] Cleland LG, James MJ, Neumann MA, et al. Linoleate inhibits EPA incorporation from dietary fish oil supplements in human subjects. Am J Clin Nutr 1992;55:395–9.
[33] Mozaffarian D, Ascherio A, Hu FB, et al. Interplay between different polyunsaturated fatty acids and risk of coronary heart disease in men. Circulation 2005;111:157–64.
[34] Cleland LG, James MJ, Proudman SM. Fish oil: what the prescriber needs to know. Arthritis Res Ther 2005;8:202.
[35] Cleland LG, Proudman SM, Hall C, et al. A biomarker of n-3 compliance in patients taking fish oil for rheumatoid arthritis. Lipids 2003;38:419–24.
[36] Cleland LG, Caughey GE, James MJ, et al. Reduction of cardiovascular risk factors with longterm fish oil treatment in early rheumatoid arthritis. J Rheumatol 2006;33:1973–9.
[37] Proudman SM, Keen HI, Stamp LK, et al. Response-driven combination therapy with conventional disease-modifying antirheumatic drugs can achieve high response rates in early rheumatoid arthritis with minimal glucocorticoid and nonsteroidal anti-inflammatory drug use. Semin Arthritis Rheum 2007;37:99–111.

[38] Maradit-Kremers H, Crowson CS, Nicola PJ, et al. Increased unrecognized coronary heart disease and sudden deaths in rheumatoid arthritis: a population-based cohort study. Arthritis Rheum 2005;52:402–11.

[39] Maradit-Kremers H, Nicola PJ, Crowson CS, et al. Cardiovascular death in rheumatoid arthritis: a population-based study. Arthritis Rheum 2005;52:722–32.

[40] Hippisley-Cox J, Coupland C. Risk of myocardial infarction in patients taking cyclo-oxygenase-2 inhibitors or conventional non-steroidal anti-inflammatory drugs: population based nested case-control analysis. BMJ 2005;330:1366–72.

[41] Chan AT, Manson JE, Albert CM, et al. Nonsteroidal antiinflammatory drugs, acetaminophen, and the risk of cardiovascular events. Circulation 2006;113:1578–87.

[42] Caughey GE, Cleland LG, Penglis PS, et al. Roles of cyclooxygenase (COX) -1 and -2 in prostanoid production by human endothelial cells: selective upregulation of prostacyclin synthesis by COX-2. J Immunol 2001;167:2831–8.

[43] Bombardier C, Laine L, Reicin A, et al. Comparison of upper gastrointestinal toxicity of rofecoxib and naproxen in patients with rheumatoid arthritis. N Engl J Med 2000;343:1520–8.

[44] Solomon SD, McMurray JJ, Pfeffer MA, et al. Cardiovascular risk associated with celecoxib in a clinical trial for colorectal adenoma prevention. N Engl J Med 2005;352:1071–80.

[45] Nussmeier NA, Whelton AA, Brown MT, et al. Complications of the COX-2 inhibitors parecoxib and valdecoxib after cardiac surgery. N Engl J Med 2005;352:1081–91.

[46] FitzGerald GA, Patrono C. The coxibs, selective inhibitors of cyclooxygenase-2. N Engl J Med 2001;345:433–42.

[47] Grosser T, Fries S, FitzGerald GA. Biological basis for the cardiovascular consequences of COX-2 inhibition: therapeutic challenges and opportunities. J Clin Invest 2006;116:4–15.

[48] Kromann N, Green A. Epidemiological studies in the Upernavik district, Greenland. Acta Med Scand 1980;208:401–6.

[49] Bang HO, Dyerberg J, Sinclair HM. The composition of Eskimo food in North Western Greenland. Am J Clin Nutr 1980;33:2657–61.

[50] Kromhout D, Bosschieter EB, de Lezenne Coulander C. The inverse relation between fish consumption and 20-year mortality from coronary heart disease. N Engl J Med 1985;312: 1205–9.

[51] Daviglus ML, Stamler J, Orencia AJ, et al. Fish consumption and the 30-year risk of fatal myocardial infarction. N Engl J Med 1997;336:1046–53.

[52] Albert CM, Hennekens CH, O'Donnell CJ, et al. Fish consumption and risk of sudden cardiac death. JAMA 1998;279:23–8.

[53] Hu FB, Bronner L, Willett WC, et al. Fish and omega-3 fatty acid intake and risk of coronary heart disease in women. JAMA 2002;287:1815–21.

[54] Dolecek TA, Grandits G. Dietary polyunsaturated fatty acids and mortality in the multiple risk factor intervention trial (MRFIT). World Rev Nutr Diet 1991;66:205–16.

[55] Burr ML, Fehily AM, Gilbert JF, et al. Effect of changes in fat, fish, and fibre intakes on death and myocardial reinfarction: diet and reinfarction trial (DART). Lancet 1989;334: 757–61.

[56] GISSI Prevenzione Investigators. Dietary supplementation with n-3 polyunsaturated fatty acids and vitamin E after myocardial infarction: results of the GISSI-Prevenzione trial. Lancet 1999;354:447–55.

[57] Siscovick DS, Raghunathan TE, King I, et al. Dietary intake and cell membrane levels of long-chain n-3 polyunsaturated fatty acids and the risk of cardiac arrest. JAMA 1995;274: 1363–7.

[58] Albert CM, Campos H, Stampfer MJ, et al. Blood levels of long-chain n-3 fatty acids and the risk of sudden death. N Engl J Med 2002;346:1113–8.

[59] Kris-Etherton PM, Harris WS, Appel LJ. Fish consumption, fish oil, omega-3 fatty acids, and cardiovascular disease. Circulation 2002;106:2747–57.

[60] Studer M, Briel M, Leimenstoll B, et al. Effect of different antilipidemic agents and diets on mortality: a systematic review. Arch Intern Med 2005;165:725–30.

ELSEVIER
SAUNDERS

Rheum Dis Clin N Am
34 (2008) 481–505

RHEUMATIC
DISEASE CLINICS
OF NORTH AMERICA

New Horizons in Pharmacologic Treatment for Rheumatic Disease Pain

Andy Dray, PhD

AstraZeneca Research & Development, 7171 Frederick Banting Street, Montreal, QC H4S 1Z9, Canada

Rheumatic disease pain, encompassing the major segments of rheumatoid arthritis (RA), osteoarthritis (OA), and low back pain (LBP), is by far the biggest chronic pain area where current therapies are suboptimal. Indeed, there are no approved therapies for LBP [1–4]. All three of these major segments represent chronic states of progressive and destructive damage to soft tissues, as well as joints and the spinal column. There is often chronic or episodic inflammation. Inflammation is beneficial in and of itself, causing orchestrated, targeted, destruction of foreign bodies and damaged tissues followed by assisted repair [5]. Sympathetic and sensory neurones are recruited to this process, causing for example changes in blood flow, vascular permeability, and also signal pain [6–8]. Dysregulated inflammation causes its own pathophysiology, resulting in chronic changes in neural function as well as destruction of normal tissue, including neurones, raising the specter of an associated nerve injury-induced pain [9–11]. Contributing to this are a number of secondary changes in central nervous system (CNS) pain processing caused by neuroimmune interactions [10,12] These processes are the basis of chronic pain in rheumatic disease, but the clinical picture is further complicated by the fact that pain frequency and intensity are related to other diverse factors, including comorbidities (eg, obesity and sleep disorders), socioeconomic factors, and education, as well as psychologic factors, such as anxiety, depression, and locus of control [13,14].

Pain mechanisms

It is important to distinguish between physiologic and pathophysiologic (chronic) pain. Physiologic pain is part of our normal defense mechanism,

E-mail address: andy.dray@astrazeneca.com

doi:10.1016/j.rdc.2008.04.005

is essential for survival, and is related directly to the degrees of existing or imminent tissue damage. Chronic pain has little defensive function, as neither the intensity nor quality of pain can be related to the degree of tissue injury. Indeed, pain may persist for many years after the resolution of any initial injury [15]. It is recognized that both chronic pains (nociceptive and neuropathic) result from aberrant functioning of a pathologically altered nervous system, similar to other neurologic and psychiatric disease states. Rheumatic pain, like other chronic pain conditions, is a complex integration of sensory, affective, and cognitive processes that involve a number of abnormal cellular mechanisms at both peripheral (eg joints) and central (spinal and supraspinal) levels of the nervous system (summarized in Fig. 1). Relative contribution of these processes in the population appears to be strongly segmented. For example, intra-articular anaesthetic studies in hip and knee OA support a peripheral drive to pain in approximately 60% to 80% of patients, depending on the affected joint [16,17]. However, in some individuals central mechanisms, such as dysfunction of descending inhibitory control [18,19] or altered cortical processing of noxious information, may play a greater role [19,20]. Furthermore, is has been highlighted that some prevalent chronic pain states (LBP, fibromyalgia and possibly more) may also present with secondary CNS neurodegeneration [21,22].

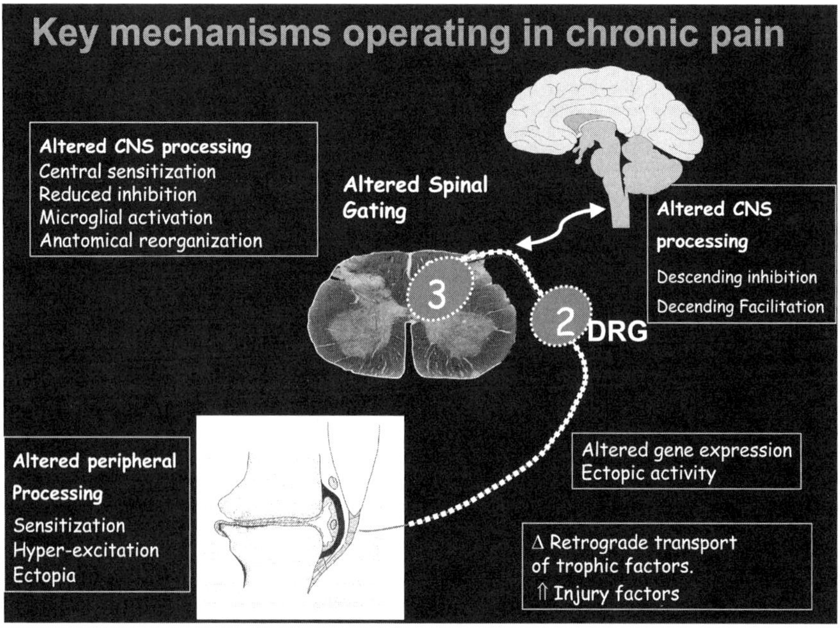

Fig. 1. Summary of key peripheral and CNS mechanisms operating in chronic pain in joints. DRG, dorsal root ganglia (2); spinal cord of CNS (3).

Mechanisms and models

Mechanistic and molecular-based understanding of chronic pain has relied heavily on animal studies for predicting efficacy of novel targets in patients. Model development has been driven by the desire to replicate the disease state (eg, LBP [23,24]), or more pragmatically to replicate a desirable clinical mechanism [25,26]. Mechanism-related laboratory models have emphasized key symptomatic characteristics, such as thermal hyperalgesia or mechanical allodynia. Earlier animal models of inflammatory pain were used to assess anti-inflammatory drug activity, such as edema and pain, using reflex limb withdrawal to a mechanical stimulation. The lack of activity of nonsteroidal anti-inflammatory drugs (NSAIDs) in acute models, such as the tail-flick and hot plate assays, raised an awareness that a sensitized and hyperexcitable state was induced by inflammation (or nerve damage), which differed from normal animals. In a similar vein, models of neuropathic pain have involved peripheral nerve lesions [25,26]. Such studies have allowed the systematic mechanistic exploration of excitability changes in pain pathways and provided the key building blocks for rational translation of findings in animal models into the clinical domain (eg, pharmacodynamic and pharmacokinetic). Supported by emerging human genetic and empirical clinical observations, these studies have highlighted a number of emerging therapeutic opportunities. These include the reduction of hyperexcitability in pain pathways (blocking inflammatory mediators or neuronal ion channels), direct inhibition of excitability (via G protein-coupled receptors), or restoring neural phenotype and metabolism through regulation of neurotrophins.

Pain therapy and challenges

There are a number of ongoing approaches that address rheumatic disease and associated pain. Disease modifying approaches are being aggressively pursued: for example, to attenuate chronic inflammation or resolve joint or cartilage degeneration. This may also impact on rheumatic pain [3,27]. Emerging pain pharmacology however, is driven by neural mechanism-based approaches and is seen primarily in terms of symptomatic treatment (through modulation of aberrant function, such as neural sensitization and excitability). This is the context in which new therapies are being developed and is the focus of this article.

Current treatments

Paracetamol is recommended as first-line treatment in mild to moderate pain, with the view that it has an improved safety profile relative to anti-inflammatory drugs, such as cyclo-oxygenase (COX) and COX-2 selective drugs. NSAIDs generally exhibit improved pain relief compared to paracetamol, but within this class there is little efficacy differentiation between nonselective and COX-2 selective NSAIDs. In terms of safety liability, increased selectivity for COX-1 is associated with increased gastrointestinal risk, and selectivity for COX-2 is associated with increased cardiovascular risk, predominantly myocardial infarction, stroke, hypertension, and congestive heart failure [1,3].

Tramadol, with properties of a weak opioid agonist, as well as serotonin norepinephrine reuptake inhibitor (SNRI), is also used widely as an adjunct in pain therapy. Limitations include the adverse effects of dizziness, nausea, and constipation [2]. The use of more potent opioids remains controversial because of side-effect limitations (constipation, nausea, somnolence) and abuse potential, but may be of use in patients where NSAIDs or other combinations, such as tramadol plus NSAIDs, are contraindicated. Finally, anti-tumor necrosis factor (TNF)-α treatment (etanerecept, infliximab) is being used to modulate disease activity in a number of inflammatory diseases, such as RA and the spondyloarthropies, but is also reported to produce significant pain relief [28].

At the core of present therapies are concerns of safety with anti-inflammatory drugs. These concerns are manifold with the elderly, who may be willing to forgo efficacy in favor of a lower perceived safety burden [29].

The identification of effective pharmacologic agents is fraught with issues because of patient heterogeneity and the belief that there are heterogenous mechanisms and molecular diversities of pain. Biomarker development and patient stratification will need to progress in parallel, to ensure "tailor-made treatment." More narrow titration of preclinical activities (eg, animal models, in vitro assays, and so forth) to specific patient subsets may also be required to improve predictability in man. Rational mechanistic approaches addressing sensory changes, such as sensitization (reduced threshold for stimulation), hyperexcitability (amplification or prolongation of nerve discharge), or spontaneous nerve activity can be associated with specific molecular changes.

Ultimately, in any patient, multiple algogenic mechanisms may underpin the pain experience. The paradigm in pain management is now showing a shift towards combination treatments rather than depending upon a single pharmacologic molecule. Combinations of pharmacologic approaches may therefore be a requirement for effective pain management. However, the concept of combination treatment will need to be balanced against cumulative safety burden of the treatments. Indeed, OA patients (particularly the elderly) may be willing to forgo efficacy in favor of lower adverse event risk [29].

Reduction of sensitization and hyperexcitability

Hyperexcitability in small and large peripheral sensory nerves acts as an important driving mechanism for chronic pain and can account for the initiation and maintenance of central hyperexcitability [30]. Thus, attenuation of local excitability by blocking mediators or by direct neural interactions appears as a valuable way forward (see Fig. 1). For example, the local anesthetic, lidocaine, reverses primary and secondary allodynia in neuropathic pain [31] at concentrations that do not affect normal nerve conduction. This is because of the well-known activity-dependent increase in voltage-gated ion (sodium and calcium) channel affinity for local anaesthetics. Additionally, intra-articular anesthetic studies in hip and knee OA support a peripheral drive to pain in approximately 60% to 80% of patients, depending on the affected joint [16,17].

Blocking the inflammatory mediators

The prostanoid family

The prostanoids, particularly prostaglandin E2 (PGE2), are considered to be the major contributor to inflammatory pain associated with a variety of cyclo-oxygenase enzyme products (PGE2, PGD2, PGF 2alpha, thromboxane, PGI2) produced during inflammation. Thus, blocking the major synthetic enzymes (COX-1 and COX-2) or inhibition of prostanoid receptors continues to be an important approach. PGE2 exerts its effects via a variety of EP receptors (EP1, -2, -3, -4) present in peripheral sensory neurones and in the spinal cord. Receptor activation produces nociceptor sensitization caused by ion channel phosphorylation. In the spinal cord, prostaglandin-induced hyperexcitability was enhanced via increased spinal cord expression of COX-1 (glia) and COX-2 (ventral horn cells) and EP receptor activation. Several mechanisms have been proposed, including receptor activation and spinal release of glutamate, as well as loss of spinal glycine receptor mediated inhibition [32]. In keeping with this, several NSAIDs have been shown to reduce inflammatory hyperalgesia via inhibition of spinal COX activity [33]. However, pain sensitivity was reduced by an EP3alpha agonist (ONO-AE-248), suggesting a balanced prostanoid regulation of pain [32].

Another COX isoform, COX-3, has been identified [34], and several NSAIDs (diclofenac, phenacetin) and acetaminophen show low efficacy but some degree of selectivity for COX-3. As COX-3 has low enzymic capacity and low abundance in the CNS and in the periphery, it is a less compelling target.

COX-2 selectivity has been associated with cardiovascular risk and many key questions remain unanswered concerning the mechanism of cardiovascular risk (see [35] for review). Despite these clinical concerns, development of COX-2 selective inhibitors still continues (eg, GW406381), reflecting the attraction of this pathway and the requirement for newer drugs with an improved overall safety profile.

The blockade of prostaglandin E synthase (PGES) offers an alternative route to PGE2 inhibition. Two isoforms of the enzyme have been identified, membrane or microsomal associated (mPGES-1) and a cytosolic enzyme (cPGES/p23), which are linked with COX-2 and COX-1 dependent PGE2 production, respectively [36,37]. Both isoforms are upregulated by inflammatory mediators. Gene deletion studies in mice indicate an important role for mPGES in acute and chronic inflammation and inflammatory pain [38]. Blocking of mPGES is thought to be an attractive possibility for PGE2 regulation without cardiovascular risk because PGI2 production would not be affected.

Bradykinin

Bradykinin is an important mediator of inflammatory pain, causing nociceptor activation and sensitization via B2 receptors [39]. The abundant metabolite of bradykinin, des Arg^9 bradykinin (kallidin), activates B1 receptors, which occur in low abundance, in the periphery and CNS [40–42].

B2 receptors undergo desensitization following prolonged kinin exposure, whereas B1 receptors do not desensitize rapidly and are dramatically upregulated in many tissues following injury [43–46], exposure to interleukin-1 beta (IL-1β), or the neurotrophin glial-derived neurotrophic factor (GDNF) [44,47]. Kinins cause a cascade of secondary changes, including prostanoid and nitric oxide production, phosphorylation of signaling proteins such as protein kinase-C, and the sensitization of sensory transducers, such as the transient receptor potential (TRP) V-1 receptor [48]. These events are linked with heat and mechanical hyperalgesia [49,50]. In keeping with this, B2 (eg, Icatibant, bradyzide) and the B1 antagonist (des Arg10 HOE-140; SSR240612) produce robust antihyperalgesic effects in models of nerve injury-induced pain [51–54]. Importantly, intra-articular administration of Icatibant (HOE 140) in OA patients was shown to reduce pain intensity at rest and during activity [55]. Other bradykinin antagonists in development include Amgen's AMG379 and Sanofi-Aventis SSR240612, both antagonists at the B1 receptor.

Cytokines, chemokines

These molecules and their receptors provide a complexity of interactions involved in chronic pain. Among the many players are TNF-α, interleukins, chemokines, nerve growth factor (NGF), sympathetic amines, leukotrienes, and prostaglandins. Cytokines induce hyperalgesia by a number of direct and indirect actions. Thus, IL-1β activates nociceptors directly via intracellular kinase activation, but it may also cause indirect nociceptor sensitization via the production of kinins and prostanoids [56]. TNF-α also activates sensory neurones directly via TNFR1 and TNFR2 receptors, and initiates a cascade of inflammatory reactions through the production of IL-1, IL-6 and IL-8 [57,58]. Notably, direct TNF-α application induces neuropathic pain behaviour that is blocked by ibuprofen and celecoxib [59], while nerve ligation causes increased TNF-α in damaged, as well as adjacent undamaged axons [60]. Interestingly, anti-TNF-α treatment with TNF antibodies produced a reduction of pain symptoms in an LBP model and in rheumatoid disease [28,61,62].

It should be noted that chemokines are important in orchestrating leucocyte migration but have also been implicated in brain development, neurodegenerative conditions, and synapse activity. Receptors have been detected throughout the CNS in the macrophage "like" microglial cells, astrocytes, oligodendrocytes, and neurons [12], as well as in primary afferent neurons and dorsal root ganglia (DRG) [63]. The major chemokines and their respective receptors are monocyte chemotactic protein (MCP)1/CCR2, macrophage-derived chemokine/CCR4, RANTES (regulated upon activation, normal T cell expressed and secreted)/CCR5, fractalkine/CX3CR1, and stromal cell-derived factor-1 alpha (SDF-1α)/CXCR4 . Specific chemokines, such as TNF-α, IL-8, and patterns of chemokine release [63,64], have been strongly associated with a number of neuropathic pain conditions. With respect to chemokine receptors, CCR2, CXCR4, CCR4, and CX3 CR1 have been shown to be expressed in glial and sensory neurons. Chemokines can contribute directly to hyperalgesia through G-protein coupled sensitization of ligand gated channels, such as TRPV1, heterologous desensitization of opioid receptors, and sensitization of sensory neurones [65,66]. Preliminary data have shown that blocking of CX3CR1 by a receptor-neutralizing antibody induces powerful antiallodynic effects. In addition, CCR2 has emerged as an important target, being powerfully expressed in spinal glia and DRG after peripheral nerve injuries, and is activated by its ligand MCP-1 to activate microglia and increase sensory fiber excitability [67]. In support of this, deletion of the CCR2 gene blocks glial cell recruitment and attenuates neuropathic pain [67]. While these preclinical data seem compelling, it should be noted that CCR2 antagonists have been in development (INCB3284, Pfizer/Incyte, and MK-0812 Merck) for treatment of rheumatoid arthritis but have not proved to be clinically efficacious.

Neuroimmune modulation is emerging as a key process in the etiology of chronic pain. Thus, neuroglial cells (microglia, astrocytes, DRG satellite cells, Schwann cells) have been highlighted as key cellular elements in these processes. Importantly, both trafficking of peripheral leukocytes into the CNS and activation of resident glial cells contribute in the etiology of neuropathic pain. Glial cell activity is important in pain amplification, as many of these cell-types regulate neuronal activity but also make close-junctional connections with each other, providing a means of spreading excitability changes beyond the boundaries of spinal segmental input. Also of importance is that glia secrete a number of mediators (nitric oxide, neurotrophins, IL1β, TNF-α, free radicals), some of which are associated with synaptogenesis but also with the plasticity that causes changes in spinal and afferent neuronal excitability, including secondary neurodegeneration and the loss of inhibitory interneurons [68].

The release of inflammatory mediators is regulated via glial receptors for adenosine triphosphate (ATP), kinins, prostanoids, N-methyl D-aspartate

(NMDA), and a variety of chemokine receptors that may also modulate spinal excitability [69,70]. A number of compounds claimed to stabilize and reduce glial activity have been shown to attenuate evoked pain in animal models. These include propentofylline [71,72], minocycline [69] and acetyl-L carnitine. Ibudilast (Avigen 411), a drug used clinically for respiratory disorders, has recently been shown to be efficacious in neuropathic pain [73] through reduction of neuroglial activation. For the most part, the actions of the aforementioned drugs that attenuate glial activity are not well understood.

Glial regulation may also be achieved through receptor modulation. In this respect a number of purinergic [74] receptors have been highlighted. For example, P2X7 and P2X4 receptors are expressed in microglia and satellite cells and are upregulated after peripheral nerve injuries [75,76]. Deletion of the P2X7 receptor-gene produced a complete absence of mechanical and thermal pain in mice [75], while the selective P2X4 antagonist trinitrophenylated-ATP attenuated mechanical allodynia [76].

While many cytokines appear to have a detrimental role in initiation and maintenance of neuropathic pain, some cytokines appear to be beneficial. Thus, a gene therapy approach, using viral and nonviral vectors (AV-333), has been used to increase spinal IL-10 production. This experimental treatment reversed the mechanical allodynia evoked in a model of neuropathic pain [77]. These are instructive observations, as they suggest that care must be given to maintaining a positive therapeutic balance when modulating the neuroimmune products that regulate chronic pain.

Modulation of excitability via ion channels

Acid sensing ion channels

Acid solutions produce prompt activation of sensory fibers through acid sensing ion channels (ASICs) and evoke a sensation of burning pain. This may be of pathopysiologic significance, as inflamed and necrotic tissues have an acidic environment. Several arthritidies, including OA, are associated with decreases in local pH during osteoclastic bone resorption, inflammation, and during tissue hypoxia [78]. H^+ ions can directly activate nociceptors via multiple mechanisms, such as TRPV1 channels.

Several types of ASICs have been identified (ASIC 1a and 1b, ASIC 2a and 2b, and ASIC 3). These are ubiquitously distributed throughout the nervous system, but specific channels (DRASIC) have been localized to small sensory neurons [79]. ASICs are sodium (Na^+) channels related to the degenerin/epithelial amiloride-sensitive Na+ channel superfamily of cation channels. A novel blocker (A-317567) of peripheral ASIC 1, -2, and -3 channels has been described [80]. This reduces hyperalgesia in models of inflammatory and postoperative pain, but there have been no reports of therapeutic advances with ASIC inhibitors.

Sodium channels

Sodium channels are characterized by their primary structure and sensitivity to tetrodotoxin (TTX). A variety of TTX sensitive (NaV1.3, Nav1.7) and TTX insensitive (NaV 1.8, NaV1.9) channels are involved in regulating sensory neural excitability [81,82]. Changes in the expression, trafficking, and redistribution of NaVs following inflammation or nerve injury are considered to account for unstable oscillations of membrane potential, abnormal firing, and the generation of ectopic activity in afferent nerves [83,84]. Mutations of NaV1.7 have been identified as the cause of burning pain in erythromelalgia [85], while loss or function mutations in these channels leads to complete ablation of pain perception in human beings, without any other notable pathology. Similar ablation of pain sensation has been observed in mice with NaV1.7-deficient sensory neurons [86].

NaV1.8 is uniquely expressed in small sensory neurones. These channels are regulated by inflammatory mediators and nerve injury [87,88]. NaV1.8 appears important for the generation of spontaneous activity in damaged sensory axons [82] and knockdown of NaV1.8 in models of neuropathic pain produces a marked reduction in abnormal pain responsiveness [89]. Recently, a NaV1.8 selective compound (A-803467) has been described [90] with a profile of activity in a variety of chronic pain models, but was surprisingly ineffective in models of acute pain, suggesting that this channel makes little contribution to nociception in the physiologic range.

NaV1.3 is also over expressed in large Ab fibers from chronic pain patients and in the spinal cord of pain models [87,88]. This channel may also be an important substrate for oscillations in peripheral and central neuron excitability, which is considered to be important for neuropathic pain.

Cardiovascular (via Nav1.5) and CNS sedation (via NaV1.2) are among the safety challenges associated with selective Na channel pharmacology. Emerging oral treatments include new sodium channel blockers, such as lacosamide (also called Vimpat or harkoseride, Schwarz Pharma) and ralfinamide (NW-1029, Alipamide, Newron Pharma), with activity at both TTX-sensitive and TTX-resistant channels. These drugs have been shown to be antihyperalgesic in models of inflammatory and neuropathic pain [91–93].

Ralfinamaide is another analgesic in advanced development. This acts via blocking Na-ion channels and by inhibiting the enzyme monoamine oxidase. This compound has shown a robust activity in a number of preclinical pain models. Clinical reports also suggest good tolerability overall, with positive outcome in a mixed population of neuropathic pain patients [93].

Voltage-gated calcium channels

Voltage-gated calcium channels are subdivided into, low voltage-activated calcium channels (T-type channels), and high voltage-activated channels (L-, N-, R-, P-, and Q-types). Several have been shown to be prominently involved in pain regulation [94]. N-type channels are unique to neurons and critical for pain neurotransmission. Thus, deletion of the N-channel gene caused a reduction in inflammatory and neuropathic pain [95], while intra spinal block with the snail conopeptide Ziconotide (Prialt: Elan/Esei) [96] or channel block with the orally available small molecule NMED-160 (Merck/Neuromed) [97] have shown efficacy across a range of chronic pain conditions.

The anticonvulsants gabapentin and pregabalin, commonly used for neuropathic pain therapy, target the alpha-2 delta-1 calcium channel subunit. This subunit is important for channel assembly, and its overexpression in small DRGs and spinal neurons is associated with allodynia in a number of specific pain models [98,99]. The exact mechanism of action of gabapentin is unknown, although block of N-channel regulated-release of CNS neurotransmitters has been considered to be critical. Recent evidence shows that gabapentin is transported into neurons via an L-neutral amino acid transporter and acts to displace an endogenous ligand, affecting the trafficking of alpa-2 delta-1 to the neural membrane [100].

Finally, low voltage-activated T channels also appear important for pain transmission and as targets for pain therapy. They are expressed in superficial laminae of the spinal cord and in DRG neurones [94] and play a prominent role in regulating spinal excitability following repetitive C-fiber stimulation [101,102]. Moreover, nerve injury-induced hyper-responsiveness was reported to be blocked by the T-channel blocker ethosuximide, which also attenuated mechanical allodynia in animal models of vincristine and paclitaxel-induced neuropathic pain [103].

Ligand-gated ion channels

A variety of ligand-gated ion channels are also being explored as targets for pain therapy. Foremost are the TRP channels. They are subdivided into six subfamilies (for review see [107]), but attention has been focussed mainly on TRPV1, TRPV3, TRPA1, and TRPM8. Many TRP channels are localized to sensory neurones and nearby keratinocytes, acting as temperature and mechanical transduction proteins. TRPV1 has been characterized in detail. This is a nonselective cation channel, gated by capsaicin, noxious heat ($>45°C$), acidic pH (<5.3), and is regulated by a variety of inflammatory mediators (eg, bradykinin, PGE2) and neuroregulators (anandamide, NGF). It is emerging as an important molecular focal point that is thought to play an important role in neural sensitization caused by mediators of inflammation and nerve injury [104,105].

Current analgesia strategies aim to develop either TRPV1 agonists or antagonist drugs to attenuate excitability in sensory fibers. TRPV1 agonists induce receptor desensitization or a reversible sensory nerve terminal degeneration because of prolonged cation influx into the nerve, osmotic damage, and metabolic collapse [106]. In this regard, topical formulation of high-dose capsaicin (eg, Transacin from NeurogesX) has been shown to be efficacious in a number of pain conditions [107].

Antagonists aim to attenuate peripheral nerve fiber sensitivity by blocking TRPV1 signal transduction. Supporting these approaches, competitive (AMG-9810, AMG 628) [108,109] and noncompetitive TRPV1 antagonists (DD161515) [110] block chemical and thermal pain sensitivity. Recent clinical studies in volunteers have also shown that oral SB705498 (GSK) attenuated capsaicin and ultraviolet C irradiation–induced pain and hyperalgesia [111], without notable side effects. These studies herald the way for a number of phase II trials for competing antagonists (eg, GRC 6211 Lilly/Glenmark; NDG6243 Merck/Neurogen; AZD1386, AstraZeneca; Amgen 517). However, others have noted the occurrence of acetaminophen-sensitive hyperthermia with this class of antagonists both in animal and human volunteer studies [112,113].

Other TRP channels (TRPV3, TRPV4, TRPA1, TRPM8) are also temperature transducers but appear to be important in pain transduction, particularly when sensitized by a pathophysiologic environment. TRPA1 is co-localized with TRPV1, is activated by capsaicin, and like TRPM8 can also be sensitized by inflammatory mediators and nerve injury to produce cold-induced burning pain [114–116]. TRPA1 selective antagonist HC030031 has been claimed to reduce pain signaling in animal models [117]. Interestingly, TRPV3 is also found in keratinocytes and sensory neurones [118,119], suggesting an interesting but indirect capacity to modulate sensor neural excitability.

Neuronal nicotinic receptors (NNRs) are part of a complex family of ligand-gated ion channels and include 5-hydroxytryptamine 3 and gamma-aminobutyric acid-A receptors. Chronic pain models reveal a significant overexpression of key NNR subunits, including the alpha-7 NNR as well as alpha-4 and alpha-5 subunits, supporting the therapeutic potential of NNRs in pain control [120,121]. In keeping with this, NNR agonists (epibatidine, ABT-594, Abbott) selective for these subunits have shown antinociception in several models of pain [122]. Several sites of action have been proposed, including supraspinal sites via descending monoaminergic and muscarinic pathways, as well direct actions via peripheral sensory neurones. Earlier clinical evaluation of ABT-594 revealed inadequate tolerability but more recent compounds, such as TC 6499 (GSK/Targacept) and ABT-894 (Abbott Pharma) are progressing in clinical phase I and II trials, respectively.

Glutamate

Glutamate excitation plays an important role in the initiation and maintenance of chronic pain. Glutamate acts through several receptors: the alpha-amino-3-hydroxy-5-methylisoxazole-4-proprionate (AMPA)/kinate receptors, ionotropic glutamate receptors (iGluRs) and G protein-coupled receptors, metabotropic glutamate receptors (mGluRs) coupled with ligand-gated ion channels. Injections of glutamate or metabolically stable receptor-selective agonists, such as NMDA, AMPA, and kainate, cause a pronociceptive response, while the administration of iGluR and mGluR antagonists attenuate pain [123,124]. Tezampanel (NGX426, TorreyPines), an AMPA kinate antagonist formulated for intravenous administration because of poor bioavailability, has shown positive outcome in several clinical trials [125,126] but with dose-limiting side effects, including blurred vision and sedation. The development of an oral prodrug is in progress, with the promise of improved bioavailability.

NMDA antagonists also show robust attenuation of pain in animal models but induce a number of side effects (sedation, confusion, motor incoordination), and thus appear to have insufficient therapeutic margin [127]. Avoidance of these side effects has been claimed via specific blockers of NMDA-receptor subtypes (NR1 and NR2) directed at the strychnine-insensitive $glycine_B$ modulatory site. This site modulates the NMDA channel during the sustained stimulation of the receptor, which is considered to occur during chronic pain. Selective NR1-Gly antagonists have been reported to reduce pain with reduced side effects [128,129]; however, clinical experience has not confirmed this. GV196771 (GSK) did not show efficacy against clinical pain, possibly because of inadequate penetration into the CNS [130].

An alternative NMDA approach has targeted the NR2B receptor [131], which has a specific distribution in sensory pathways. Blockade of this receptor produces anti-nociception (ifenprodil, traxoprodil, CP-101,606) with reduced side effects [132]. To date, traxoprodil has advanced into phase I safety and efficacy study for acute ischemic stroke and there is little information about possible development in pain. On the other hand, other NR2B programs, including RGH 896 (Gideon Richter) and EVT101 (Evotec), are continuing phase II trials [131].

Metabotropic glutamate receptors, particularly mGluR5, is thought to play a key role in central sensitization in chronic pain. Thus, spinal administration of selective agonists, such as dihydroxy-phenyl-glycine, produced pain hypersensitivity, while mGluR5 has been shown to be significantly overexpressed in some chronic pain models [132,133]. Several mGluR5 antagonists (MPEP, SIB 1747) have shown robust efficacy in pain models [134,135], while several compounds (ADX 10059, ADX 4861) have provided clinical validation of this target in several pain conditions, including migraine and fibromyalgia [136].

Enhancing inhibition: opioids, cannabinoids and monoamine modulation

Other emerging approaches to attenuate hyper-excitability in pain circuitry are to enhance cellular inhibitory mechanisms. These include targeting cannabinoid receptors or enhancing central monoaminergic inhibitory control.

Opiates

Opiate analgesia is frequently employed to treat OA pain in patients who do not respond to or have contraindications to NSAIDs. Opiates owe their profound and diverse effects through actions at peripheral, spinal, and supraspinal sites [80]. In the periphery, inflammation enhances the apparent potency of opioid agonists, in particular agonists at the mu-receptor. This may be the result of changes in receptor density, affinity, and recruitment of endogenous opioid-expressing leukocytes to the site of injury. In the periphery, opioids hyperpolarize sensory neurones and attenuate nerve hyperexcitability caused by inflammation or injury [137–139]. Localized, intra-articular delivery of morphine supports the concept that peripherally restricted opiate analgesia is plausible in OA and may overcome the common adverse events of centrally penetrating opiates [140]. Several pharma are investigating peripheral restricted mu-opioid agonists, which have shown efficacy in pain models [140,141], such as DiPOA (Perdue), a selective mu-receptor agonist and ADL-2-1294 (Adolor), a topical and intra-articular formulation of loperamide for local delivery [141–143].

Delta opioid receptor (DOR) agonists may provide analgesic efficacy without the confounding side effects of mu-opioid agonists, such as morphine (see [144] for review). Delta opioid analgesia has been shown in primate and nonprimate pain models with several ligands, such as D-Pen2, D-Pen5, enkephalin (DPDPE), SNC80, ARM-390. Emerging DOR biology has indicted that stimulus-dependent (pain, inflammation) trafficking of DOR from cytoplasm to cell surface appears to modulate apparent efficacy of agonists. Thus, delta ligands have low analgesic efficacy in acute pain models but show robust analgesia efficacy in a variety of chronic pain conditions accompanied by inflammation [145]. Following this, several DOR agonists are starting clinical evaluation (ADL-5859 ADL-5747; Adolor).

Cannabionoids

Cannabionoids act as pain modulation via two major receptors, CB1 and CB2. CB1 receptors are widely distributed in the CNS and in peripheral sensory neurons, while CB2 receptors have been found mainly in peripheral tissues, including tissues of the immune system and keratinocytes, with limited expression in sensory and CNS cells [146]. Several fatty acids (eg, anandamide, 2-arachidonylglycerol, and palmitoylethanolamide) have been identified as the endogenous ligands for these receptors, while specific antagonists (eg, SR141716A, SR147778 for CB1 and SR144428 for CB2) have been used to characterize receptor functions and support the validation of CBs in models of chronic pain [146].

The efficacy of cannabinoids for pain modulation are mediated mainly through CB1 receptors located in both the peripheral and CNS. Several clinical studies have show that cannabinoids, such as delta (9)-tetrahydrocannabinol (THC) or Sativex (THC plus cannabidiol: GW Pharma) reduce neuropathic pain, but these compounds also produce adverse effect,s such as euphoria, dizziness, and sedation at therapeutic concentrations [147]. Side effects may be limited by selective targeting of the peripheral cannabinoid CB1 receptors while maintaining significant pain relief. Studies in which the central CB1-receptor was deleted suggest significant analgesic efficacy can be retained through peripheral CB1 activation [148]. Supporting this hypothesis, localized or topical administration of nonselective agonists, such as HU210 or KDS2000 (Kadmus Pharma), or the oral administration of a CB1 agonist with limited CNS availability (ajulemic acid, CT3: Indevus Pharma), produced analgesia both in pain models [149,150] and in the clinic at a dose that caused minimal CNS side effects [151].

Interestingly, CB2 selective agonists (eg, HU-308, CP55940, AM1241, and GW405833) have also been shown to modulate chronic pain [152–154]. It is unclear how the analgesic effects of CB2 agonists are produced, because few CB2 receptors are found in the CNS or on sensory neurons [155]. However, de novo expression of CB2 receptors occurs in central glial cells after peripheral nerve lesions [156]. It is therapeutically significant that CB2 agonists have not shown CB1-like side effects.

Alternatively, the endogenous cannabinoid systems may be harnessed for pain control via inhibition of fatty acid amide hydrolysis, the major degradation pathway for endogenous cannabinoids [157]. Data supporting this show that mice lacking this enzyme [158], or treatment with fatty acid amide hydrolysis inhibitors, such as URB597 and OL135, significantly elevated brain anandamide and increased the pain threshold in pain models [159].

Monoamine receptors

Monoamine-containing sympathetic postganglionic neurons provide a rich innervation to the joint capsule, synovium, and bone. A dynamic interplay exists between sympathetic innervation and the control of vascular tone, bone turnover, inflammatory status, and sensory innervation in the joint.

Increased expression of alpha-1 and alpha-2 adrenergic receptors on sensory neurons or on postganglionic sympathetic terminal occurs following nerve injury and inflammation. This is accompanied by excitability changes driven by sympathetic transmitters [160,161]. Sympathomimetics, such as clonidine, and other alpha-2 agonists, such as dexmedetomidine, produce analgesia via their major site of action in the spinal cord by blocking of pre- and postsynaptic excitability. However, sedation and hypotension are target-related systemic side effects of these compounds. It is possible that these side effects can be avoided by direct intra-articular joint administration.

The successful treatment of neuropathic pain with amitriptyline and duloxetine has stimulated further interest in exploring mechanisms and drugs (eg, Venlafaxine, Bicifidine) that enhance monoamine pathways in the CNS. Because the effects of these SNRI drugs, in chronic neuropathic pain, appear to be independent of antidepressant activity, an attractive hypothesis is that they reinforce descending inhibitory pain circuitry. Other types of monoamine inhibitors, such as SRNI (fluoxetine, paroxetine), selective serotonin reuptake inhibitors (mirtazapine), or nonadrenergic reuptake inhibitors (reboxetine) require further evaluation [14]. However, it has been concluded that antidepressants represent useful tools in chronic situations, but must be evaluated against other analgesics in a clinically meaningful setting [162].

Restoring neural phenotype

Many changes in cellular phenotype have been identified during chronic pain because of disruption of regulators such as neurotrophins. These changes drive alterations in the expression of membrane receptor and ion channel proteins, alterations in cellular neurochemistry, and patterns of released transmitters, as well as synaptic reorganizations that impact on normal sensory functions. These changes can be regarded as critical elements of the disease processes that maintain the chronic pain state. Modulation of neurotrophins is seen as an attractive therapeutic possibility to address both chronic pain symptoms and disease progression.

Neurotrophins and their receptors

Neurotrophins represent an important family of regulatory proteins essential for sensory nerve development, survival, and the determination of neurochemical phenotypes critical for the regulation of excitability [163,164]. Neurotrophins include nerve growth factor, brain derived growth factor (BDNF), and neurotrophins (NT) 3, 4, and 5. Each neurotrophin binds with high affinity to a receptor tyrosine kinases (trk): NGF to trkA, BDNF and NT4/5 to trkB, and NT3 to trKC. NT3 also binds with trKA and trKB. Mature neurotrophins also bind to a structurally distinct receptor p75, which affects neuronal development through downstream signaling. Neurotrophins arise from proneurotrophin precursors following extracellular cleavage by metalloproteinases and plasmin. It is notable that proneurotrophins may signal through the p75 receptor in a manner that opposes the effects of neurotrophins, for example, to produce apoptosis rather than cell survival [165].

NGF is one of the most studied neurotrophins. It is a key regulator of sensory neurone excitability and an important mediator of injury-induced nociceptive and pain [166–168]. NGF activates a number of kinase-pathways (eg, p38 kinase) to alter gene transcription and regulate the synthesis of sensory neuropeptides (substance P, calcitonin gene-related peptide), ion channels (TRPV1, NaV1.8, ASIC3, P2X3), membrane receptors (bradykinin and P2X3), and structural molecules [169–172]. Increased expression and release of NGF have been demonstrated, for example, in ultraviolet and surgical injury [163], as well as in diseases including arthritis, cystitis, prostatitis, and headache [173–175]. Localized administration of exogenous NGF induces thermal and mechanical hyperalgesia in animals and in human beings [176,177], considered to be caused in part by mast cell degranulation and by directly increasing sensory neuronal excitability.

Few therapeutic NGF antagonists have been reported, but ALE0540 and PD90780, which inhibit NGF binding to TrK A and p75 respectively, have shown efficacy in chronic pain models [178,179]. In addition, the therapeutic utility of targeting NGF has also received clinical confirmation, because humanized anti-NGF monoclonal antibody (mAb) RN624 (Pfizer/Rinat) and AMG 403 (Amgen) has been reported to be efficacious in reducing pain and improved mobility in OA [180]. Anti-NGF mAb therapy thus appears as an attractive therapeutic approach, with further validation being pursued in other indications, including postherpetic neuralgia and low back pain.

BDNF is another important neurotrophin released from neuroglial and sensory cells and whose expression can be regulated by NGF following painful nerve injury [181]. In the spinal dorsal horn, BDNF increases spinal excitability [182] by direct neural excitation, phophorylation of NMDA receptors, and via altered regulation of the neural chloride-ion transporter In addition, spinally administered BDNF causes thermal and mechanical allodynia, whereas anti-BNDF neutralization or trK-B IgG administration reduces nerve injury hypersensitivity in animal models [181,183].

GDNF represents an extensive family of ligands and membrane receptor complexes that have an important role in regulating peripheral and central neural phenotypes. GDNF related ligands include neurturin and artemin, which act via the complex RET tyrosine kinase receptor and coreceptors GFRalpha-1, alpha-2, alpha-3, and alpha-4. GDNF has been shown to have neuroprotective and restorative properties in a number of neurodegenerative and neuropathic pain states [181]. Specifically, GDNF, and more recently artemin treatment, has been shown to restore peripheral sensory neurone function [184], including peptide and ion channel expression patterns, following peripheral nerve injury accompanied by an attenuation of pain behaviors [181]. Clinical observations using GDNF have shown unacceptable side effects, such as weight loss and allodynia, which has discouraged therapeutic development [185].

Summary

Rheumatic disease is associated with progressive and destructive damage to soft tissues as well as peripheral and spinal joints. Chronic pain is a major concern to patients but current therapies are suboptimal. There appears to be a complex spectrum of neurologic changes, manifesting both nociceptive and neuropathic pain. These are driven by joint pathophysiology and abnormal excitability in peripheral and central pain pathways. A variety of mechanisms have been identified and there is a belief that rheumatic disease pain patients can be segmented according to their molecular mechanistic signatures. This offers a multiplicity of possible intervention points for pain therapy, supported by a mechanisms-based focus on the key molecular drivers of neural excitability. A rich and diverse series of molecular events has been identified in the pathophysiology of chronic pain, representing most families of regulatory proteins. Emerging therapies are designed to reduce abnormal neural sensitization and excitability by targeting inflammatory mediators (kinins, prostanoids, mPGES, cytokines, chemokines) as well as ligand (TRPV1, NNRs, NMDA, mGluR) and voltage-regulated (NaV1.7, NaV1.8, CaV2.2) ion channels. Alternatively, inhibitory mechanisms are being enhanced through monoaminergic modulation using receptor agonists or through block of monoamine reuptake. Neurotrophic abnormalities, which cause the dysregulation of excitability and alterations of neural phenotype, are being restored through the modulation of specific neurotrophins such NGF and GDNF. There is great optimism that these initiatives, most often derived from studies in animal models and supported by greater clinical understanding of the neurologic changes in pain patients, will enable confident translation through clinical development to bring new generations of drugs to the rheumatic disease pain patient.

References

[1] Dray A, Read SJ. Future targets to control osteoarthritis pain. Arthritis Res Ther 2007;9:212.
[2] Kidd BL, Langford RM, Wodehouse T. Current approaches in the treatment of arthritic pain. Arthritis Res Ther 2007;9:214.
[3] Read SJ, Dray A. Osteoarthritic pain: a review of current, theoretical and emerging therapeutics. Expt Opin Invest Drugs 2008;17:616–40.
[4] Ruspe H. Management of chronic low back pain in 2007–2008. Curr Opin Rheumatol 2008;20:276–81.
[5] Nathan C. Points of control in inflammation. Nature 2002;420:846–52.
[6] Hunt SP, Mantyh P. The molecular dynamics of pain control. Nat Rev Neurosci 2001;2:83–91.
[7] Scholz J, Woolf CJ. Can we conquer pain? Nat Neurosci 2002;5:1062–5.
[8] Woolf CJ, Ma Q. Nociceptors-noxious stimulus detectors. Neuron 2007;55:353–64.
[9] Dray A. The pharmacology of inflammatory pain. In: Mersky H, Loeser JD, Dubner R, editors. The pathways of pain 1975–2005. Seattle (WA): IASP Press; 2005. p. 177–90.
[10] Scholz J, Woolf CJ. The neuropathic pain triad: neurons, immune cells and glia. Nat Neurosci 2007;10:1361–8.
[11] Hucho T, Levine JD. Signaling pathways in sensitization: towards a nociceptor cell biology. Neuron 2007;55:365–76.
[12] Watkins LR, Maier S. Beyond neurons: evidence that immune and glial cells contribute to pathological pain states. Physiol Rev 2002;82:981–1011.
[13] Ferrer-Garcia MD, Wernicke JF, Detke MJ, et al. The depression-pain complex: overlap between the two problems and implications for neuropathic pain. In: Campbell JN, Basbaum AI, Dray A, et al, editors. Emerging strategies for the treatment of neuropathic pain. Seattle (WA): IASP Press; 2006. p. 307–25.
[14] McQuay HJ, Moore RA. Antidepressants and chronic pain. BMJ 1997;314:763–4.
[15] Campbell JN, Basbaum AI, Dray A, et al, editors. Emerging strategies for the treatment of neuropathic pain. Seattle (WA): IASP Press; 2006.
[16] Creamer P, Hunt M, Dieppe P. Pain mechanisms in osteoarthritis of the knee: effect of intra-articular anaesthetic. J Rheumatol. 1996;23:1031–6.

[17] Crawford RW, Gie GA, Ling RS, et al. Diagnostic value of intra-articular anaesthetic in primary osteoarthritis of the hip. J Bone Joint Surg Br 1998;80:279–81.
[18] Kosek E, Ordeberg G. Lack of pressure pain modulation by heterotopic noxious conditioning stimulation in patients with painful osteoarthritis before, but not following, surgical pain relief. Pain 2000;88:69–78.
[19] Buffington AL, Hanlon CA, McKeown MJ. Acute and persistent pain modulation of attention-related anterior cingulated fMRI activations. Pain 2005;113:172–84.
[20] Rowbotham MC, Kidd BL, Porreca F. Role of central sensitization in chronic pain: osteoarthritis and rheumatoid arthritis compared to neuropathic pain. In: Flor H, Kalso E, Dostrovsky J, editors. Proceedings of the 11th World Congress on Pain. Seattle (WA): IASP Press; 2006. p. 231–49.
[21] Baliki MN, Gehe PY, Apkarain AV, et al. Beyond feeling: chronic pain hurts the brain, disrupting the default mode network dynamics. J Neurosci 2008;28:1398–403.
[22] Kuchinad A, Schweinhardt P, Wood P, et al. Accelerated brain gray-matter loss in fibromyalgia patients: premature aging of the brain? J Neurosci 2007;27:4004–7.
[23] Gu X, Yang L, Wang S. A rat model of radicular pain induced by chronic compression of lumbar dorsal root ganglia with SURGIFLO. Anesthesiology 2008;108:113–21.
[24] Alini M, Eisenstein SM, Ito K, et al. Are animal models useful for studying human disc disorders/degeneration? Eur Spine J 2008;17:2–19.
[25] Le Bars D, Gozariu M, Cadden SW. Animal models of nociception. Pharmacol Rev 2001; 53:597–652.
[26] Gold MS, Chessell I, Devor M, et al. Peripheral nervous system targets: Rapporteur report. In: Campbell JN, Basbaum AI, Dray A, et al, editors. Emerging strategies for the treatment of neuropathic pain. Seattle (WA): IASP Press; 2006. p. 3–36.
[27] Ikeda K, Cox S, Emery P. Biological therapy in early arthritis—overtreatment or the way to go? Arthritis Res Ther 2007;9:211.
[28] Fedmann M, Maini RN. Anti-TNF a therapy of rheumatoid arthritis: what we learned? Annu Rev Immunol 2001;19:163–9.
[29] Fraenkel M, Bogardus ST, Concato J, et al. Treatment options in knee OA. Arch Intern Med 2004;164:1299–304.
[30] Woolf CJ, Salter MW. Neuronal plasticity: increasing the gain in pain. Science 2000;288: 1765–9.
[31] Gracely RH, Lynch SA, Bennett GJ. Painful neuropathy: altered central processing maintained dynamically by peripheral input. Pain 1992;51:175–94.
[32] Bar KJ, Natura G, Telleria-Diaz A, et al. Changes in the effect of spinal prostaglandin E2 during inflammation: prostaglandin E9(EP1-EP4) receptors in spinal nociceptive processing of input from the normal and inflamed knee joint. J Neurosci 2004;24:642–51.
[33] Yaksh TL, Dirig DM, Conway CM, et al. The acute hyperalgesic action of non-steroidal, anti-inflammatory drugs and release of spinal prostaglandin E2 is mediated by the inhibition of constitutive spinal cyclooxygenase-2 (COX-2) but not COX-1. J Neurosci 2001;21: 5847–53.
[34] Chandrasekharan NV, Dai H, Roos KL, et al. COX-3, a cyclooxygenase-1 variant inhibited by acetaminophen and other analgesic/antipyretic drugs: cloning, structure, and expression. Proc Natl Acad Sci 2002;99:13926–31.
[35] Mitchell JA, Warner TD. COX isoforms in the cardiovascular system: understanding the activities of non-steroidal anti-inflammatory drugs. Nat Rev Drug Discov 2006;5:75–85.
[36] Jakobsson PJ, Thoen S, Morgenstern R, et al. Identification of human prostaglandin E synthase: a microsomal, glutathione-dependent, inducible enzyme, constituting a potential novel drug target. Proc Natl Acad Sci 1999;96:7220–5.
[37] Claveau D, Sirinyan M, Guay J, et al. Microsomal prostaglandin synnthase-1 is a major terminal synthase that is selectively upregulated during cyclooxygenase-2-dependent prostaglandin E2 production in the rat adjuvant-arthritis model. J Immunol 2003;170: 4738–44.

[38] Trebino CE, Stock JL, Gibbons CP, et al. Impaired inflammatory and pain responses in mice lacking an inducible prostaglandin E synthase. Proc Natl Acad Sci 2003;100:9044–9.
[39] Dray A. Kinins and their receptors in hyperalgesia. Can J Physiol Pharmacol 1997;75: 704–12.
[40] Dray A, Perkins MN. Bradykinin and inflammatory pain. Trends Neurosci 1993;16: 99–104.
[41] Wotherspoon G, Winter J. Bradykinin B1 receptor is constitutively expressed in the rat sensory nervous system. Neurosci Lett 2000;294:175–8.
[42] Shughrue PJ, Ky B, Austin CP. Localization of B1 bradykinin receptors mRNA in the primate brain and spinal cord: an in situ hybridization study. J Comp Neurol 2003;46: 372–84.
[43] Levy D, Zochodne DW. Increased mRNA expression of the B1 and B2 bradykinin receptors and antinociceptive effects of their antagonists in an animal model of neuropathic pain. Pain 2000;86:265–71.
[44] Fox A, Wotherspoon G, McNair K, et al. Regulation and function of spinal and peripheral neuronal B(1) bradykinin receptors in inflammatory mechanical hyperalgesia. Pain 2003; 104:683–91.
[45] Ferreira J, Beirith A, Mori MAS, et al. Reduced nerve injury induced neuropathic pain in kinin B1 receptor knock-out mice. J Neurosci 2005;25:2405–12.
[46] Eisenbarth H, Rukwied R, Petersen M, et al. Sensitization to bradykinin B1 and B2 receptor activation in UV-B irradiated human skin. Pain 2004;110:197–204.
[47] Vellani V, Zachrisson O, McNaughton PA. Functional bradykinin B1 receptors are expressed in nociceptive neurons and are upregulated by the neurotrophin GDNF. J Physiol 2004;560:391–401.
[48] Marceau F, Hess JF, Bachvarov DR. The B1 receptors for kinins. Pharmacol Rev 1998;50: 357–86.
[49] Liang YF, Haake B, Reeh PW. Sustained sensitization and recruitment of rat cutaneous nociceptors by bradykinin and a novel theory of its excitatory action. J Physiol 2001;532: 229–39.
[50] Fox A, Kaur S, Li B, et al. Antihyperalgesic activity of a novel nonpeptide bradykinin B1 receptor antagonist in transgenic mice expressing the human B1 receptor. Br J Pharmacol 2005;144:889–99.
[51] Stewart JM. Bradykinin antagonists: discovery and development. Peptides 2004;25:527–32.
[52] Burgess GM, Perkins MN, Rang HP, et al. Bradyzide, a potent nonpeptide B2 bradykinin receptors antagonist with long lasting oral activity in animal models of inflammatory hyperalgesia. Br J Pharmacol 2000;129:77–86.
[53] Gougat J, Ferrari B, Lionel S, et al. SSR240612 [(2R)-2-[((3R0-3-(1,3-benzodiol-5-yl)-3-{[(6-methoxy-2-napthyl)sulfonyl]amino}propanoyl)amino]-3-(4-{[2R,6S)-2,6-dimethylpiperidyl] methyl} phenyl} -N-isoproyl-Nmethylpropanamide hydrochloride], a new nonpeptide antagonist of the bradykinin B1 receptor: biochemical and pharmacological characterization. J Pharmacol Exp Ther 2005;309:661–9.
[54] Gabra BH, Sirois P. Beneficial effects of chronic treatment with the selective bradykinin B1 receptor antagonists, R-715 and R-953, in attenuating streptozotocin-diabetic thermal hyperalgesia. Peptides 2003;24:1131–9.
[55] Flechtenmacher J, Talke M, Veith D, et al. Icatibant induces pain relief in patients with osteoarthritis of the knee. Proceedings of the 9th World Congress on Osteoarthritis (ORSI). Osteo Arthritis Res Soc Int 2004;12:P332.
[56] Sommer C, Kress M. Recent findings on how proinflammatory cytokines cause pain: peripheral mechanisms in inflammatory and neuropathic hyperalgesia. Neurosci Lett 2004; 361(1–3):184–7.
[57] Ohtori S, Takahashi K, Moriya H, et al. TNF-alpha and TNF-alpha receptor type 1 upregulation in glia and neurons after peripheral nerve injury: studies in murine DRG and spinal cord. Spine 2004;29:1082–8.

[58] Pollock J, McFarlane SM, Connell MC, et al. TNF-alpha receptors simultaneously activate Ca2+ mobilisation and stress kinases in cultured sensory neurons. Neuropharmacology 2002;42:93–106.
[59] Schafers M, Marziniak M, Sorkin LS, et al. Cyclooxygenase inhibition in nerve-injury and TNF-induced hyperalgesia in the rat. Exp Neurol 2004;185(1):160–8.
[60] Schafers M, Sorkin LS, Geis C, et al. Spinal ligation induces transient upregulation of tumor necrosis factor receptors 1 and 2 in injured and adjacent uninjured dorsal root ganglia of rat. Neurosci Lett 2003;347:179–82.
[61] Grunke M, Schulze-Koops H. Successful treatment of inflammatory knee osteoarthritis with tumour necrosis factor blockade. Ann Rheum Dis 2006;65:555–6.
[62] Nobuhisa S, Kikuchi S-I, Konno S-I, et al. Anti-TNF-[alpha] antibody reduces pain behavioral changes induced by epidural application of nucleus pulposus in a rat model depending on the timing of administration. Spine 2007;32:413–6.
[63] Kotani N, Kudo R, Sakurai Y, et al. Cerebrospinal fluid interleukin 8 concentrations and the subsequent development of postherpetic neuralgia. Am J Med 2004;116:318–24.
[64] Lindenlaub T, Sommer C. Cytokines in sural nerve biopsies from inflammatory and noninflammatory neuropathies. Acta Neuropathol 2003;105:593–602.
[65] Zhang N, Inan S, Cowan A, et al. A proinflammatory chemokine, CCL3, sensitizes the heat- and capsaicin-gated ion channel TRPV1. Proc Natl Acad Sci 2005;102:4536–41.
[66] Oh SB, Tran PB, Gillard SE, et al. Chemokines and glycoprotein 120 produce pain hypersensitivity by directly exciting primary nociceptive neurons. J Neurosci 2001;21:5027–35.
[67] Abbadie C, Lindia JA, Cumiskey AM, et al. Impaired neuropathic pain responses in mice lacking the chemokine receptor CCR2. Proc Natl Acad Sci 2003;100:7947–52.
[68] Moore KA, Kohno T, Karchewski LA, et al. Partial peripheral nerve injury promotes a selective loss of GABAergic inhibition in the superficial dorsal horn of the spinal cord. J Neurosci 2002;22:6724–31.
[69] Watkins LR, Maier SF. Glia: a novel drug discovery target for clinical pain. Nat Rev Drug Discov 2003;2:973–85.
[70] White FA, Jung H, Miller R. Chemokines and the pathophysiology of neuropathic pain. Proc Natl Acad Sci U S A 2007;104:20151–8.
[71] Sweitzer SM, Pahl JL, DeLeo JA. Propentofylline attenuates vincristine-induced peripheral neuropathy in the rat. Neurosci Lett 2006;400:258–61.
[72] Ledeboer A, Liu T, Shumilla JA, et al. The glial modulatory drug AV411 attenuates mechanical allodynia in rat models of neuropathic pain. Neuron Glia Biol 2007;10:1–13.
[73] Raghavendra V, Tanga F, Rutkowski MD, et al. Anti-hyperalgesic and morphine-sparing actions pf propentofylline following peripheral nerve injury in rats: mechanistic implications of spinal glia and proinflammatory cytokines. Pain 2003;104:655–64.
[74] Donelly-Roberts D, McGaraughty S, Shieh CC, et al. Painful purinergic receptors. J Pharmacol Exp Ther 2008;324:409–15.
[75] Chessell IP, Hatcher JP, Davey PT, et al. Disruption of the P2x7 purinoceptor gene abolishes chronic inflammatory and neuropathic pain. Nature 2005;114:386–96.
[76] Tsuda M, Shigemoto-Mogami Y, Koizumi S, et al. P2X4 receptors induced in spinal microglia gate tactile allodynia after nerve injury. Nature 2003;424:778–83.
[77] Milligan ED, Langer SJ, Sloane EM, et al. Controlling pathological pain by adenovirally driven spinal production of the anti-inflammatory cytokine, interleukin-10. Eur J Neurosci 2005;21:2136–48.
[78] Giatromanolaki A, Sivridis E, Maltezos E, et al. Upregulated hypoxia inducible factor-1alpha and -2alpha pathway in rheumatoid arthritis and osteoarthritis. Arthritis Res Ther 2003;5(4):R193–201.
[79] Leffler A, Monter B, Koltzenburg M. The role of the capsaicin receptor TRPV1 and acid sensing ion channels (ASICs) in proton sensitivity of subpopulation of primary nociceptive neurons in rats and mice. Neuroscience 2006;139:699–709.

[80] Dube GR, Lehto SG, Breese NM, et al. Electrophysiological and in vivo characterization of A-317567, a novel blocker of acid sensing ion channels. Pain 2005;117:88–96.
[81] Eglen RM, Hunter JC, Dray A. Ions in the fire: recent ion-channel research and approaches to pain therapy. Trends Pharmacol Sci 1999;8:337–42.
[82] Matzner O, Devor M. Hyperexcitability at sites of nerve injury depends on voltage sensitive – sodium channels. J Neurophysiol 1994;72:349–59.
[83] Devor M. Sodium channels and mechanisms of neuropathic pain. Pain 2005;7(Suppl 1): S3–12.
[84] Amir R, Liu CN, Devor M. Oscillatory mechanisms in primary sensory neurones. Brain 2002;125:421–35.
[85] Waxman SG, Dib-Hajj S. Erythermalgia: molecular basis for an inherited pain syndrome. Trends Mol Med 2005;11:555–62.
[86] Nassar MA, Stirling LC, Forlani G, et al. Nociceptor-specific gene deletion reveals a major role for Na_v1.7 (PN1) in acute and inflammatory pain. Proc Natl Acad Sci U S A 2004;101: 12706–11.
[87] Coward K, Plumpton C, Facer P, et al. Immunolocalization of SNS/PN3 and NaN/SNS2 sodium channels in human pain states. Pain 2000;85:41–50.
[88] Hains BC, Klein JP, Saab CY, et al. Upregulation of sodium channel NaV 1.3 and functional involvement in neuronal hyperexcitability associated with central neuropathic pain after spinal cord injury. J Neurosci 2003;23:8881–92.
[89] Roza C, Laird JM, Souslova V, et al. The tetrodotoxin-resistant Na channel NaV1.8 is essential for the expression of spontaneous activity in damaged sensory axons of mice. J Physiol 2003;550(3):921–6.
[90] Jarvis MF, Honore P, Shieh CC, et al. A-803467 a potent and selelctive NaV1.8 sodium channel blocker, attenuates neuropathic and inflammatory pain in the rat. Proc Natl Acad Sci U S A 2007;104:8520–5.
[91] Beyreuther B, Callizot N, Stohr T. Antinociceptive efficacy of lacosamide in a rat model for painful diabetic neuropathy. Eur J Pharmacol 2006;539:64–70.
[92] Hao JX, Stohr T, Selve N, et al. Lacosamide, a new anti-epileptic, alleviates neuropathic pain-like behaviors in rat models of spinal cord or trigeminal nerve injury. Eur J Pharmacol 2006;553:135–40.
[93] Cattabeni F. Ralfinamide. Newron Pharamaceuticals. I Drugs 2004;7:935–9.
[94] Yaksh TL. Calcium channels as therapeutic targets in neuropathic pain. Pain 2006; 7(Suppl 1):S13–30.
[95] Saegusa H, Kurihara T, et al. Suppression of inflammation and neuropathic pain symptoms in mice lacking the N-type Ca2+ channel. EMBO J 2001;20:2349–56.
[96] Miljanich GP. Ziconitide: neuronal calcium channel blocker for treating severe chronic pain. Curr Med Chem 2004;11:3029–40.
[97] Snutch TP. Targeting chronic and neuropathic pain: the N-type calcium channel comes of age. NeuroRx 2005;2:662–70.
[98] Kim C, Jun K, Lee T, et al. Altered nociceptive responses in mice deficient in the alpha1δ subunit of the voltage dependent calcium channel. Mol Cell Neurosci 2001;18:235–45.
[99] Luo ZD, Calcutt NA, Higuera ES, et al. Injury type-specific calcium channel alpha (2) delta-1 subunit up-regulation in rat neuropathic pain. J Pharmacol Exp Ther 2002;303: 1199–205.
[100] Hendrich J, Van Winh AT, Heblich F, et al. Pharmacological disruption of calcium channel trafficking by the alpha2 delta ligand gabapentin. Proc Natl Acad Sci U S A 2008;105: 3628–33.
[101] Ikeda H, Heinke B, Ruscheweyh R, et al. Synaptic plasticity in spinal lamina 1 projection neurons that mediate hyperalgesia. Science 2003;299:1237–40.
[102] Matthews EA, Dickenson AH. Effects of spinally delivered N-and P-type voltage dependent calcium channel antagonists on dorsal horn neuronal responses in a rat model of neuropathy. Eur J Pharmacol 2001;415:141–9.

[103] Flatters SJ, Bennett GJ. Ethosuximaide reverses paclitaxel and vincristine-induced painful peripheral neuropathy. Pain 2004;109:150–61.
[104] Ramsey IS, Delling M, Clapham DE. An introduction to TRP channels. Annu Rev Physiol 2006;68:619–47.
[105] Vellani V, Mappleback S, Moriondo A, et al. Protein kinase C activation gating of the vanilloid receptor VR1 by capsaicin, protons, heat and anandamide. J Physiol 2001;534: 813–25.
[106] Szallasi A, Blumberg PM. Vanilloid (Capsaicin) receptors and mechanisms. Pharmacol Rev 1999;51(2):159–212.
[107] Bley KR. Recent developments in transient receptor potential vanilloid receptor 1 agonist-based therapies. Expert Opin Investig Drugs 2004;13:1445–56.
[108] Gavva NR, Tamir R, Qu Y, et al. AMG 9810 [(E) –3- (4-t- butylphenyl)-N-(2,3-dihydrobenzo[b][1,4] dioxin-6-yl)acrylamide], a novel vanilloid receptor 1 (TRPV1) antagonist with antihyperalgesic properties. J Pharmacol Exp Ther 2005;313:473–84.
[109] Wang HL, Katon J, Balan C, et al. Vanilloid receptor-1 antagonists: 3. The identification of a second-generation clinical candidate with improved physicochemical and pharmacokinetic properties. J Med Chem 2007;50:3528–39.
[110] Garcia-Martinez C, Humet M, Planells-Casas R, et al. Attenuation of thermal nociception and hyperalgesia by VR1 blockers. Proc Natl Acad Sci U S A 2002;99:2374–9.
[111] Chizh BA, O'Donnell MB, Napoltano A, et al. The effects of the TRPV1 antagonist SB-705498 on TRPV1 receptor-mediated activity and inflammatory hyperalgesia in humans. Pain 2007;132:132–41.
[112] Gavva NR, Bannon AW, Howland DN, et al. Repeated administration of vanilloid receptor TRPV1 antagonist attenuates hyperthermia elicited by TRPV1 blockade. J Pharmacol Exp Ther 2007;323:128–37.
[113] Gavva NR, Treanor JS, Garami A, et al. Pharmacological blockade of the vanilloid receptor TRPV1 elicits marked hyperthermia in humans. Pain 2008;136:202–10.
[114] Bandell M, Story GM, Hwang SW, et al. Noxious cold ion channel TRPA1 is activated by pungent compounds and bradykinin. Neuron 2004;41:849–53.
[115] Obata K, Katsura H, Mizushima T, et al. TRPA1 induced in sensory neurons contributes to cold hyperalgesia after inflammation and nerve injury. J Clin Invest 2005;115: 2393–401.
[116] Proudfoot CJ, Garry EM, Cottrell DF, et al. Analgesia mediated by the TRPM8 cold receptor in chronic neuropathic pain. Curr Biol 2006;16:1591–609.
[117] McNamara CR, Mandel-Brehm J, Bautista DM, et al. TRPA1 mediates formalin-induced pain. Proc Natl Acad Sci U S A 2007;104:13525–30.
[118] Koizumi S, Fujishita K, Inoue K, et al. Ca^{2+} waves in keratinocytes are transmitted to sensory neurons: the involvement of extracellular ATP and P2Y2 receptor activation. Biochem J 2004;380:329–38.
[119] Peier AM, Reeve AT, Andersson DA, et al. A heat sensitive TRP channel expressed in keratinocytes. Science 2002;296:2046–9.
[120] Decker MW, Meyer MD, Sullivan JP. The therapeutic potential of nicotinic acetylcholine receptor agonist for pain control. Expert Opin Investig Drugs 2001;10:1819–30.
[121] Vincler M. Neuronal nicotinic receptors as targets for novel analgesics. Expert Opin Investig Drugs 2005;14:1191–8.
[122] Meyer MD. Neuronal nicotinic acetylcholine receptors as a target for the treatment of neuropathic pain. Drug Devolpment Research 2006;67:355–9.
[123] Neugebauer V. Glutamate receptor ligands. Handb Exp Pharmacol 2007;177:217–49.
[124] Szekely JI, Torok K, Mate G. The role of ionotropic glutamate receptors in nociception with special regard to the AMPA binding sites. Curr Pharm Des 2002;8(10):887–912.
[125] Sang CN, Hostetter MP, Gracely RH, et al. AMPA/Kainate antagonist LY293558 reduces capsaicin-evoked hyperalgesia but not pain in normal skin in humans. Anesthesiology 1998;89:1060–7.

[126] Sang CN, Ramadan NM, Wallihan RG, et al. LY293558, a novel AMPA/GluR5 antagonist, is efficacious and well-tolerated in acute migraine. Cephalalgia 2004;24:596–602.
[127] Olney JW, Farber NB. NMDA antagonists as neurotherapeutic drugs, psychotogens, neurotoxins, and research tools for studying schizophrenia. Neuropsychopharmacology 1995; 13:335–45.
[128] Danysz W, Parsons CG. GlycineB recognition site of NMDA receptors and its antagonists. Amino Acids 1998;14:205–6.
[129] Quartaroli M, Fasdelli N, Bettelini L, et al. GV196771A, an NMDA receptor/glycine site antagonist, attenuates mechanical allodynia in neuropathic rats and reduces tolerance induced by morphine in mice. Eur J Pharmacol 2001;430:219–27.
[130] Wallace MS, Rowbotham MC, Katz NP, et al. A randomized, double blind, placebo-controlled trial of a glycine antagonist in neuropathic pain. Neurology 2002;59:1694–700.
[131] Gogas KR. Glutamate-based therapeutic approaches: NR2B receptor antagonists. Curr Opin Pharmacol 2006;6:68–74.
[132] Hudson LJ, Bevan S, McNair K, et al. Metabotropic glutamate receptor 5 up-regulation in A-fibers after spinal nerve injury: 2-Methyl-6-(phenylethynyl)-pyridine (MPEP) reverses the induced thermal hyperalgesia. J Neurosci 2002;22:2660–8.
[133] Zhu CZ, Wilson SG, Mikusa JP, et al. Assessing the role of metabotropic glutamate receptor 5 in multiple nociceptive modalities. Eur J Pharmacol 2004;506:107–18.
[134] Taniguchi K, Shinjo K, Mizutani M, et al. Antinociceptive actions of CP-101, 606, an NMDA receptor NR2B subunit antagonist. Br J Pharmacol 1997;12:809–12.
[135] Dogrul A, Ossipov MH, Lai J, et al. Peripheral and spinal antihyperalgesic activity of SIB-1757, a metabotropic glutamate receptor (mGluR5) antagonist, in experimental neuropathic pain in rats. Neurosci Lett 2000;292:115–8.
[136] Jaeschke G, Wettstein JG, Nordquist RE, et al. mGlu5 receptor antagonists and their therapeutic potential. Expert Opinion Therapeutic Patents 2008;18:123–42.
[137] Yaksh TL. Pharmacology and mechanisms of opioid analgesic activity. Acta Anaesthesiol Scand 1997;41:94–111.
[138] Hurley RW, Hammond DL. The analgesic effects of supraspinal μ and δ opioid receptor agonists are potentiated during persistent inflammation. J Neurosci 2000;20:1249–59.
[139] Sawynok J. Topical and peripherally acting analgesics. Pharmacol Rev 2003;55:1–20.
[140] Likar R, Schafer M, Paulak F, et al. Intraarticular morphine analgesia in chronic pain patients with osteoarthritis. Anesth Analg 1997;84:1313–7.
[141] Menendez L, Lastra A, Meana A, et al. Analgesic effects of loperamide in bone cancer pain in mice. Pharmacol Biochem Behav 2005;81:114–21.
[142] Whiteside GT, Boulet JM, Walker K. The role of central and peripheral mu opioid receptors in inflammatory pain and edema: a study using morphine and DiPOA ([8-(3,3-diphenyl-propyl)-4-oxo-1-phenyl-1,3,8-triaza-spiro[4.5]dec-3-yl]-acetic acid). J Pharmacol Exp Ther 2005;314:1234–40.
[143] Valenzano KJ, Miller W, Chen Z, et al. DiPOA ([8-(3,3-diphenyl-propyl)-4-oxo-1-phenyl-1,3,8-triaza spiro[4.5]dec-3-yl]-acetic acid), a peripherally-acting mu opioid agonist with anti-hyperalgesic properties. J Pharmacol Exp Ther 2004;310:783–729.
[144] Dray A. Alternatives to mu-opioid analgesics: delta-opioid and galanin-receptor selective compounds. In: Kalso E, McQuay HJ, Wiesenfeld-Hallin Z, editors. Progress in pain research and management. Seattle (WA): IASP Press; 1999. p. 269–80.
[145] Cahill CM, Morinville A, Lee M-C, et al. Prolonged morphine treatment targets δ-opioid receptors to neuronal plasma membranes and enhances δ-mediated antinociception. J Neurosci 2001;21:7598–607.
[146] Fox A, Bevan S. Therapeutic potential of cannabinoid receptor agonists as analgesic agents. Expert Opin Investig Drugs 2005;14:695–703.
[147] Campbell FA, Tramer MR, Carroll D, et al. Are cannabinoids an effective and safe treatment option in the management of pain? A quantitative systematic review. BMJ 2001;323: 13–6.

[148] Agarwal N, Pacher P, Tegeder I, et al. Cannabinoid mediated analgesia largely via peripheral type 1 cannabinoid receptors in nociceptors. Nat Neurosci 2007;7:870–9.
[149] Dyson A, Peacock M, Chen A, et al. Antihyperalgesic properties of the cannabinoid CT-3 in chronic neuropathic and inflammatory pain states in the rat. Pain 2005;116:129–37.
[150] Richardson JD, Kilo S, Hargreaves KM. Cannabinoids reduce hyperalgesia and inflammation via interactions with peripheral CB1 receptors. Pain 1998;75:111–9.
[151] Karst M, Salim K, Burstein S, et al. Analgesic effect of the synthetic cannabinoid CT-3 on chronic neuropathic pain: a randomized controlled trial. JAMA 2003;290:1757–62.
[152] Labuda CJ, Koblish M, Little PJ. Cannabinoid CB2 receptor agonist activity in the hindpaw incision model of postoperative pain. Eur J Pharmacol 2005;527:172–5.
[153] Malan TP Jr, Ibrahim MM, Lai J, et al. CB2 cannabinoid receptor agonists: pain relief without psychoactive effects? Curr Opin Pharmacol 2003;3(1):62–7.
[154] Valenzano KJ, Tafesse L, Lee G, et al. Pharmacological and pharmacokinetic characterization of the cannabinoid receptor 2 agonist GW405833,utilizing rodent models of acute and chronic pain, anxiety, ataxia and catalepsy. Neuropharmacology 2005;48:658–72.
[155] Sokal DM, Elmes SJR, Kendall DA, et al. Intraplantar injection of anandamide inhibits mechanically-evoked responses of spinal neurons via activation of CB2 receptors in anaesthetized rats. Neuropharmacology 2003;45:404–11.
[156] Zhang J, Hoffert C, Vu K, et al. Induction of CB2 receptor expression in the rat spinal cord of neuropathic but not inflammatory chronic pain models. Eur J Neurosci 2003;17:2750–4.
[157] Cravatt BF, Lichtman AH. The endogenous cannabinoid system and its role in nociceptive behavior. J Neurobiol 2004;61:149–60.
[158] Cravatt BF, Demarest K, Patricelli MP, et al. Supersensitivity to anandamide and enhanced endogenous cannabinoid signaling in mice lacking fatty acid amide hydrolyse. Proc Natl Acad Sci 2001;98:9371–6.
[159] Lichtman AH, Leung D, Shelton CC, et al. Reversible inhibitors of fatty acid amide hydrolase that promote analgesia: evidence for an unprecedented combination of potency and selectivity. J Pharmacol Exp Ther 2004;311:441–8.
[160] Sato J, Perl ER. Adrenergic excitation of cutaneous pain receptors induced by peripheral nerve injury. Science 1991;251:1608–10.
[161] Lee DH, Liu X, Kim HT, et al. Receptor subtype mediating the adrenergic sensitivity of pain behavior and ectopic discharges in neuropathic Lewis rats. J Neurophysiol 1999;81:2226–33.
[162] Sundrup SH, Otto M, Finnerup NB, et al. Antidepressants in the treatment of neuropathic pain Basic Clin Pharmacol. Toxicol 2005;96:399–409.
[163] Griffin JW. The roles of growth factors in painful length-dependent axonal neuropathies. In: Campbell JN, Basbaum AI, Dray A, editors. Emerging strategies for the treatment of neuropathic pain. Seattle (WA): IASP Press; 2006. p. 271–90.
[164] Zweifel LS, Kuruvilla R, Ginty DD. Functions and mechanisms of retrograde neurotrophin signaling. Nat Rev Neurosci 2005;6:615–25.
[165] Lu B, Pang PT, Woo NH. The yin and yang of neurotrophin action. Nat Rev Neurosci 2005;6:603–14.
[166] Hefti FF, Rosenthal A, Walicka PA, et al. Novel class of pain drug based on antagonism of NGF. Trends in Pharmacological Sciences 2005;27:85–91.
[167] Theodosiou M, Rush RA, Zhou XF, et al. Hyperalgesia due to nerve damage: role of nerve growth factor. Pain 1999;81:245–55.
[168] Ro LS, Chen ST, Tang LM, et al. Effect of NGF and anti-NGF on neuropathic pain in rats following chronic constriction injury of the sciatic nerve. Pain 1999;79:265–74.
[169] Fjell J, Cummings TR, Fried K, et al. In vivo NGF deprivation reduces SNS expression and TTX-R sodium currents in IB4-negative DRG neurons. J Neurophysiol 1999;81:803–10.
[170] Ji RR, Samad TA, Jin SX, et al. P38 MAPK activation by NGF in primary sensory neurons after inflammation increases TRPV1 levels and maintains heat hyperalgesia. Neuron 2002;36:57–68.

[171] Mamet J, Lazdunski M, Voilley N. How nerve growth factor drives physiological and inflammatory expression of acid-sensing ion channels 3 in sensory neurons. J Biol Chem 2003;278:48907–13.
[172] Ramer MS, Bradbury EJ, McMahon SB. Nerve growth factor induces P2X(3) expression in sensory neurons. J Neurochem 2001;77:864–75.
[173] Halliday DA, Zettler C, Rush RA, et al. Elevated growth factor levels in the synovial fluid of patients with inflammatory joint disease. Neurochem Res 1998;23:919–22.
[174] Discou E, Perrot S, Menkes CJ, et al. Nerve growth factor (NGF) Autoantibodies and NGF in the synovial fluid: Implications in spondylarthropathies. Autoimmunity 1996; 24:1–9.
[175] Sarchielli P, Alberti A, Floridi A, et al. Levels of nerve growth factor in cerebrospinal fluid of chronic headache patients. Neurology 2001;57:132–4.
[176] Andreev N, Dimitrieva N, Kolzenburg M, et al. Peripheral administration of nerve growth factor in the adult rat produces a thermal hyperalgesia that requires the presence of sympathetic post-ganglionic neurones. Pain 1995;63:109–15.
[177] Svensson P, Cairns B, Wang K, et al. Injection of nerve growth factor into human masseter muscle evokes long-lasting mechaniscal allodynia and hyperalgesia. Pain 2003;104:241–7.
[178] Colquhoun A, Lawrance GM, Shamovsky IL, et al. Differential activity of the nerve growth factor (NGF) antagonist PD90780 [7-(benzoylamino)-4,9-dihydro-4methyl-8-oxo-pyrazolo-[5,1-b]-quinazoline-2-carboxylic acid] suggest altered NGF-p75NTR interactions in the presence of trkA. J Pharmacol Exp Ther 2004;310:505–11.
[179] Owolabi JB, Rizkalla G, Tehim A, et al. Characterization of antiallodynic actions ALE-0540, a novel nerve growth factor receptor antagonist, in the rat. J Pharmacol Exp Ther 1999;289:1271–6.
[180] Lane N, Webster L, Shiao-Ping L, et al. RN624 (Anti NGF) improves pain and function in subjects with moderate knee osteoarthritis: a phase 1 study. Arthritis Rheum 2005;52:S461.
[181] Sah DW, Ossipov MH, Porecca F. Neurotrophic factors as novel therapeutics for neuropathic pain. Nat Rev Drug Discov 2003;2:460–72.
[182] Kerr BJ, Bradbury EJ, Bennett DL, et al. Brain derived neurotrophic factor modulates nociceptive sensory neurone input and NMDA-evoked responses in the rat spinal cord J Neurosci 1999;19:5136–49.
[183] Deng YS, Zhong JH, Zhou XF. Effects of endogenous neurotrophin on sympathetic sprouting in the dorsal root ganglia and allodynia following spinal nerve injury. Exp Neurol 2000;164:344–50.
[184] Wang R, King T, Ossipov MH, et al. Restoration of sensory function by immediate or delayed systemic artemin after dorsal root injury. Nat Neurosci 2008;11:488–96.
[185] Nutt JG, Burchiel KJ, Comella CL, et al, ICV GDNF Study Group. Implanted intracerebroventricular. Glial cell line-derived neurotrophic factor. Randomized, double-blind trial of glial cell line-derived neurotrophic factor (GDNF) in PD. Neurology 2003;60:69–73.

ELSEVIER
SAUNDERS

Rheum Dis Clin N Am
34 (2008) 507–513

RHEUMATIC
DISEASE CLINICS
OF NORTH AMERICA

Index

Note: Page numbers of article titles are in **boldface** type.

doi:10.1016/S0889-857X(08)00055-0